Endometrium and Related Endouterine Pathologies

An Essential Examination for a Modern and Integrated Approach

nova
Medicine & Health
New York

Obstetrics and Gynecology Advances Series

Navigating Pregnancy Challenges: Policies, Programs, and Protections
Javier Giles (Editor)
ISBN: 979-8-89530-857-8
eBook ISBN: 979-8-89530-924-7

Exploring Menopause from a Multidisciplinary Perspective: Biology, Psychosocial Factors, and Clinical Insights
Nazan Yurtcu, MD,
Dilay Karademir, MD
and Fatih Durmuşoğlu (Editors)
ISBN: 979-8-89530-001-5
eBook ISBN: 979-8-89530-108-1

Pregnancy-Associated Pelvic Girdle Pain: A Single Entity or an "Umbrella Term?"
Noa Martonovich, MD,
Sharon Perlman, MD,
Ophir Blickstein, MD
and Ran Thein, MD
eBook ISBN: 979-8-89530-050-3

Preterm Delivery: Prevalence, Risk Factors and Related Complications
Llanos Belmonte Andujar, PhD
and Ana Fuentes Rozalen, MD
ISBN: 979-8-89113-664-9
eBook ISBN: 979-8-89113-754-7

Polycystic Ovarian Syndrome (PCOS) and Our Biological Clock
Arpita Roy, PhD,
Gowhar Rashid, PhD
and Nihad Ashraf Khan (Editors)
ISBN: 979-8-89113-100-2
eBook ISBN: 979-8-89113-212-2

Holistic Approach to Assisted Reproductive Technology
Kenan Demir
and Rumeysa Göç (Editors)
ISBN: 979-8-89113-017-3
eBook ISBN: 979-8-89113-064-7

More information about this series can be found at
https://novapublishers.com/product-category/series/obstetrics-and-gynecology-advances/

Liliana Mereu
Salvatore Giovanni Vitale
Editors

Endometrium and Related Endouterine Pathologies

An Essential Examination for a Modern and Integrated Approach

nova
Medicine & Health
New York

DOI: https://doi.org/10.52305/IWIX5130

NOTICE TO THE READER

Library of Congress Cataloging-in-Publication Data

ISBN: 979-8-89530-818-9 (Hardcover)
ISBN: 979-8-89530-972-8 (eBook)

Published by Nova Science Publishers, Inc. † New York

Contents

Foreword

The endometrium, the thin inner lining of the uterus, is a dynamic tissue essential for female reproductive health. It is subject to a wide range of alterations, which can vary from benign conditions, such as hyperplasia and polyps, to malignant diseases, such as endometrial carcinoma, one of the most common neoplasms in women.

Endometrial pathology represents a diagnostic and therapeutic challenge for clinicians and researchers. Its complexity lies in the diversity of clinical manifestations, the need for accurate and timely diagnosis, and the selection of a personalized treatment approach based on the specific characteristics of each patient.

This book aims to provide a comprehensive and up-to-date overview of both benign and malignant endometrial pathology. The most recent knowledge and the strongest scientific evidence have been gathered to offer readers a useful and practical tool.

The text is divided into chapters that address the various pathological entities, from the most common to the rarest, with a particular focus on diagnosis, clinical management, and therapeutic strategies. Considerable space has been dedicated to imaging, facilitating the understanding of histopathological and clinical aspects.

It is intended for gynecologists, pathologists, oncologists, radiologists, and all healthcare professionals involved in the diagnosis and treatment of women with endometrial disorders. I am confident that it will serve as a valuable support in daily clinical practice and as a stimulus for further research and in-depth study.

I extend my congratulations to all those who contributed to the realization of this work: the authors, for their expertise and dedication; the collaborators, for their invaluable assistance; and the editors, for their professionalism and sensitivity.

Aware that medicine is constantly evolving and that new discoveries and scientific advances will necessitate a future revision of this text, I am nonetheless certain that this first edition represents an important reference for the scientific community and a tangible contribution to improving women's health.

Paolo Scollo
Full Professor of Obstetrics and Gynecology,
Rector, University of Enna "Kore," Enna, Italy

About the Editors

Liliana Mereu, MD, PhD

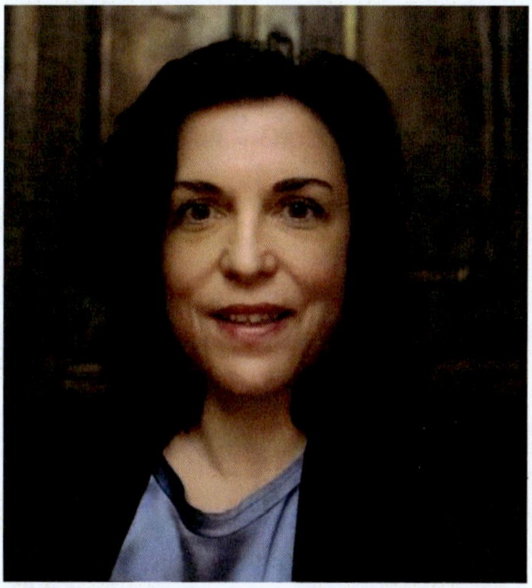

Professor Liliana Mereu, graduated in medicine and surgery in 2000 and specialized in Ob&Gyn in 2005 with top marks from the University of Pavia. In 2015, she obtained a doctorate in biotechnology in Ob&Gyn at the University of Siena. She is currently an Associate Professor of Obstetrics and Gynecology, on the Faculty of Medicine and Surgery of the University of Catania, Department of General Surgery and Medical-Surgical Specialties, and is Director of the Obstetrics and Gynecology Unit of the "*Gaspare Rodolico-San Marco*" University Hospital in Catania.

Professor Mereu is the author of over 180 published works. She participates in numerous national and international research groups in the field of gynecological oncology, endometriosis, urogynecology and new minimally invasive surgical technologies.

She has been elected to the boards of national and international scientific societies. She is a director of a level II master's degree program and a member of a doctorate teaching council. She has won national and international recognition awards in the gynaecologic field and minimally invasive surgery. She has participated as scientific director, scientific committee, speaker, moderator, expert, live surgery operator in more than 200 national and international conferences.

She has focused her activity on minimally invasive surgery thanks also to her attendance at national and international institutes. The high level she has achieved is demonstrated by her numerous attendances at national and international conferences Over the years, she has dedicated herself to teaching the most advanced surgical techniques through teaching positions at national and international schools.

Salvatore Giovanni Vitale, MD, PhD

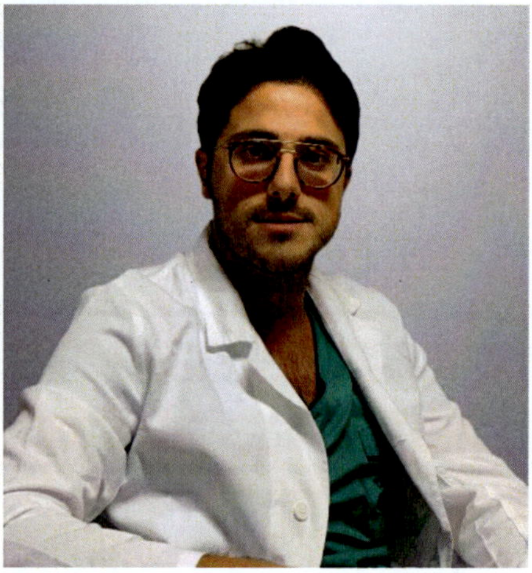

Salvatore Giovanni Vitale is Professor of Obstetrics and Gynecology in the Faculty of Medicine and Surgery at the University of Catania (Italy), Department of General Surgery and Medical-Surgical Specialties, and Consultant in the Obstetrics and Gynecology Unit at the "*Gaspare Rodolico-San Marco*" University Hospital in Catania. Born in Catania, Italy, on August 30, 1984, he earned a *Cum Laude* degree in medicine and surgery from the University of Catania (Italy) in 2009, where he also specialized with honors in Gynecology and Obstetrics in 2015, before completing a PhD in Medical and Surgical Biotechnologies at the University of Messina (Italy) in 2018.

His main clinical and research interests include intracavitary uterine pathologies, hysteroscopy and minimally invasive surgery, female infertility, and gynecological endocrinology. He has patented several hysteroscopic mechanical instruments, among which the "*biopsy snake grasper sec. VITALE*" stands out, successfully marketed and distributed worldwide. During the 15th Congress of the European Society of Gynecology (ESG) held in Amsterdam, he was awarded the *Alice and Albert Netter Prize* for developing this innovative device, recognizing him as the best young European researcher for his scientific and clinical merits, as well as for his contribution to technological advancement in hysteroscopic instrumentation.

He has been and continues to serve as Principal Investigator (PI) and Co-Investigator in numerous national and international research projects, many of which have been funded by prestigious Research Institutes and Universities through rigorous peer review. He has authored over 300 papers published in PubMed-indexed international peer-reviewed journals, as well as several monographs and chapters in international medical textbooks.

The excellence of his scientific output has earned him continuous inclusion, since 2019, in the "*World's Top 2% Scientists,*" a ranking compiled by Stanford University (Ioannidis et al.) in collaboration with Elsevier (Scopus).

He is also an advisor and reviewer for prestigious national and international Research Institutes and currently serves as an editor for several high-impact gynecologic journals, including *Archives of Gynecology and Obstetrics*, *International Journal of Women's Health*, *Gynecologic and Obstetric Investigation*, Minimally Invasive Therapy and Allied Technologies (MITAT) and *Advances in Therapy*, among others.

Introduction

Liliana Mereu[*], MD, PhD
and Salvatore Giovanni Vitale, MD, PhD
Obstetrics and Gynecology Unit, "*Gaspare Rodolico*" University Hospital,
Department of General Surgery and Medical Surgical Specialties,
University of Catania, Catania, Italy

The endometrium, a dynamic and multifunctional tissue, is the cornerstone of female reproductive health. It is uniquely capable of undergoing cyclical regeneration, differentiation, and shedding in response to hormonal cues, ensuring its readiness to support implantation and pregnancy [1]. This adaptability highlights the remarkable complexity of the endometrium, which balances intricate molecular and cellular processes to maintain its function. However, this very complexity also makes it vulnerable to a wide spectrum of pathological conditions that can disrupt its physiological roles, leading to significant clinical challenges [2].

Endometrial health is central to menstruation, fertility, and overall gynecological well-being. It acts as a responsive interface, dynamically interacting with systemic hormonal signals and local immune environments [3, 4]. These interactions are essential for normal endometrial function but also create opportunities for dysregulation [2]. Disorders of the endometrium, ranging from benign lesions to malignant transformations, illustrate the delicate balance required for its optimal performance [2]. Understanding this balance and the factors that disturb it is crucial for advancing diagnostic and therapeutic strategies.

Endometrial disorders are among the most common reasons for gynecological consultations, impacting millions of women globally. Abnormal uterine bleeding (AUB), for example, is reported in up to one-third

[*] Corresponding Author's Email: liliana.mereu@unict.it

of women during their reproductive years and is particularly prevalent during the perimenopausal transition [5, 6]. AUB is a symptom rather than a disease and is frequently associated with underlying conditions such as endometrial polyps, fibroids, adenomyosis, or hormonal imbalances [7]. Chronic anovulation, a key contributor to AUB, is closely linked to conditions like polycystic ovary syndrome (PCOS), which affects approximately 10% of women of reproductive age worldwide [8]. These conditions highlight the interconnected nature of endometrial health and systemic hormonal regulation.

Among the common structural abnormalities, endometrial polyps and uterine fibroids illustrate the localized impact of hormonal and molecular dysregulation on the endometrium.

Endometrial polyps, benign overgrowth of the endometrial lining, are detected in 8-35% of women, with a higher incidence in perimenopausal and postmenopausal populations [9]. Although often asymptomatic, polyps can contribute to abnormal bleeding and infertility [6, 9]. Their pathogenesis involves localized hormonal dysregulation and angiogenesis, making them a focal point for diagnostic and therapeutic advancements [10]. Hysteroscopy, the gold standard for polyp detection and removal, exemplifies the role of minimally invasive techniques in modern gynecology [11–14].

Similarly, uterine fibroids, the most prevalent benign tumors in reproductive-age women, are influenced by genetic, hormonal, and environmental factors [15]. These tumors, affecting up to 20-50% of reproductive-age women, can lead to heavy menstrual bleeding, pelvic pain, and reproductive dysfunction [16]. Advances in imaging techniques, such as three-dimensional ultrasound and MRI, have enhanced our ability to classify fibroids and tailor management strategies [17]. Treatments now range from pharmacological options, such as selective progesterone receptor modulators, to surgical interventions, including minimally invasive myomectomy and uterine artery embolization [18, 19]. In addition to these well-established methods, emerging technologies are broadening the therapeutic landscape for uterine fibroids and other structural abnormalities. Techniques such as laser ablation and radiofrequency ablation (RFA) have gained attention for their ability to target fibroid tissue with precision while minimizing damage to surrounding healthy tissue [20, 21].

Adenomyosis, a disorder involving the invasion of endometrial tissue into the myometrium, bridges structural and inflammatory pathologies. This condition, historically underdiagnosed, is now recognized for its significant impact on dysmenorrhea, heavy bleeding, and infertility, particularly in women in their fourth and fifth decades of life [22].

Recent advances in diagnostic imaging, particularly high-resolution transvaginal ultrasound and MRI, have improved detection rates [23]. Understanding the molecular underpinnings of adenomyosis, including its inflammatory and angiogenic pathways, has opened avenues for targeted therapies aimed at reducing symptoms and preserving fertility [23, 24]. Emerging treatments, such as uterine-sparing techniques and hormonal modulators, offer new hope for affected women. [25, 26]

Intrauterine adhesions (IUA), further illustrate how structural and inflammatory factors converge to disrupt endometrial function. These adhesions often arise from uterine trauma, including surgical interventions like curettage or hysteroscopic procedures performed to treat polyps, fibroids, or retained products of conception [27]. By disrupting the endometrial lining, they can impair uterine receptivity, leading to infertility or recurrent pregnancy loss [28, 29]. Advances in hysteroscopic techniques have revolutionized their management, enabling precise adhesiolysis and the use of barrier methods to prevent recurrence [30]. The development of biodegradable adhesion barriers and anti-inflammatory treatments offers additional preventive options, reducing the likelihood of recurrence [31].

Chronic endometritis, an inflammatory condition linked to microbial dysbiosis or persistent infections, highlights the role of the endometrial immune environment in pathology [32, 33]. Affecting up to 30% of women with unexplained infertility or recurrent miscarriage, chronic endometritis is often associated with microbial dysbiosis or persistent infections [34]. The application of next-generation sequencing to study the endometrial microbiome has provided valuable insights into its role in reproductive health, while hysteroscopic-guided biopsies have enhanced diagnostic accuracy [35, 36]. Antibiotic regimens tailored to microbial profiles have shown promising results in restoring endometrial function [37].

Beyond addressing benign or inflammatory conditions, gynecologists must also consider the endometrium's potential for malignant transformation. Persistent inflammation or hormonal imbalances, if left untreated, can alter the cellular microenvironment, increasing the risk of endometrial hyperplasia or cancer [38]. For example, unopposed estrogen exposure, often exacerbated by conditions such as obesity or metabolic syndrome, plays a key role in driving hyperplasia, a recognized precursor to endometrial malignancy [39]. Epidemiological data indicate that women with obesity are three to five times more likely to develop endometrial hyperplasia or cancer compared to those with a healthy weight [39]. Molecular studies have identified genetic mutations, such as PTEN alterations, that not only enhance our understanding of its pathogenesis but also inform targeted therapeutic strategies [40]. Management of endometrial hyperplasia focuses on preventing progression to cancer. For hyperplasia without atypia, progestin therapy, administered orally, intrauterinely, or parenterally, is the cornerstone of treatment. However, atypical hyperplasia, with its higher malignant potential, often requires more aggressive management, such as hysterectomy [41]. Lifestyle modifications addressing obesity and metabolic syndrome are integral to reducing estrogenic stimulation and mitigating disease progression [41, 42].

Endometrial cancer, the most common gynecological malignancy in developed nations, represents the potential endpoint of unchecked proliferative dysregulation. In 2020, it accounted for approximately 417,000 new cases globally [43]. Its rising incidence is closely tied to the same risk factors that drive hyperplasia, including obesity, diabetes, and an aging population [44, 45]. Advances in molecular classification have further refined our understanding of endometrial cancer's progression. The Cancer Genome Atlas (TCGA) has identified four distinct subtypes of endometrial cancer, offering a framework for personalized diagnostic and therapeutic approaches [46]. These insights are driving the development of innovative treatments, including immunotherapy and molecularly targeted agents like PD-1 inhibitors, which have shown promise in managing advanced or recurrent disease [47]. Recent clinical trials have demonstrated the efficacy of combination therapies that integrate immunotherapeutics with standard chemotherapy protocols, providing hope for improved survival rates [47].

The intricate interplay of hormonal, structural, and molecular factors underlying endometrial pathologies demands innovative approaches to diagnosis and treatment. Conditions such as polyps, fibroids, and hyperplasia often coexist or progress along shared pathways, highlighting the need for management strategies that address this interconnected spectrum. Advances in minimally invasive technologies and personalized medicine have transformed the way these disorders are managed, providing precision and efficacy across the continuum of benign, precancerous, and malignant conditions. Minimally invasive techniques, such as hysteroscopy, laparoscopy, and robotic surgery, have revolutionized the treatment of structural abnormalities like polyps and fibroids, while also enabling early intervention in precancerous conditions such as hyperplasia [48]. These tools not only offer precision and reduced recovery times but also play a critical role in managing the progression from benign to malignant states by facilitating timely and targeted therapeutic actions.

This book aims to serve as a comprehensive guide to the complexities of endometrial health and its related pathologies, offering a valuable resource for healthcare professionals committed to improving diagnostic accuracy, therapeutic approaches, and patient outcomes. By bringing together the latest scientific evidence, clinical insights, and technological advances, it seeks to address the challenges posed by this intricate and multifaceted field.

The endometrium, with its complex physiological processes and essential reproductive role, is susceptible to a spectrum of disorders which, as we have mentioned, range from benign growths like polyps and fibroids to inflammatory, precancerous, and malignant conditions. This book delves into these issues, highlighting their interconnected nature and the shared mechanisms—hormonal, structural, and molecular—that drive their development and progression.

Each section provides a detailed examination of individual pathologies, delving into their prevalence, underlying causes, clinical presentation, diagnostic approaches, and available treatments. Particular emphasis is placed on the role of emerging tools and techniques, such as minimally invasive surgeries and personalized medicine, in revolutionizing the management of these disorders. Through this exploration, readers will gain insights into how innovative approaches are being employed to improve outcomes, whether addressing structural issues like fibroids or polyps, managing inflammatory conditions, or preventing progression to malignancy.

The book also underscores the importance of a collaborative and integrated approach to patient care. By fostering partnerships between specialists (gynecologists, radiologists, pathologists, and reproductive health experts) clinicians can better navigate the complexities of endometrial disorders and tailor treatments to the unique needs of each patient. This multidisciplinary perspective is essential to advancing care in a way that is both modern and effective.

Rather than being a mere repository of knowledge, this book aspires to be a practical and inspiring tool for those working in gynecology and reproductive medicine. It invites readers to explore the complexities of endometrial physiology and pathology from multiple angles, equipping them with the knowledge and strategies needed to address both common and complex cases. By doing so, it contributes to the broader goal of enhancing women's health and ensuring that advancements in research translate into meaningful improvements in clinical practice.

References

[1] Maybin JA, Critchley HOD. Menstrual physiology: implications for endometrial pathology and beyond. *Hum Reprod Update.* 2015;21(6):748–61.

[2] Dallenbach-Hellweg G, Schmidt D, Dallenbach F. *Atlas of Endometrial Histopathology.* 3rd ed. Vol. IX. Berlin, Heidelberg: Springer; 2010.

[3] Mihm M, Gangooly S, Muttukrishna S. The normal menstrual cycle in women. *Anim Reprod Sci.* 2011;124(3):229–36.

[4] Vitale SG, Corrado F, Caruso S, Di Benedetto A, Giunta L, Cianci A, D'Anna R. Myo-inositol supplementation to prevent gestational diabetes in overweight non-obese women: bioelectrical impedance analysis, metabolic aspects, obstetric and neonatal outcomes - a randomized and open-label, placebo-controlled clinical trial. *Int J Food Sci Nutr.* 2021;72(5):670–9.

[5] Vitale SG, Angioni S, D'Alterio MN, Ronsini C, Saponara S, De Franciscis P, Riemma G. Risk of endometrial malignancy in women treated for breast cancer: the BLUSH prediction model–evidence from a comprehensive multicentric retrospective cohort study. *Climacteric.* 2024;27(5):482–8.

[6] Dreisler E, Frandsen CS, Ulrich L. Perimenopausal abnormal uterine bleeding. *Maturitas.* 2024;184:107944.

[7] Vitale SG, Riemma G. Risk of endometrial cancer in asymptomatic postmenopausal women in relation to ultrasonographic endometrial thickness: look but do not overlook. *Am J Obstet Gynecol.* 2023;229(1):86–7.

[8] Ali DES, Shah M, Ali A, Malik MO, Rehman F, Badshah H, Ehtesham E, Vitale SG. Treatment with Metformin and Combination of Metformin plus Pioglitazone on Serum Levels of IL-6 and IL-8 in Polycystic Ovary Syndrome: A Randomized Clinical Trial. *Horm Metab Res.* 2019;51(11):714–22.

[9] AAGL practice report: practice guidelines for the diagnosis and management of endometrial polyps. *J Minim Invasive Gynecol.* 2012;19(1):3–10.

[10] King AE, Critchley HO. Oestrogen and progesterone regulation of inflammatory processes in the human endometrium. *J Steroid Biochem Mol Biol.* 2010;120:116.

[11] Vitale SG, Angioni S, Saponara S, Sicilia G, Etrusco A, D'Alterio MN, Cobellis L, De Franciscis P, Riemma G. TikTok as a platform for hysteroscopy information: An analytical video-based cross-sectional study to assess quality, reliability, and accuracy. *Int J Gynecol Obstet.* 2025;168(1):353–61.

[12] Vitale SG, Angioni S, Saponara S, Sicilia G, Mignacca A, Caiazzo A, De Franciscis P, Riemma G. Hysteroscopic metroplasty and its reproductive impact among the social networks: A cross-sectional analysis on video quality, reliability and creators' opinions on YouTube, TikTok and Instagram. *Int J Med Inform.* 2025;195:105776.

[13] Florio P, Puzzutiello R, Filippeschi M, D'Onofrio P, Mereu L, Morelli R, Marianello D, Litta P, Mencaglia L, Petraglia F. Low-dose spinal anesthesia with hyperbaric bupivacaine with intrathecal fentanyl for operative hysteroscopy: a case series study. *J Minim Invasive Gynecol.* 2012;19(1):107–12.

[14] Török P, Molnár S, Herman T, Jashanjeet S, Lampé R, Riemma G, Vitale SG. Fallopian tubal obstruction is associated with increased pain experienced during office hysteroscopy: a retrospective study. *Updates Surg.* 2020;72(1):213–8.

[15] Vitale SG, Saponara S, Sicilia G, Klarić M, Sorrentino F, D'Alterio MN, Nappi L, Angioni S. Hysteroscopic diode laser myolysis: from a case series to literature review of incisionless myolysis techniques for managing heavy menstrual bleeding in premenopausal women. *Arch Gynecol Obstet.* 2024;309(3):949–59.

[16] Baird DD, Dunson DB, Hill MC, Cousins D, Schectman JM. High cumulative incidence of uterine leiomyoma in black and white women: Ultrasound evidence. *Am J Obstet Gynecol.* 2003;188(1):100–7.

[17] Munro MG, Critchley HOD, Fraser IS. The two FIGO systems for normal and abnormal uterine bleeding symptoms and classification of causes of abnormal uterine bleeding in the reproductive years: 2018 revisions. *Int J Gynecol Obstet.* 2018;143(3):393–408.

[18] Sohn GS, Cho SH, Kim YM, Cho CH, Kim MR, Lee SR. Current medical treatment of uterine fibroids. *Obstet Gynecol Sci.* 2018;61(2):192.

[19] Mencaglia L, Carri G, Prasciolu C, Giunta G, Albis Florez ED, Cofelice V, Mereu L. Feasibility and complications in bipolar resectoscopy: preliminary experience. *Minim Invasive Ther Allied Technol.* 2013;22(1):50–5.

[20] Vitale SG, Saponara S, Succu AG, Sicilia G, Martsidis K, D'Alterio MN, Angioni S. Efficacy and Safety of Non-Ablative Dual Wavelength Diode Laser Therapy for Genitourinary Syndrome of Menopause: A Single-Center Prospective Study. *Adv Ther.* 2024;41(12):4617–27.

[21] Vitale SG, Moore O, Riemma G, Carugno J, Yarto ML, Haimovich S. Hysteroscopic laser ablation of symptomatic uterine fibroids: insights from a prospective study. *Climacteric.* 2023;26(5):497–502.

[22] Saponara S, Angioni S, Parry JP, Pacheco LA, Carugno J, Moawad N, Haimovich S, Lasmar RB, Dealberti D, Aksakal E, Urman B, Nappi L, Vitale SG. The Pivotal role of hysteroscopy in diagnosing subtle uterine lesions in infertile patients: Seeing the unseen can make the difference. *Eur J Obstet Gynecol Reprod Biol.* 2025;305:132–41.

[23] Vannuccini S, Petraglia F. Recent advances in understanding and managing adenomyosis. *F1000Research.* 2019;8:F1000 Faculty Rev-283.

[24] Chiofalo B, Palmara V, Vilos GA, Pacheco LA, Lasmar RB, Shawki O, Giacobbe V, Alibrandi A, Di Guardo F, Vitale SG. Reproductive outcomes of infertile women undergoing "see and treat" office hysteroscopy: a retrospective observational study. *Minim Invasive Ther Allied Technol.* 2021;30(3):147–53.

[25] Landi S, Mereu L, Pontrelli G, Stepniewska A, Romano L, Tateo S, Dorizzi C, Minelli L. The influence of adenomyosis in patients laparoscopically treated for deep endometriosis. *J Minim Invasive Gynecol.* 2008;15(5):566–70.

[26] Restaino S, Mereu L, Finelli A, Spina MR, Marini G, Catena U, Turco LC, Moroni R, Milani M, Cela V, Scambia G, Fanfani F. Robotic surgery vs laparoscopic surgery in patients with diagnosis of endometriosis: a systematic review and meta-analysis. *J Robot Surg.* 2020;14(5):687–94.

[27] Vitale SG, Parry JP, Carugno J, Cholkeri-Singh A, Della Corte L, Cianci S, Schiattarella A, Riemma G, De Franciscis P. Surgical and Reproductive Outcomes after Hysteroscopic Removal of Retained Products of Conception: A Systematic Review and Meta-analysis. *J Minim Invasive Gynecol.* 2021;28(2):204–17.

[28] Vitale SG, Laganà AS, Török P, Lasmar RB, Carugno J, Palumbo M, Tesarik J. Virtual sonographic hysteroscopy in assisted reproduction: A retrospective cost-effectiveness analysis. *Int J Gynaecol Obstet.* 2022;156(1):112–8.

[29] Vitale SG, De Angelis MC, Della Corte L, Saponara S, Carugno J, Laganà AS, Török P, Tinelli R, Pérez-Medina T, Ertas S, Urman B, Angioni S. Uterine cervical stenosis: from classification to advances in management. Overcoming the obstacles to access the uterine cavity. *Arch Gynecol Obstet.* 2024;309(3):755–64.

[30] Vitale SG, Riemma G, Carugno J, Perez-Medina T, Alonso Pacheco L, Haimovich S, Parry JP, Di Spiezio Sardo A, De Franciscis P. Postsurgical barrier strategies to avoid the recurrence of intrauterine adhesion formation after hysteroscopic adhesiolysis: a network meta-analysis of randomized controlled trials. *Am J Obstet Gynecol.* 2022;226(4):487-498.e8.

[31] Urman B, Yakin K, Ertas S, Alper E, Aksakal E, Riemma G, Angioni S, Vitale SG. Fertility and anatomical outcomes following hysteroscopic adhesiolysis: An 11-year retrospective cohort study to validate a new classification system for intrauterine adhesions (Urman-Vitale Classification System). *Int J Gynecol Obstet.* 2024;165(2):644–54.

[32] Kitaya K, Takeuchi T, Mizuta S, Matsubayashi H, Ishikawa T. Endometritis: new time, new concepts. *Fertil Steril.* 2018;110(3):344–50.

[33] Shi Y, Zhu Y, Fan S, Vitagliano A, Liu X, Liao Y, Liang Y, Vitale SG. Clinical Characteristics and Antifungal Susceptibility of Candida nivariensis from Vulvovaginal Candidiasis. *Gynecol Obstet Invest.* 2020;85(1):88–93.

[34] Cicinelli E, Ziegler D, Nicoletti R, Tinelli R, Saliani N, Resta L. Poor reliability of vaginal and endocervical cultures for evaluating microbiology of endometrial cavity in women with chronic endometritis. *Gynecol Obs Invest.* 2009;68(2):108–115.

[35] Vitale SG, Laganà AS, Caruso S, Garzon S, Vecchio GM, La Rosa VL, Casarin J, Ghezzi F. Comparison of three biopsy forceps for hysteroscopic endometrial biopsy in postmenopausal patients (HYGREB-1): A multicenter, single-blind randomized clinical trial. *Int J Gynecol Obstet.* 2021;155(3):425–32.

[36] Vitale SG. The Biopsy Snake Grasper Sec. VITALE: A New Tool for Office Hysteroscopy. *J Minim Invasive Gynecol.* 2020;27(6):1414–6.

[37] Cicinelli E, Matteo M, Tinelli R, Lepera A, Alfonso R, Indraccolo U, Marrocchella S, Greco P, Resta L. Prevalence of chronic endometritis in repeated unexplained implantation failure and the IVF success rate after antibiotic therapy. *Hum Reprod.* 2015;30(2):323–30.

[38] Lacey J V., Chia VM. Endometrial hyperplasia and the risk of progression to carcinoma. *Maturitas.* 2009;63(1):39–44.

[39] Schmandt RE, Iglesias DA, Co NN, Lu KH. Understanding Obesity and Endometrial Cancer Risk: Opportunities for Prevention. *Am J Obstet Gynecol.* 2011;205(6):518.

[40] Mutter GL, Monte NM, Neuberg D, Ferenczy A, Eng C. Emergence, involution, and progression to carcinoma of mutant clones in normal endometrial tissues. *Cancer Res.* 2014;74(10):2796–802.

[41] Management of Endometrial Intraepithelial Neoplasia or Atypical Endometrial Hyperplasia: ACOG Clinical Consensus No. 5. *Obstet Gynecol.* 2023;142(3):735–44.

[42] Vitale SG, Caruso S, Rapisarda AMC, Valenti G, Rossetti D, Cianci S, Cianci A. Biocompatible porcine dermis graft to treat severe cystocele: impact on quality of life and sexuality. *Arch Gynecol Obstet.* 2016;293(1):125–31.

[43] Sung H, Ferlay J, Siegel RL, Laversanne M, Soerjomataram I, Jemal A, Bray F. Global Cancer Statistics 2020: GLOBOCAN Estimates of Incidence and Mortality Worldwide for 36 Cancers in 185 Countries. *CA Cancer J Clin.* 2021;71(3):209–49.

[44] Corrado G, Vizza E, Cela V, Mereu L, Bogliolo S, Legge F, Ciccarone F, Mancini E, Gallotta V, Baiocco E, Monterossi G, Perri MT, Zampa A, Pasciuto T, Scambia G. Laparoscopic versus robotic hysterectomy in obese and extremely obese patients with endometrial cancer: A multi-institutional analysis. *Eur J Surg Oncol.* 2018;44(12):1935–41.

[45] Corrado G, Mereu L, Bogliolo S, Cela V, Gardella B, Sperduti I, Certelli C, Pellegrini A, Posar G, Zampa A, Tateo S, Gadducci A, Spinillo A, Vizza E. Comparison between single-site and multiport robot-assisted hysterectomy in obese patients with endometrial cancer: An Italian multi-institutional study. *Int J Med Robot.* 2020;16(2):e2066.

[46] Gaffney D, Matias-Guiu X, Mutch D, Scambia G, Creutzberg C, Fotopoulou C, Berek JS, Concin N. 2023 FIGO staging system for endometrial cancer: The evolution of the revolution. *Gynecol Oncol.* 2024;184:245–53.

[47] Mirza MR, Sharma S, Herrstedt J, Shahin MS, Cibula D, Fleming E, Raspagliesi F, Buscema J, Hanker LC, Coleman RL, Boere IA, Schneider K, Gilbert L, Slomovitz BM, Teneriello MG, Powell MA, Ghosh S, Stevens S, Ring K, Stuckey A. 740MO Dostarlimab + chemotherapy for the treatment of primary advanced or recurrent endometrial cancer (pA/rEC): Analysis of progression free survival (PFS) and overall survival (OS) outcomes by molecular classification in the ENGOT-EN6-NSGO/GOG-3031/RUBY trial. *Ann Oncol.* 2023;34:S507.

[48] Corrado G, Vizza E, Perrone AM, Mereu L, Cela V, Legge F, Hilaris G, Pasciuto T, D’Indinosante M, La Fera E, Certelli C, Bruno V, Kogeorgos S, Fanfani F, De Iaco P, Scambia G, Gallotta V. Comparison Between Laparoscopic and Robotic Surgery in Elderly Patients With Endometrial Cancer: A Retrospective Multicentric Study. *Front Oncol.* 2021;11:724886.

Chapter 1

Endometrium: The Keystone

Thozhukat Sathyapalan*, MD, PhD
and Elizabeth Pond, MD
Academic Endocrinology, Diabetes and Metabolism, Hull York Medical School, Hull, UK

Abstract

The endometrium is a vital tissue in the female reproductive system, uniquely capable of cyclic regeneration without scarring. It plays a pivotal role in preparing for and supporting potential pregnancy through growth, differentiation, and shedding processes. These cyclical changes are regulated by the hypothalamic-pituitary-ovarian (HPO) axis, which coordinates hormonal, vascular, and cellular events to maintain endometrial functionality. The menstrual cycle is divided into distinct phases (menstrual, proliferative, ovulatory, and luteal), each characterized by specific hormonal and structural changes. Additionally, abnormalities in these processes can lead to conditions such as abnormal uterine bleeding (AUB), which significantly impacts women's health and quality of life. Understanding the endometrium's physiology, structure, and pathological alterations is essential for addressing reproductive health challenges and advancing clinical approaches.

Keywords: endometrium, menstrual cycle, abnormal uterine bleeding, endometrial physiology, decidualization

---

* Corresponding Author's Email: thozhukat.sathyapalan@hyms.ac.uk

In: Endometrium and Related Endouterine Pathologies
Editors: Liliana Mereu and Salvatore Giovanni Vitale
ISBN: 979-8-89530-818-9

Introduction

The endometrium is a highly specialized and dynamic tissue, integral to the female reproductive system. Its primary role is to prepare for and support potential pregnancy by undergoing cyclical growth, differentiation, and shedding processes. This tissue uniquely regenerates itself each menstrual cycle without fibrosis or scarring, ensuring its sustained functionality throughout reproductive life [1].

In this chapter, we examine the endometrium's physiological and histopathological characteristics, focusing on the phases of the menstrual cycle and their hormonal regulation by the hypothalamic-pituitary-ovarian (HPO) axis. Furthermore, we explore the clinical relevance of endometrial pathophysiology in the context of abnormal uterine bleeding (AUB), an issue with significant implications for women's health globally. The chapter comprehensively explains the endometrium's role in health and disease by analyzing these aspects.

1.1. Histopathological Characteristics: Structure and Microstructure

Anatomically, the endometrium is divided into two layers (Figure 1):

1) *Stratum Functionalis*: This superficial layer undergoes cyclic changes regulated by ovarian steroid hormones. It is composed of a surface epithelial lining and an underlying stroma. The epithelial component includes luminal and glandular epithelium, while the stroma contains fibroblasts, immune cells, extracellular matrix, and spiral arteries. These arteries play a crucial role in nourishing the endometrium and undergo extensive remodeling during the menstrual cycle. The functional layer is shed during menstruation if implantation does not occur [2, 3].
2) *Stratum Basalis*: The basal layer lies adjacent to the myometrium and serves as a reservoir for endometrial regeneration. It contains endometrial progenitor and stem cells, critical for reconstituting the functional layer after menstruation. Unlike the stratum functionalis, this layer does not respond dynamically to hormonal fluctuations [2, 3].

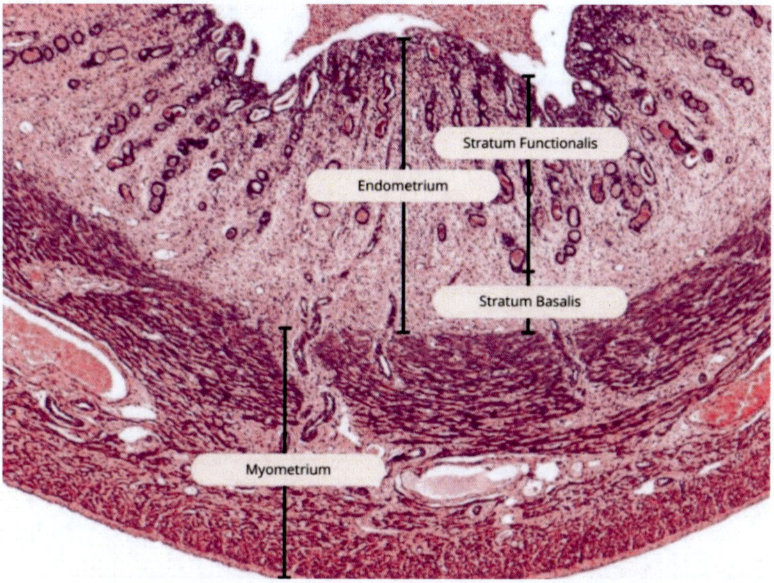

Figure 1. Histological cross-section of the uterus showing the key layers of the uterine wall. The outer muscular layer, the *Myometrium*, is composed of smooth muscle fibers responsible for uterine contractions. The innermost layer, the *Endometrium*, is divided into two sublayers: the *Stratum Basalis*, a regenerative layer that remains intact during the menstrual cycle, and the *Stratum Functionalis*, which undergoes cyclical changes and is shed during menstruation.

From a histological perspective, the functional layer comprises simple columnar epithelium that overlies the multicellular stroma. These epithelial stromal cells are targets for progesterone [2, 3].

The basal layer is composed of endometrial progenitor/stem cells [4]. Recent studies highlight the importance of stem cell populations within the basal layer in maintaining the regenerative capacity of the endometrium, an attribute unique among human tissues [4].

The process that the dynamic endometrium undergoes during the menstrual cycle can be defined into three phases: the proliferative phase, the secretory phase, and the menstrual phase [1]. The menstrual phase marks the first day of the endometrial cycle, where desquamation occurs and the endometrial lining is shed, provided no pregnancy has occurred. Menstruation lasts on average five days, and subsequently this is followed by the proliferative phase which continues until ovulation. The endometrial secretory phase follows this, corresponding to the luteal phase in the ovary [1].

1.2. Physiology of Menstruation

The physiology of menstruation is a cornerstone of female reproductive health, reflecting the intricate coordination of the hypothalamic-pituitary-ovarian (HPO) axis [5]. The menstrual cycle is characterized by hormonal, vascular, and cellular events that prepare the endometrium for potential implantation. If fertilization does not occur, the functional layer of the endometrium is shed, initiating a new cycle [1].

This process is carefully regulated by the hypothalamic-pituitary-ovarian (HPO) axis, all three elements working collectively via a feedback loop. Dysfunction of any of these will result in a disrupted menstrual cycle, reducing the chances of pregnancy and can be detrimental to overall health [5].

Menstruation is a cyclical process typically lasting 21 to 35 days, with an average duration of 28 days [6]. It is not unusual for prolonged anovulatory cycles to occur in the first years after the onset of menarche, lasting 45 days or more. However, regular ovulatory cycles usually occur in 45% of females by 2 years after menarche and in 80% by 5 years [7].

1.2.1. Endocrine Regulation of the Menstrual Cycle

The menstrual cycle is regulated by the hypothalamic-pituitary-ovarian (HPO) axis, which coordinates hormonal signals to drive the cyclical changes in the endometrium [5].

1.2.1.1. Hypothalamus and Pituitary

The hypothalamus releases gonadotropin-releasing hormone (GnRH) in a pulsatile manner, which stimulates the anterior pituitary to secrete follicle-stimulating hormone (FSH) and luteinizing hormone (LH) [5]. The frequency and amplitude of GnRH pulses vary across the menstrual cycle, with high-frequency, small-amplitude pulses favoring LH secretion during the follicular phase and low-frequency, high-amplitude pulses promoting FSH release during the luteal phase [5].

Neuroendocrine modulators, such as leptin and kisspeptin, regulate GnRH secretion. Adverse conditions, including low body mass index (BMI), inadequate caloric intake, and stress, can suppress GnRH pulsatility, leading to decreased FSH and LH production and, ultimately, anovulation or amenorrhea [8].

The hypothalamic-hypophyseal portal system connects the hypothalamus to the anterior pituitary, enabling efficient hormone transfer [9]. In the anterior pituitary, FSH and LH synthesis occurs in gonadotroph cells, comprising 5–

15% of the pituitary population. These gonadotropins share a common alpha subunit but differ in their beta subunits, which confer their unique biological activities [10].

1.2.1.2. Ovaries

The ovaries are the primary target of gonadotropins and play a crucial role in the menstrual cycle [9]. During fetal development, the ovaries house millions of oogonia, which undergo mitosis and differentiate into oocytes [11]. By birth, these oocytes are arrested in prophase I of meiosis, and their numbers decline significantly over time, with fewer than one million remaining at puberty and approximately 500 ovulated during a woman's reproductive lifespan [9]. The decline in oocyte quantity and quality with age increases the risk of chromosomal abnormalities. Ovarian follicles, which consist of theca cells, granulosa cells, and an oocyte, are the functional units of the ovary (Figure 2) [8].

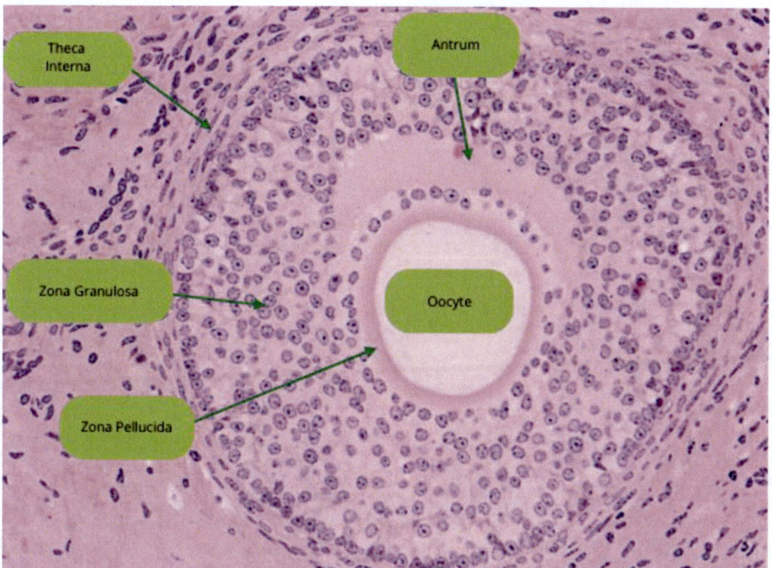

Figure 2. Histological section of a developing ovarian follicle showing its key structural components. The central *Oocyte* is surrounded by the *Zona Pellucida*, a glycoprotein layer. The *Zona Granulosa* comprises granulosa cells that support follicular development. The fluid-filled cavity, the *Antrum*, is visible within the follicle. Surrounding the follicle, the *Theca Interna* is a layer of stromal cells involved in hormone production.

FSH stimulates granulosa cells to secrete estrogen, while LH induces theca cells to produce androstenedione, which is converted to estrogen by the enzyme aromatase. Estrogen levels rise during the follicular phase, promoting endometrial proliferation, while the luteal phase is dominated by progesterone, secreted by the corpus luteum [8].

These intricate hormonal interactions ensure the successful progression of the menstrual cycle and prepare the endometrium for potential implantation.

1.2.2. Phases of the Menstrual Cycle

The menstrual cycle is a dynamic and multifaceted process characterized by physiological changes that prepare the endometrium for potential implantation [1]. These changes are classified into distinct phases, each marked by specific hormonal and structural events (Table 1) (Figure 3).

Table 1. Phases of the menstrual cycle

Phase of the Menstrual Cycle	Description	Endometrial Events	Involved Hormones
Menstrual Phase	Beginning of the cycle (days 1-5), characterized by the shedding of the functional layer of the endometrium due to the absence of pregnancy.	Shedding of the functional layer, triggered by the decline in estrogen and progesterone levels.	Decline in progesterone and estrogen
Follicular Phase	Proliferative phase (days 6-14), during which the endometrium regenerates under the influence of estrogen.	Regeneration of the functional layer, proliferation of stromal and epithelial cells, formation of new spiral arteries.	Estrogen (produced by granulosa cells)
Ovulation	Release of the mature oocyte from the dominant follicle, typically around day 14 in a 28-day cycle.	Preparation for implantation.	LH surge, high levels of estrogen
Luteal Phase	Secretory phase (days 15-28), during which the corpus luteum produces progesterone to prepare the endometrium for implantation.	Decidualization of stromal cells, secretion of nutrients by endometrial glands, formation of coiled spiral arteries.	Progesterone (from the corpus luteum), moderate estrogen levels

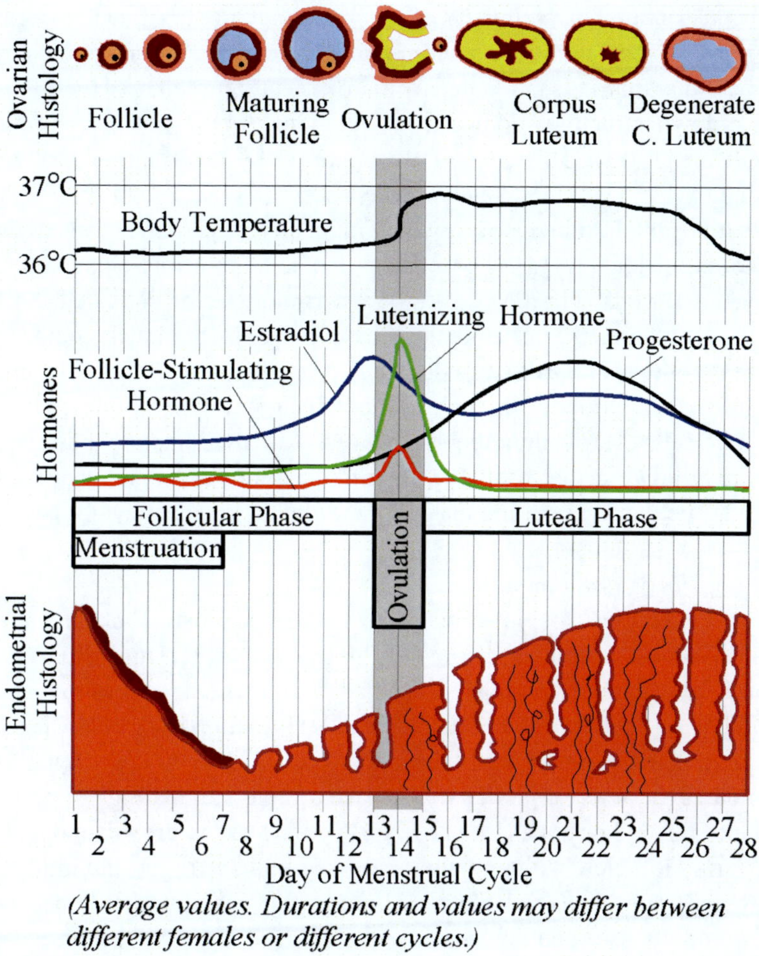

Figure 3. Overview of the menstrual cycle depicting changes in ovarian histology, hormonal levels, body temperature, and endometrial histology over a 28-day cycle *(©2017 From Wikimedia Commons image. Licensed under cc-by-sa 3.0 license)*.

1.2.2.1. Menstrual Phase

The menstrual phase marks the first phase of the menstrual cycle and begins on day one, lasting approximately 3 to 7 days. This phase is characterized by the shedding of the functional layer of the endometrium, the stratum functionalis, which occurs when pregnancy has not been established [1]. The collapse of the corpus luteum from the previous cycle leads to a sharp decline in progesterone and estrogen levels. This hormonal withdrawal triggers vasoconstriction of spiral arteries, resulting in localized hypoxia and subsequent necrosis of the endometrial tissue [12]. The degradation of the extracellular matrix is facilitated by matrix metalloproteinases (MMPs), which break down structural components, allowing for tissue disintegration and expulsion [1, 13]. This process is supported by an inflammatory response mediated by cytokines, cyclooxygenase-2 (COX2), and prostaglandins, particularly PGF2α and PGE2, which induce uterine contractions to facilitate tissue expulsion [1, 13]. The nuclear factor kappa-light-chain-enhancer of activated B cells (NFκB) is a key transcription factor activated during this phase, regulating the inflammatory cascade [13]. Previously suppressed by progesterone, NFκB activity rises after progesterone withdrawal, promoting the influx of immune cells such as macrophages and neutrophils [13]. These immune cells clear cellular debris and secrete growth factors to initiate tissue repair. Following the resolution of inflammation, angiogenesis restores the vascular network, preparing the endometrium for the next cycle [14].

1.2.2.2. Follicular Phase

The follicular phase begins concurrently with the menstrual phase and extends until ovulation, lasting approximately 10 to 21 days [1]. During this phase, the ovaries and endometrium are prepared for potential conception under the hypothalamic-pituitary-ovarian (HPO) axis regulation [10]. Pulsatile secretion of gonadotropin-releasing hormone (GnRH) from the hypothalamus stimulates the anterior pituitary to release follicle-stimulating hormone (FSH) and luteinizing hormone (LH) [10]. FSH promotes the growth and maturation of ovarian follicles, with granulosa cells secreting estrogen and inhibin A and B [8]. LH stimulates the theca cells to produce androstenedione, which is converted to estrogen by aromatase produced by granulosa cells [6, 8]. Estrogen exerts a proliferative effect on the endometrium, marking the beginning of *the proliferative phase* [1]. During this time, the endometrium regenerates its functional layer, driven by the proliferation of stromal and epithelial cells. The glands elongate and spiral arteries reform, creating a new vascular network. The endometrium, initially thin, becomes thicker and pseudo-stratified, with increased responsiveness to estrogen [1]. Progesterone receptors (PR-A and PR-B) are expressed in stromal cells but remain largely inactive until the subsequent phase. This phase concludes with selecting a dominant follicle, which produces sufficient estrogen to trigger ovulation [10, 11].

1.2.2.3. Ovulation

Ovulation occurs midway through the menstrual cycle, typically around day 14 in a 28-day cycle, but its timing depends on the maturation of the dominant follicle. Usually, rising oestrogen levels will suppress the release of FSH and LH via negative feedback. However, the large amounts of oestrogen produced by the granulosa cells, once sustained at a level over 200-300pg/ml over a period of 48 hours, will cause positive feedback on the hypothalamus and pituitary [1]. This positive feedback encourages the release of both FSH and LH from the anterior pituitary. However, FSH is relatively suppressed due to inhibin, also produced by the granulosa cells [10, 11]. Inhibin does not have the same suppressive effect on LH, hence the large surge in LH [15]. This LH surge triggers enzymatic activity within the follicle, breaking down its wall and releasing the oocyte into the fallopian tube. The granulosa and theca cells of the ruptured follicle luteinize, forming the corpus luteum, which begins secreting progesterone [16]. Although ovulation marks the luteal phase's transition, the endometrium's structural and vascular changes remain pivotal for implantation readiness.

1.2.2.4. Luteal Phase

The luteal phase spans from ovulation to the end of the cycle and typically lasts 14 days in a standard 28-day cycle. During this phase, the corpus luteum secretes high levels of progesterone, which acts on the endometrium, transitioning it into the secretory phase [1].

It Is also responsible for uterine muscle quiescence, preventing any implanted embryo from being expelled from uterine smooth muscle contractions.

The corpus luteum also secretes lower estrogen levels; however, progesterone is released in the highest quantities. This in turn causes negative feedback to suppress FSH and LH [8]. The corpus luteum will also produce inhibin, which prevents FSH release and any further follicles developing at this time [8].

The endometrium, primed by rising estrogen levels earlier in the cycle, begins to differentiate under the influence of progesterone, preparing for the potential blastocyst implantation. The stratum functionalis undergoes noticeable stromal changes, including the development of coiled spiral arteries, stromal edema, and the accumulation of stroma around spiral arterioles. These structural modifications enhance the endometrium's receptivity to an implanting embryo.

During the late luteal phase, or secretory phase, the endometrial stromal cells undergo decidualisation, transforming into decidual stromal cells (DSCs) [17]. This process is regulated intracellularly by cyclic adenosine monophosphate (cAMP), resulting in elongated cells expressing progesterone-dependent proteins [18]. Decidualisation, a unique feature of the human endometrium, occurs cyclically and independently of conception. It is vital for adequate trophoblast invasion and the establishment of a successful pregnancy [18]. Poor decidualisation has been associated with complications such as miscarriage, pre-eclampsia, and intrauterine growth restriction [19]. This process also facilitates immune tolerance by altering the function of immune cells, including natural killer (NK) cells in the stroma, which develop connections between themselves and other stromal cells [20].

By the mid-luteal phase, the endometrium reaches its peak receptivity, known as the 'window of implantation', typically occurring between days 19 and 21 of the cycle [18]. During this period, the glandular epithelium secretes glycogen and other nutrients to sustain the embryo, while the stromal environment becomes supportive of trophoblast invasion. Attempted implantation outside this critical window is often unsuccessful. Techniques to accurately identify the 'window of implantation' are under active exploration in the field of assisted reproductive technology (ART) [21].

If implantation occurs, the developing embryo secretes human chorionic gonadotropin (hCG), which maintains the corpus luteum and its progesterone production [6]. This ensures the continued maintenance of the endometrium until the placenta assumes this role during the first trimester. However, in the absence of pregnancy, the corpus luteum regresses, leading to a decline in progesterone and estrogen levels. Although the corpus luteum suppresses FSH and LH, it requires LH for survival. When hormonal suppression persists, the corpus luteum atrophies, resulting in hormonal withdrawal that triggers endometrial shedding [6]. Consequently, this marks the onset of the menstrual phase, and the cycle restarts as GnRH, FSH, and LH levels rebound to stimulate follicular development anew [6].

1.3. Practical Assessment and Measurement of Abnormal Uterine Bleeding

The complex physiology of menstruation forms a foundation for understanding disorders like abnormal uterine bleeding (AUB), which often arises from disruptions in these processes. The precise orchestration of hormonal regulation, tissue remodeling, and inflammation underscores the need for accurate diagnostic frameworks and effective interventions.

Abnormal uterine bleeding confers a significant burden across the world, with the vast majority of complaints being heavy menstrual bleeding (HMB) [22] It has been shown that out of the 1.2 million referrals made to gynaecology in the UK, 20% have been for HMB [23]. A US study quantified the financial losses from HMB as $2000 per patient per year, largely due to lost working days [24]. A European Study conducted by Fraser et al. found that as little as 6% of women seek medical support for HMB, with many unaware that their suffering is both abnormal and able to be treated [25].

However, the noticeable increase in women seeking treatment is not surprising, given the increasing awareness of menstrual problems and public health promotion enabling women to seek medical support for problems previously deemed taboo [24]. Additionally, in the past, women could expect to have around 40 periods in their lifetime with significant periods of amenorrhoea due to repeated pregnancies and lactation [1]. However, in present times, with improved family planning options, career prioritisation, and starting families later in life, women can now expect to have up to 400 periods in their lifetime [1]. This, therefore, amounts to a significant amount of potential lost working hours, relationship difficulties and morbidity that comes with HMB.

Management expectations have changed over recent decades, with fertility ending treatment not an option for many women [22]. Indeed, according to the UK Office for National Statistics, in 2015, the largest percentage increase in fertility rate was for women over 40, with the fertility rate in this age group greater than those under 20 years old in 2015 [26].

In order to meet these expectations and to manage AUB as effectively as possible, with little disruption to fertility and quality of life, it is imperative to determine the underlying cause of the AUB. For many years, varying terminology was used across the globe to describe and diagnose AUB. Terms such as menorrhagia, dysfunctional uterine bleeding and oligomenorrhoea have been found to be unclear and potentially confusing, leading to underreporting or underdiagnosing certain complaints [22].

In 2011, FIGO produced guidance that revolutionised the terminology used in AUB, creating standardised terms that can be understood and used worldwide, such as Heavy Menstrual Bleeding instead of menorrhagia [27]. FIGO also produced guidance on the structured assessment of AUB, diagnosis and management. This was updated in 2018 and is used globally [28].

Arguably, the most useful of these updates from FIGO is the PALM-COIEN classification for diagnosis of AUB causes [28]. PALM denotes structural causes, while COIEN covers non-structural causes. It is important to note that causes of AUB are not mutually exclusive, and patients can have multiple pathologies contributing to their symptoms [28] (Figure 4).

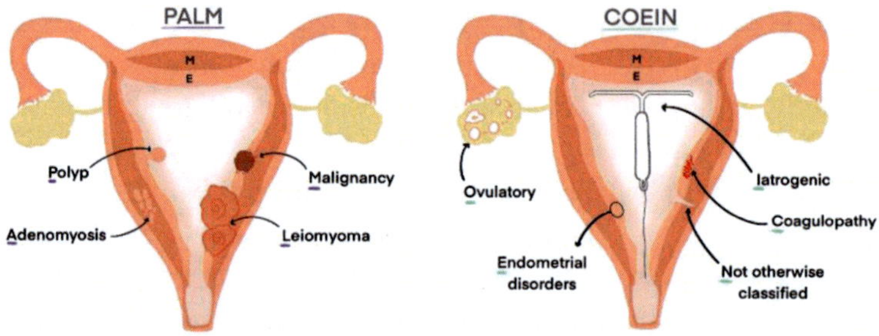

Figure 4. Classification of abnormal uterine bleeding (AUB) using PALM-COEIN *(©2024 Modified from Maybin JA et al. COVID-19 and abnormal uterine bleeding: potential associations and mechanisms. Licensed under the Creative Commons Attribution 4.0).*

1.3.1. Structural Causes (PALM)

1.3.1.1. Polyps

These benign proliferations of endometrial tissue are often asymptomatic; however, they can present with irregular uterine bleeding [29]. These can be ruled in or out with simple ultrasound or hysteroscopy imaging. The advantage of hysteroscopy for the diagnosis of endometrial polyps is that the vast majority can be surgically removed in the same appointment [30].

1.3.1.2. Adenomyosis

The diagnosis of adenomyosis can be difficult due to varied reporting and experience among patients [31]. The presence of endometrial glands and stroma in the myometrium causes cyclical pain and heavy bleeding, with a prevalence of between 7-27% [32]. Adenomyosis shows a resistant to medical treatments, with surgery often unacceptable to patients due to the usual age of presentation being in the reproductive years and preservation of fertility paramount [33, 34].

A proposed cause for this resistance to medical management is decreased progesterone receptor levels in the endometrium of those with adenomyosis and, therefore, a reduced response to any progesterone hormone treatment [33]. It is also hypothesised that estrogen receptors in the endometrium of these patients might increase, with less suppression of estrogen by progesterone in the proliferative phase, thereby contributing to HMB [13].

1.3.1.3. Leiomyomas (Fibroids)

These are the most common benign tumors in women of reproductive age, with a lifetime risk of up to 80%. Smooth muscle cells and collagen undergo excessive proliferation, producing the smooth whorls that define uterine leiomyomas. Fifty percent of women with leiomyoma will be symptomatic, either with pressure symptoms due to the size/position of the leiomyoma or AUB [23, 29].

Leiomyomas causing AUB are in the main submucosal, causing a defect in the secretory endometrium. This impacts endometrial function during menstruation, leading to increased blood loss [35]. It is thought that impairment in vasoconstriction can significantly increase menstrual blood loss [36].

Treatment options for uterine leiomyomas include medical therapies, minimally invasive procedures, and surgical interventions [37, 38]. The choice of treatment should be individualized based on symptom severity, fibroid characteristics, patient age, reproductive desires, and overall health [39].

1.3.1.4. Malignancy

Abnormal uterine bleeding (AUB) is the most common symptom of endometrial cancer [40]. While the prevalence of endometrial cancer increases with age, approximately 25% of new diagnoses occur in patients younger than 55 years [41]. Long-term unopposed estrogen exposure is a primary risk factor for the development of endometrial carcinoma [42]. Bleeding patterns in patients with uterine malignancy are highly variable, underscoring the importance of thorough evaluation of any abnormal bleeding, regardless of patient age [43, 44].

1.3.2. Non-Structural Causes (COIEN)

1.3.2.1. Coagulopathies

By far, the most common coagulopathy in women presenting with AUB is von Willebrand, with this disorder affecting 12-14% of these patients [23, 29]. The following specific set of screening questions can be used to diagnose AUB secondary to a coagulation disorder.

1.3.2.1.1. Ovulatory Disorders

These disorders disrupt regular ovulation and hence affect the normal menstrual cycle, leading to unpredictable and often heavy bleeding. While ovulatory problems are common at extremes of reproductive age, the conditions throughout reproductive life can cause significant problems for patients, with examples such as hyperprolactinemia and polycystic ovarian syndrome (PCOS) [45]. This chapter will discuss the normal menstrual cycle in further detail.

1.3.2.1.2. Endometrial Dysfunction

There is no specific 'test' to make this diagnosis; hence, it is an exclusion diagnosis. Most importantly, malignancy needs to be excluded. Endometrial dysfunction can occur primarily due to disturbances in the molecular pathways, including tissue fibrinolytic activity, prostaglandins and other inflammatory and vasoactive mediators [22]. There has been some evidence to suggest that subclinical chlamydia trachomatis infection may have a disruptive effect on these pathways, however further research into this is required [29].

1.3.2.1.3. Iatrogenic

Iatrogenic causes of AUB are vast, however, they are mainly due to the exogenous administration of hormones and sex-steroids, as well as GnRH agonists. 'Break through' bleeding that can occur as a result of these treatments can be significantly problematic for patients and lead to poor compliance and reduced quality of life [46, 47]. Additionally, drugs that affect hepatic enzyme activity can contribute to AUB, for example anti TB drug Rifampicin and certain antiepileptics [47].

1.3.2.1.4. Not Otherwise Classified

This group comprises endometriosis and more uncommon pathologies such as uterine arteriovenous malformations [48].

1.3.3. Diagnosis and Management

The approach to the patient with AUB requires a structured history thorough and appropriate examination, followed by any necessary investigations. The examination should come before investigations, as examination is not complete with just pelvic examination and speculum alone. A general examination searching for signs of anemia, evidence of thyroid disease or PCOS and abdominal palpation for masses can direct the investigations and prevent unnecessary and potentially time-consuming tests [23]. If acceptable to the patient, a speculum and pelvic examination should be completed. In those who it would be deemed inappropriate, e.g., virgo intacta, young adolescents and those who do not consent, diagnosis should be attempted to be reached without this examination [23].

A thorough history should include the duration and frequency of AUB and the volume of blood loss. Previously, patients would be asked to quantify their blood loss in milliliters, using teaspoons, tablespoons and egg cups as examples for patients to relate to. This was because the definition of HMB was more than 80ml per cycle [25]. Due to the subjectivity of heavy menstrual loss between patients, and the lack of correlation between objective measures and symptomatology, the clinical definition of HMB has been standardised as follows: "*excessive menstrual blood loss which interferes with a woman's physical emotional, social and material quality of life and which occurs alone or in combination with other symptoms*" [49]. Using this definition, the patient's history can address these points and determine whether bleeding is excessive or abnormal.

The prevalence of iron deficiency anemia is 30% of menstruating women worldwide, with 60% having iron deficiency without anemia [25]. Because of this large proportion of women being iron deficient without objective anemia, this condition goes largely underdiagnosed. Routine ferritin measurement is not recommended routinely in many countries, hence, if the hemoglobin is normal, iron deficiency can go unnoticed [23]. Ferritin is an acute phase protein, so that chronic HMB iron studies can be more informative.

If the patient describes regular cycles in both duration and frequency, they are likely ovulatory, with less frequent and irregular cycles likely anovulatory. Measuring progesterone can be helpful when confirming ovulation, however timing is critical, with the test performed seven days before the next cycle [50]. Further investigations comprising prolactin, FSH/LH and androgens should be considered if the cycles are deemed anovulatory [50].

Medical therapies can be considered prior to further imaging if the patient has no risk factors for malignancy [51] (Table 2). A reasonable approach to management in these cases is a 3–6-month trial of medical therapy, with further investigations should this fail. Tranexamic acid can reduce blood loss by up to 50% [52]. This is often used alongside mefenamic acid, which, while reducing blood loss by 25-50%, has the added benefit of analgesia [52]. Hormonal treatment may be commenced, with the combined oral contraceptive pill (COCP) being preferred, provided the patient has no risk factors for its use [52].

Table 2. Risk Factors for endometrial malignancy

Risk Factors for endometrial malignancy
Obesity
Chronic anovulation
Early menarche
Late menopause
Unopposed exogenous oestrogen therapy
Tamoxifen use
Lynch Syndrome

For those in whom medical treatments fail, or for those who have higher risk of significant pathology, transvaginal ultrasound is the preferred imaging assessment, provided the patient is agreeable. Assessment of endometrial thickness in post-menopausal women is far more reliable when compared to pre-menopausal patients, as the endometrium changes significantly during the cycle [43]. Intra-operator differences and patient factors such as BMI can affect the reliability of pelvic ultrasound. If symptoms persist despite a normal ultrasound or there are risk factors for malignancy present, then endometrial sampling, ideally by hysteroscopy, is the most appropriate next step [53]. Hysteroscopy is minimally invasive and can exclude and confirm pathologies requiring further treatment [54, 55]. If ultrasound shows endometrial polyps or fibroids distorting the endometrial cavity or more than 3cm in size, referral to secondary care can be recommended, as AUB is likely to continue unless these pathologies are adequately managed, most likely surgically [56].

The management of AUB is beyond the scope of this chapter, however the mainstay of treatment is to reduce the bleeding and improve quality of life. Wish for fertility, patient preferences, and co-morbidities should be central to any management. Excellent patient counseling and effort to understand their expectations can help ensure compliance, especially as many treatments can take up to 6 months to fully effect. This is particularly important considering an audit by the Royal College of Obstetricians and Gynaecologists (RCOG) of patients with HMB in the UK showed that 37% remained "unhappy" or "very unhappy" with ongoing symptoms [57]. An additional survey in the UK in 2021 revealed that 84% of women felt that their concerns regarding HMB had not been listened to or adequately addressed [58].

1.4. Abnormal Uterine Bleeding: What Role for the Endometrium?

Having delineated the causes of abnormal uterine bleeding, the endometrial role in AUB can be discussed further. There are many views on the endometrial factors contributing to AUB, and much research has been done to compare the functioning of the endometrium in those with AUB compared to those without, with the focus of these studies being HMB.

It has been suggested that immature endometrial vessels and, therefore, a reduction in vasoconstriction can result in a larger vessel radius during menstruation and increased blood loss [59]. Studies have demonstrated a larger vessel wall circumference in those with HMB and a reduction in vascular smooth muscle cell proliferation in spiral arterioles in the mid-luteal phase [60]. Regulators of vascular contractility and tone, smoothelin and calponin, are often dysregulated in those with HMB. For the spiral arterioles to develop normally during the cycle, coordinated maturation of vascular smooth muscle cells and endothelial cells is paramount [60]. It has been reported that in those with HMB, there are differences in the maturation of these cells, resulting in poorly formed spiral arterioles [59].

It has also been hypothesised that ineffective vasoconstriction maybe secondary to poor production of vasoactive factors PGF2a and endothelin-1 after progesterone levels decrease. Women with HMB have been shown to have a lower PGF2a/PGE2 ratio and reduced PGF factor expression compared to controls. An excess of PGE2 compared with PGF2a can disrupt the normal process of vasoconstriction [12].

The longer bleed of approximately two additional days in those with HMB, compared to those without, may be directly caused by this poor vasoconstriction [61].

Another endometrial factor hypothesised as having a role in HMB is alterations in the process of endometrial hypoxia. Endometrial hypoxia from spiral arteriole vasoconstriction is necessary for sloughing of the endometrium, however hypoxia is also seen to have a pivotal role in endometrial repair [36, 61]. This has been demonstrated with mice models, as in mice kept in hyperoxic conditions endometrial repair has been shown to be delayed [62]. In the human endometrium hypoxia inducible factor (HIF) regulates response to hypoxia at a cellular level. In hypoxic conditions, HIF enters the cell nucleus and influences the transcription of genes for processes involved in hypoxic response, such as angiogenesis and tissue remodeling. HIF-a is a subunit of HIF that remains stable only in hypoxic conditions and becomes degraded in conditions with abundant oxygen [62]. HIF-a has been detected in the endometrium immediately before menstruation, however levels have been found to be low in those with HMB, proposing a faulty response to hypoxia [62].

In endometrial repair, activation of the coagulation cascade dominates over platelet activation [13].

It has been proposed that levels of tissue plasminogen activator (t-PA) are higher on the second day of menstruation in those with HMB when compared with normal controls, perhaps pointing towards an overactive fibrinolytic system contributing to increased menstrual loss [63].

Whilst menstruation is an inflammatory process, resolution of this inflammation is key to endometrial repair and cessation of menses. Dysregulation in COX enzymes has been seen in HMB, potentially delaying the resolution of inflammation and contributing to longer bleeding [64]. Research also suggests that an increase in expression of cortisol-inactivity enzyme may be present in those with HMB, and this along with the hypothesis that cortisol promotes resolution of endometrial inflammation, may show that cortisol deficiency could contribute to increased bleeding [65]. Evidence for this however is scarce and more research is required before this theory can be safely adopted.

Conclusion

The endometrium exemplifies the complexity and resilience of the female reproductive system. Beyond its role in the menstrual cycle and potential pregnancy, it reflects broader principles of cellular regeneration, hormonal regulation, and tissue remodeling. The endometrium adapts dynamically to shifting reproductive needs by seamlessly integrating multiple physiological processes.

Abnormalities in endometrial function, such as those observed in abnormal uterine bleeding (AUB), highlight the consequences of disrupted hormonal and structural mechanisms. These conditions affect physical health and have far-reaching social and emotional implications, emphasizing the need for timely diagnosis and tailored interventions.

As modern lifestyles and reproductive choices evolve, the study of the endometrium becomes increasingly relevant. Addressing conditions associated with endometrial dysfunction requires a multidisciplinary approach, combining advances in molecular biology, imaging, and clinical practice. By continuing to explore the endometrium's unique capabilities and vulnerabilities, we can better understand its role in health and disease, ensuring improved outcomes for women worldwide.

References

[1] Maybin JA, Critchley HOD. Menstrual physiology: implications for endometrial pathology and beyond. *Hum Reprod Update.* 2015;21(6):748–61.

[2] Dallenbach-Hellweg G, Schmidt D, Dallenbach F. *Atlas of Endometrial Histopathology.* 3rd ed. Vol. IX. Berlin, Heidelberg: Springer; 2010.

[3] Dallenbach-Hellweg G. The Normal Histology of the Endometrium. In: *Histopathology of the Endometrium.* Berlin, Heidelberg: Springer; 1971. p. 22–88.

[4] Gargett CE, Schwab KE, Deane JA. Endometrial stem/progenitor cells: the first 10 years. *Hum Reprod Updat.* 2016;22(2):137–63.

[5] Naftolin F, Khafaga A, Nachtigall M. The Hypothalamic-Pituitary-Ovarian Axis and Regulation of the Menstrual Cycle. In: Berga S, Genazzani A, Naftolin F, Petraglia F, editors. *International Society of Gynecological Endocrinology Series.* Springer, Cham; 2019 [cited 2025 Jan 19]. Available from: https://link.springer.com/chapter/10.1007/978-3-030-14358-9_1. p. 1–13.

[6] Mihm M, Gangooly S, Muttukrishna S. The normal menstrual cycle in women. *Anim Reprod Sci.* 2011;124(3):229–36.

[7] Carlson LJ, Shaw ND. Development of Ovulatory Menstrual Cycles in Adolescent Girls. *J Pediatr Adolesc Gynecol.* 2019;32(3):249–53.

[8] Barbieri RL. The endocrinology of the menstrual cycle. *Methods Mol Biol.* 2014;1154:145–69.

[9] Xuereb GP, Prichard MML, Daniel PM. The Hypophysial Portal System of Vessels in Man. *Q J Exp Physiol Cogn Med Sci.* 1954;39(3):219–30.

[10] Amar AP, Weiss MH. Pituitary anatomy and physiology. *Neurosurg Clin.* 2003;14(1):11–23.

[11] Channing CP, Schaerf FW, Anderson LD, Tsafriri A. Ovarian follicular and luteal physiology. *Int Rev Physiol.* 1980;22:117–201.

[12] Maybin JA, Critchley HOD. Steroid regulation of menstrual bleeding and endometrial repair. *Rev Endocr Metab Disord* 2012 134. 2012;13(4):253–63.

[13] Watters M, Martínez-Aguilar R, Maybin JA. The Menstrual Endometrium: From Physiology to Future Treatments. *Front Reprod Heal.* 2022;3:794352.

[14] Salamonsen LA, Hutchison JC, Gargett CE. Cyclical endometrial repair and regeneration. *Dev.* 2021;148(17).

[15] Luisi S, Florio P, Reis FM, Petraglia F. Inhibins in female and male reproductive physiology: role in gametogenesis, conception, implantation and early pregnancy. *Hum Reprod Update.* 2005;11(2):123–35.

[16] Robker RL, Hennebold JD, Russell DL. Coordination of Ovulation and Oocyte Maturation: A Good Egg at the Right Time. *Endocrinology.* 2018;159(9):3209–18.

[17] Pan-Castillo B, Gazze SA, Thomas S, Lucas C, Margarit L, Gonzalez D. Morphophysical dynamics of human endometrial cells during decidualization. *Nanomedicine*. 2018;14(7):2235–45.

[18] Ng SW, Norwitz GA, Pavlicev M, Tilburgs T, Simón C, Norwitz ER. Endometrial Decidualization: The Primary Driver of Pregnancy Health. *Int J Mol Sci.* 2020;21(11):4092.

[19] Dunk C, Kwan M, Hazan A, Walker S, Wright JK, Harris LK, Jones RL, Keating S, Kingdom JCP, Whittle W, Maxwell C, Lye SJ. Failure of decidualization and maternal immune tolerance underlies uterovascular resistance in intra uterine growth restriction. *Front Endocrinol (Lausanne).* 2019;10(MAR):432963.

[20] Zhang X, Wei H. Role of Decidual Natural Killer Cells in Human Pregnancy and Related Pregnancy Complications. Front Immunol. 2021;12:728291.

[21] Enciso M, Aizpurua J, Rodríguez-Estrada B, Jurado I, Ferrández-Rives M, Rodríguez E. The precise determination of the window of implantation significantly improves ART outcomes. *Sci Rep.* 2021;11(1).

[22] Munro MG. Practical aspects of the two FIGO systems for management of abnormal uterine bleeding in the reproductive years. *Best Pract Res Clin Obstet Gynaecol.* 2017;40:3–22.

[23] MacGregor R, Jain V, Hillman S, Lumsden MA. Investigating abnormal uterine bleeding in reproductive aged women. *BMJ.* 2022;378:e07090.

[24] Schoep ME, Nieboer TE, van der Zanden M, Braat DDM, Nap AW. The impact of menstrual symptoms on everyday life: a survey among 42,879 women. *Am J Obstet Gynecol.* 2019;220(6):569.e1-569.e7.

[25] Fraser IS, Mansour D, Breymann C, Hoffman C, Mezzacasa A, Petraglia F. Prevalence of heavy menstrual bleeding and experiences of affected women in a European patient survey. *Int J Gynaecol Obs.* 2015;128(3):196–200.

[26] McLaren E. Births in England and Wales: 2015 [Internet]. Office for National Statistics. 2016 [cited 2025 Jan 19]. Available from: https://www.ons.gov.uk/people populationandcommunity/birthsdeathsandmarriages/livebirths/bulletins/birthsumm arytablesenglandandwales/2015.

[27] Munro MG, Critchley HOD, Broder MS, Fraser IS. FIGO classification system (PALM-COEIN) for causes of abnormal uterine bleeding in nongravid women of reproductive age. *Int J Gynecol Obstet.* 2011;113(1):3–13.

[28] Munro MG, Critchley HOD, Fraser IS. The two FIGO systems for normal and abnormal uterine bleeding symptoms and classification of causes of abnormal uterine bleeding in the reproductive years: 2018 revisions. *Int J Gynecol Obstet.* 2018;143(3):393–408.

[29] Marnach ML, Laughlin-Tommaso SK. Evaluation and Management of Abnormal Uterine Bleeding. *Mayo Clin Proc.* 2019;94(2):326–35.

[30] Chiofalo B, Palmara V, Vilos GA, Pacheco LA, Lasmar RB, Shawki O, Giacobbe V, Alibrandi A, Di Guardo F, Vitale SG. Reproductive outcomes of infertile women undergoing "see and treat" office hysteroscopy: a retrospective observational study. *Minim Invasive Ther Allied Technol.* 2021;30(3):147–53.

[31] Saponara S, Angioni S, Parry JP, Pacheco LA, Carugno J, Moawad N, Haimovich S, Lasmar RB, Dealberti D, Aksakal E, Urman B, Nappi L, Vitale SG. The Pivotal

role of hysteroscopy in diagnosing subtle uterine lesions in infertile patients: Seeing the unseen can make the difference. *Eur J Obstet Gynecol Reprod Biol.* 2025;305:132–41.

[32] Vercellini P, Viganò P, Somigliana E, Daguati R, Abbiati A, Fedele L. Adenomyosis: epidemiological factors. *Best Pr Res Clin Obs Gynaecol.* 2006;20(4):465–77.

[33] Szegeczki V, Fazekas L, Kulcsár M, Reglodi D, Török P, Orlik B, Laganà AS, Jakab A, Juhasz T. Endometrium as Control of Endometriosis in Experimental Research: Assessment of Sample Suitability. *Diagnostics.* 2022;12(4).

[34] Landi S, Mereu L, Pontrelli G, Stepniewska A, Romano L, Tateo S, Dorizzi C, Minelli L. The influence of adenomyosis in patients laparoscopically treated for deep endometriosis. *J Minim Invasive Gynecol.* 2008;15(5):566–70.

[35] Vitale SG, Moore O, Riemma G, Carugno J, Yarto ML, Haimovich S. Hysteroscopic laser ablation of symptomatic uterine fibroids: insights from a prospective study. *Climacteric.* 2023;26(5):497–502.

[36] Jain V, Munro M, Critchley H. Contemporary evaluation of women and girls with abnormal uterine bleeding: FIGO Systems 1 and 2. *Int J Gynecol Obstet.* 2023;162(S2):29–42.

[37] Vitale SG, Saponara S, Succu AG, Sicilia G, Martsidis K, D'Alterio MN, Angioni S. Efficacy and Safety of Non-Ablative Dual Wavelength Diode Laser Therapy for Genitourinary Syndrome of Menopause: A Single-Center Prospective Study. *Adv Ther.* 2024;41(12):4617–27.

[38] Pontis A, Sedda F, Mereu L, Podda M, Melis GB, Pisanu A, Angioni S. Review and meta-analysis of prospective randomized controlled trials (RCTs) comparing laparo-endoscopic single site and multiport laparoscopy in gynecologic operative procedures. *Arch Gynecol Obstet.* 2016;294(3):567–77.

[39] Urman B, Yakin K, Ertas S, Alper E, Aksakal E, Riemma G, Angioni S, Vitale SG. Fertility and anatomical outcomes following hysteroscopic adhesiolysis: An 11-year retrospective cohort study to validate a new classification system for intrauterine adhesions (Urman-Vitale Classification System). *Int J Gynecol Obstet.* 2024;165(2):644–54.

[40] Concin N, Matias-Guiu X, Vergote I, Cibula D, Mirza MR, Marnitz S, Ledermann J, Bosse T, Chargari C, Fagotti A, Fotopoulou C, Gonzalez Martin A, Lax S, Lorusso D, Marth C, Morice P, Nout RA, O'Donnell D, Querleu D, Raspollini MR, Sehouli J, Sturdza A, Taylor A, Westermann A, Wimberger P, Colombo N, Planchamp F, Creutzberg CL. ESGO/ESTRO/ESP guidelines for the management of patients with endometrial carcinoma. *Int J Gynecol Cancer.* 2021;31(1):12–39.

[41] National Cancer Institute. Surveillance, Epidemiology, and End Results Program. *Cancer stat facts: uterine cancer.* [Internet]. National Cancer Institute. 2024 [cited 2025 Jan 10]. Available from: https://seer.cancer.gov/statfacts/html/corp.html.

[42] Papaioannou S, Tzafettas J. Anovulation with or without PCO, hyperandrogenaemia and hyperinsulinaemia as promoters of endometrial and breast cancer. *Best Pract Res Clin Obstet Gynaecol.* 2010;24(1):19–27.

[43] Vitale SG, Angioni S, D'Alterio MN, Ronsini C, Saponara S, De Franciscis P, Riemma G. Risk of endometrial malignancy in women treated for breast cancer: the

BLUSH prediction model–evidence from a comprehensive multicentric retrospective cohort study. *Climacteric.* 2024;27(5):482–8.

[44] Bogani G, Scambia G, Cimmino C, Fanfani F, Costantini B, Loverro M, Ferrandina G, Landoni F, Bazzurini L, Grassi T, Vitobello D, Siesto G, Perrone AM, Zanagnolo V, De Iaco P, Multinu F, Ghezzi F, Casarin J, Berretta R, Capozzi VA, Zupi E, Centini G, Pellegrino A, Corso S, Stevenazzi G, Montoli S, Boschi AC, Comerci G, Greco P, Martinello R, Sopracordevole F, Giorda G, Simoncini T, Caretto M, Sartori E, Ferrari F, Cianci A, Sarpietro G, Matarazzo MG, Zullo F, Bifulco G, Morelli M, Ferrero A, Biglia N, Barra F, Ferrero S, Maggiore ULR, Cianci S, Chiantera V, Ercoli A, Sozzi G, Martoccia A, Schettini S, Orlando T, Cannone FG, Ettore G, Puppo A, Borghese M, Martinelli C, Muzii L, Di Donato V, Driul L, Restaino S, Bergamini A, Candotti G, Bocciolone L, Plotti F, Angioli R, Mantovani G, Ceccaroni M, Cassani C, Dominoni M, Giambanco L, Amodeo S, Leo L, Thomasset R, Raimondo D, Seracchioli R, Malzoni M, Gorlero F, Di Luca M, Busato E, Kilzie S, Dell'acqua A, Scarfone G, Vercellini P, Petrillo M, Dessole S, Capobianco G, Ciavattini A, Delli Carpini G, Giannella L, Mereu L, Tateo S, Sorbi F, Fambrini M, Cicogna S, Romano F, Ricci G, Trojano G, Consonni R, Cantaluppi S, Lippolis A, Tinelli R, D'ippolito G, Aguzzoli L, Mandato VD, Palomba S, Calandra D, Rosati M, Gallo C, Surico D, Remorgida V, Ruscitto F, Beretta P, Panici PB, Raspagliesi F. Characteristics and patterns of care of endometrial cancer before and during COVID-19 pandemic. *J Gynecol Oncol.* 2022;33(1):e10.

[45] Ali DES, Shah M, Ali A, Malik MO, Rehman F, Badshah H, Ehtesham E, Vitale SG. Treatment with Metformin and Combination of Metformin plus Pioglitazone on Serum Levels of IL-6 and IL-8 in Polycystic Ovary Syndrome: A Randomized Clinical Trial. *Horm Metab Res.* 2019;51(11):714–22.

[46] Vitale SG, De Angelis MC, Della Corte L, Saponara S, Carugno J, Laganà AS, Török P, Tinelli R, Pérez-Medina T, Ertas S, Urman B, Angioni S. Uterine cervical stenosis: from classification to advances in management. Overcoming the obstacles to access the uterine cavity. *Arch Gynecol Obstet.* 2024;309(3):755–64.

[47] Hickey M, Fraser IS. Iatrogenic unscheduled (breakthrough) endometrial bleeding. *Rev Endocr Metab Disord.* 2012;13(4):301–8.

[48] Angioni S, Saponara S, Succu AG, Sigilli M, Scicchitano F, D'Alterio MN. Metabolomic Characteristics in Endometriosis Patients. In: Genazzani AR, Nisolle M, Petraglia F, Taylor RN, editors. *Endometriosis pathogenesis, clinical impact and management.* ISGE series. Cham: Springer; 2021.

[49] Jain V, Chodankar RR, Maybin JA, Critchley HOD. Uterine bleeding: how understanding endometrial physiology underpins menstrual health. *Nat Rev Endocrinol.* 2022;18(5):290–308.

[50] Wu CH, Mikhail G. Plasma hormone profile in anovulation. *Fertil Steril.* 1979;31(3):258–66.

[51] Nees LK, Heublein S, Steinmacher S, Juhasz-Böss I, Brucker S, Tempfer CB, Wallwiener M. Endometrial hyperplasia as a risk factor of endometrial cancer. *Arch Gynecol Obstet.* 2022;306(2):407–21.

[52] Maybin JA, Critchley HO. Medical management of heavy menstrual bleeding. *Womens Heal.* 2016;12(1):27–34.

[53] Vitale SG, Laganà AS, Caruso S, Garzon S, Vecchio GM, La Rosa VL, Casarin J, Ghezzi F. Comparison of three biopsy forceps for hysteroscopic endometrial biopsy in postmenopausal patients (HYGREB-1): A multicenter, single-blind randomized clinical trial. *Int J Gynaecol Obstet.* 2021;155(3):425–32.

[54] Vitale SG, Laganà AS, Török P, Lasmar RB, Carugno J, Palumbo M, Tesarik J. Virtual sonographic hysteroscopy in assisted reproduction: A retrospective cost-effectiveness analysis. *Int J Gynaecol Obstet.* 2022;156(1):112–8.

[55] Florio P, Puzzutiello R, Filippeschi M, D'Onofrio P, Mereu L, Morelli R, Marianello D, Litta P, Mencaglia L, Petraglia F. Low-dose spinal anesthesia with hyperbaric bupivacaine with intrathecal fentanyl for operative hysteroscopy: a case series study. *J Minim Invasive Gynecol.* 2012;19(1):107–12.

[56] Vitale SG, Saponara S, Sicilia G, Klarić M, Sorrentino F, D'Alterio MN, Nappi L, Angioni S. Hysteroscopic diode laser myolysis: from a case series to literature review of incisionless myolysis techniques for managing heavy menstrual bleeding in premenopausal women. *Arch Gynecol Obstet.* 2024;309(3):949–59.

[57] Morrison Mckinsey SJ, Van Der Meulen J, Smith SC. National Heavy Menstrual Bleeding Audit Annual Report [Internet]. *Final Report.* 2015 [cited 2025 Jan 19]. Available from: https://www.researchgate.net/publication/257873466_National_Heavy_Menstrual_Bleeding_Audit_Annual_Report.

[58] Department of Health and Social Care. Results of the 'Women's Health – Let's talk about it' survey [Internet]. 2022 [cited 2025 Jan 19]. Available from: https://www.gov.uk/government/calls-for-evidence/womens-health-strategy-call-for-evidence/outcome/3fa4a313-f7a5-429a-b68d-0eb0be15e696.

[59] Maybin JA, Critchley HO, Jabbour HN. Inflammatory pathways in endometrial disorders. *Mol Cell Endocrinol.* 2011;335(1):42–51.

[60] Abberton KM, Taylor NH, Healy DL, Rogers PAW. Vascular smooth muscle cell proliferation in arterioles of the human endometrium. *Hum Reprod.* 1999;14(4):1072–9.

[61] Martínez-Aguilar R, Kershaw LE, Reavey JJ, Critchley HOD, Maybin JA. Hypoxia and Reproductive Health: The presence and role of hypoxia in the endometrium. *Reproduction.* 2021;161(1):F1–17.

[62] Maybin JA, Murray AA, Saunders PTK, Hirani N, Carmeliet P, Critchley HOD. Hypoxia and hypoxia inducible factor-1α are required for normal endometrial repair during menstruation. *Nat Commun.* 2018;9(1):295.

[63] Vannuccini S, Jain V, Critchley H, Petraglia F. From menarche to menopause, heavy menstrual bleeding is the underrated compass in reproductive health. *Fertil Steril.* 2022;118(4):625–36.

[64] Smith OPM, Jabbour HN, Critchley HOD. Cyclooxygenase enzyme expression and E series prostaglandin receptor signalling are enhanced in heavy menstruation. *Hum Reprod.* 2007;22(5):1450–6.

[65] Sadek S, Jacot TA, Thomas MC, Liu X, Duffy DM, Archer DF. PGE2 Regulates the Plasminogen Activator Pathway in Human Endometrial Endothelial Cells: Differences between Normal and Heavy Menstrual Bleeders. *Fertil Steril.* 2021;116(3):e306.

Chapter 2

Endometrial Polyps: From Pathogenesis to Clinical Management

Péter Török[1,*], MD, PhD
Stefania Saponara[2], MD
Liliana Mereu[3], MD, PhD
and Salvatore Giovanni Vitale[3], MD, PhD
[1]Department of Obstetrics and Gynecology, Faculty of Medicine, University of Debrecen, Debrecen, Hungary
[2]Division of Gynecology and Obstetrics, Department of Surgical Sciences, University of Cagliari, Cagliari, Italy
[3]Obstetrics and Gynecology Unit, "*Gaspare Rodolico*" University Hospital, Department of General Surgery and Medical Surgical Specialties, University of Catania, Catania, Italy

Abstract

Endometrial polyps are the most common focal lesions of the uterine cavity, often presenting with abnormal uterine bleeding, infertility, or as incidental findings during imaging. They arise from monoclonal hyperplasia of endometrial glands and stroma surrounding a central feeding vessel and are influenced by hormonal imbalances, particularly estrogen overexpression and progesterone insensitivity. Pathogenesis involves genetic, hormonal, and vascular dysregulation, with overactivation of estrogen beta receptors playing a central role. Factors such as obesity, advanced age, tamoxifen use, and inflammation further contribute to their development. Diagnosis relies on imaging modalities, including transvaginal ultrasonography, saline-infused sonohystero-

* Corresponding Author's Email: petertorokdr@gmail.com

In: Endometrium and Related Endouterine Pathologies
Editors: Liliana Mereu and Salvatore Giovanni Vitale
ISBN: 979-8-89530-818-9

graphy, and hysteroscopy, with histological assessment remaining the gold standard. Hysteroscopic techniques have revolutionized management, offering minimally invasive, precise resection methods, with advancements such as tissue removal systems, laser technology, and bipolar electrosurgery ensuring high efficacy and safety. While endometrial polyps are largely benign, certain factors like postmenopausal status, abnormal bleeding, and obesity increase the risk of malignancy, necessitating surgical intervention and histopathological evaluation.

Keywords: endometrial polyps, abnormal uterine bleeding, hysteroscopy, estrogen receptors, polypectomy

Introduction

Endometrial polyps are among the most common focal lesions of the uterine cavity, presenting a wide spectrum of clinical manifestations ranging from abnormal uterine bleeding to infertility or incidental findings during imaging studies. These growths, which arise from the endometrial lining, are influenced by complex interactions between hormonal, genetic, and vascular factors. Their pathogenesis involves the overactivation of estrogen receptors, hormonal imbalances, and dysregulated angiogenesis, while their clinical management has been revolutionized by advancements in minimally invasive hysteroscopic techniques [1].

This chapter delves into the definition, etiology, and pathogenesis of endometrial polyps, examining the intricate biological mechanisms underlying their development. Furthermore, it explores diagnostic tools and their respective accuracies, along with various therapeutic approaches, ranging from expectant management to advanced hysteroscopic interventions. By addressing the nuances of endometrial polyp classification, clinical implications, and their role in infertility, the chapter provides a comprehensive guide to understanding and managing this prevalent gynecological condition.

2.1. Definition and Etiology

Endometrial polyps are the most common focal lesions found in the uterine cavity [1]. Their incidence is higher in postmenopausal women compared to those of reproductive age and is extremely rare in adolescents. These polyps originate from the endometrium and are usually benign outgrowths, although histopathological examination may occasionally reveal premalignant or malignant changes. Microscopically, they exhibit monoclonal hyperplasia of endometrial glands and stroma surrounding a central feeding vessel, referred to as the axis or feeding artery (Figure 1). Due to the base of the polyp attaching the endometrial surface polyps can be sessile (wide base) or pedunculated (stalk). Based on their attachment to the endometrial surface, polyps are classified as sessile (broad-based) or pedunculated (stalk-like). They can develop at any location within the uterine cavity, varying greatly in size from a few millimeters to several centimeters, and may occur as single or multiple lesions [2–6].

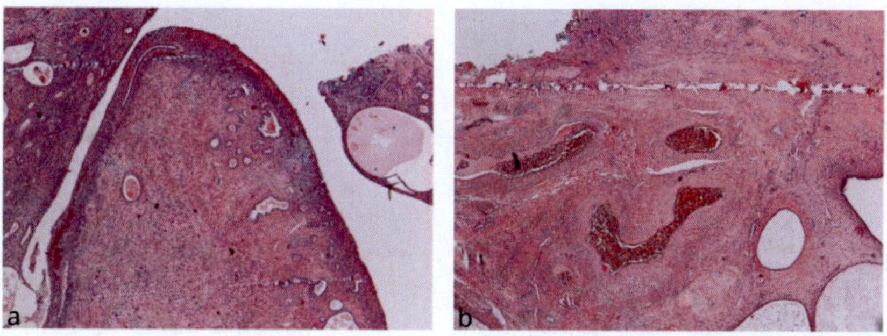

Figure 1. Histological image of an endometrial polyp, showing characteristic features such as fibrous stroma, endometrial glands, and thick-walled blood vessels.

Endometrial polyps often present with symptoms such as abnormal uterine bleeding (AUB), particularly in women undergoing evaluation for bleeding disorders. Their incidence peaks in the fifth decade of life, occurring in 10–40% of affected women [2–6]. Polyps are also associated with infertility, recurrent miscarriage, or may be incidentally found in asymptomatic patients, with a prevalence ranging from 1% to 12% [1, 3, 7]. A higher prevalence of up to 30% has been observed in infertile patients, suggesting a potential role of polyps in impaired fertility [8–11]. Prevalence of endometrial polyps in population with no symptoms found 0.5-12.1% in premenopausal patients. In asymptomatic premenopausal women, the prevalence of endometrial polyps ranges between 0.5% and 12.1%, whereas in postmenopausal women with a thickened endometrial lining, it increases to 60–70% [7, 12]. Expectant management may be an option, as spontaneous regression of polyps can occur, particularly for those smaller than 10 mm, where regression rates are higher [2]. While endometrial polyps are predominantly benign, the risk of malignancy varies between 0.5% and 5.4%, depending on the studied population [13]. Risk factors for malignant transformation include abnormal uterine bleeding, particularly in postmenopausal women, larger polyp size, obesity, and diabetes mellitus [14]. In symptomatic patients, such as those with abnormal uterine bleeding or infertility, surgical removal of endometrial polyps is recommended to alleviate symptoms and rule out malignancy [15].

2.2. Pathogenesis of Endometrial Polyps: Evidence and Hypotheses

Endometrial polyps express estrogen and progesterone receptors, which are believed to influence their development and growth [16].

Both alpha and beta estrogen receptors are expressed in the glandular and stromal cells of the endometrium. These receptor levels tend to decline in the functional layer of the endometrium during the advanced secretory phase [17]. Endometrial polyps specifically exhibit high levels of estrogen and progesterone receptors in the glandular epithelium, while the stroma shows low progesterone receptor expression and variable estrogen receptor levels [18]. A critical factor in the development of endometrial polyps is the hyperactivation of estrogen beta receptors, particularly during the proliferative and secretory phases, leading to stromal growth, increased angiogenesis, and progesterone insensitivity [19].

Hormonal imbalances significantly impact the pathogenesis of endometrial polyps. Estrogen plays a central role in facilitating endometrial growth, while progesterone works to regulate and reduce this activity. Elevated estrogen levels, as seen in cases of advanced age or obesity, are associated with a higher prevalence of polyps due to enhanced endometrial proliferation [20]. In postmenopausal women, polyps develop through mechanisms similar to premenopausal stages, albeit under altered hormonal conditions. Unbalanced receptor responses and irregular sensitivity to estrogens result in enhanced endometrial growth and reduced apoptosis, contributing to the increased prevalence of polyps in this population [21].

Excessive estrogenic stimulation, often caused by overexpression of estrogen receptors, can lead to overgrowth of endometrial tissue. Conversely, decreased levels of progesterone, particularly in anovulatory cycles such as those seen in PCOS patients, result in the absence of progesterone's modulating effect on endometrial growth. This imbalance promotes increased endometrial tissue activity. Additionally, abnormalities in the regulation of vascular development can lead to the formation of a central feeding vessel, further facilitating polyp development.

Other hypotheses suggest that modifications in the uterine environment, such as inflammation, reduced immune response, and mechanical interventions (e.g., prior intrauterine procedures), play a role in polyp formation. For instance, endometrial polyps have been linked to cesarean section scars, non-medicated intrauterine devices (IUDs), tubal ligation, chronic endometritis, and endometriosis [22].

The dysregulation of growth factors, including Fibroblast Growth Factors (FGFs), Transforming Growth Factor-beta (TGF-β), and Vascular Endothelial Growth Factors (VEGFs), further contributes to polyp formation. These growth factors, which are regulated by hormones during the secretory phase, influence cell growth, angiogenesis, differentiation, and extracellular matrix production [23].

Genetic factors are also implicated in the pathogenesis of endometrial polyps. Overexpression of genes involved in cell proliferation, such as cyclin D1, and survival, such as Bcl-2, has been observed in polyps. Dysregulation of the Bcl-2 gene indicates that polyp development may result not from excessive endometrial proliferation but from a failure of physiological apoptosis [24]. Furthermore, a connection has been proposed between the prevalence of endometrial polyps and endometriosis, a condition characterized by chronic inflammation and excessive estrogen stimulation through beta receptors. This imbalance promotes inflammation, angiogenesis, and Bcl-2 overexpression, leading to impaired apoptosis and subsequent polyp formation [25].

Tamoxifen therapy, commonly used in breast cancer patients as a selective estrogen receptor modulator (SERM), is another factor associated with the development of endometrial polyps. Tamoxifen causes relatively elevated estrogen levels, which may stimulate endometrial growth. In such cases, growth factors further establish a pathological link between angiogenesis and the growth of polyps [26].

2.3. Diagnosis

The diagnosis of endometrial polyps relies on imaging techniques and direct visualization, with confirmation achieved through histological assessment.

Transvaginal ultrasonography (TVUS) is the first-line diagnostic tool widely used by gynecologists due to its accessibility and effectiveness. Endometrial polyps typically appear as echogenic focal intrauterine lesions that may distort the endometrial lining. However, the accuracy of conventional 2D ultrasonography varies significantly in the literature, with reported sensitivity ranging from 19% to 96% and specificity from 53% to 100% [27] (Figure 2).

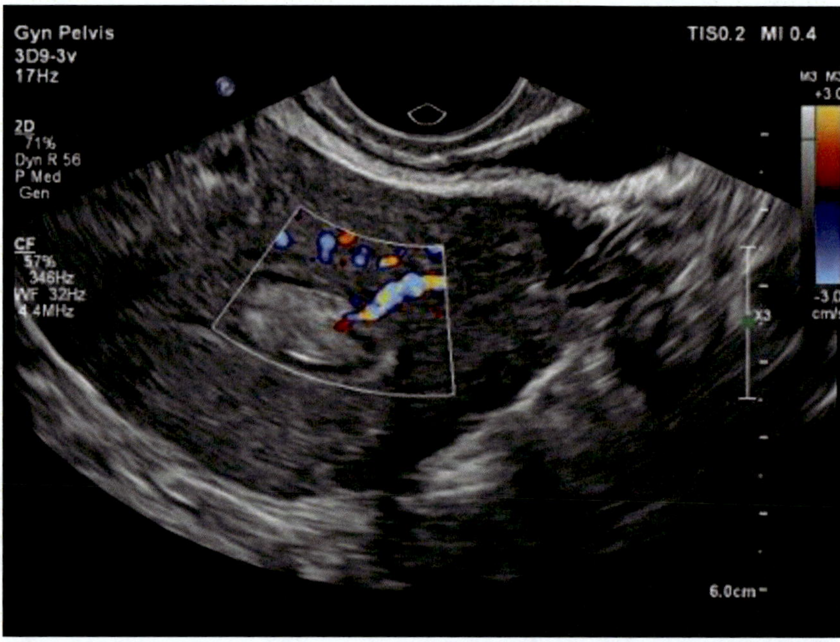

Figure 2. 2D transvaginal ultrasound and Color Doppler imaging of an endometrial polyp, highlighting the echogenic lesion and the single feeding vessel.

The addition of 3D ultrasonography improves diagnostic accuracy by enabling better visualization of the endometrial contour and polyp localization, with sensitivity and specificity reaching 65.6% and 89%, respectively [28] (Figure 3). Incorporating power Doppler allows for the identification of the central axis artery (single feeding vessel), further enhancing sensitivity and specificity to 81.2%–97% and 88.2%–100%, respectively [29, 30] (Figure 2). Saline-infused sonohysterography (SIS) is another technique that increases diagnostic precision. By injecting normal saline into the uterine cavity, the fluid surrounds and highlights the polyp, making it appear as an echogenic mass against an anechoic background (Figure 4). This approach achieves a sensitivity of 87%–93% and specificity of 81%–91% [31].

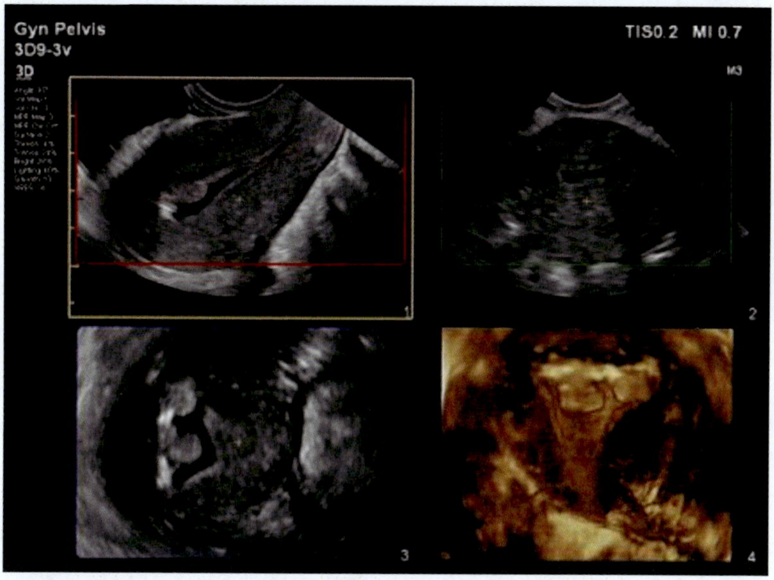

Figure 3. 3D ultrasound image of an endometrial polyp, demonstrating the detailed visualization of the endometrial contour and polyp localization.

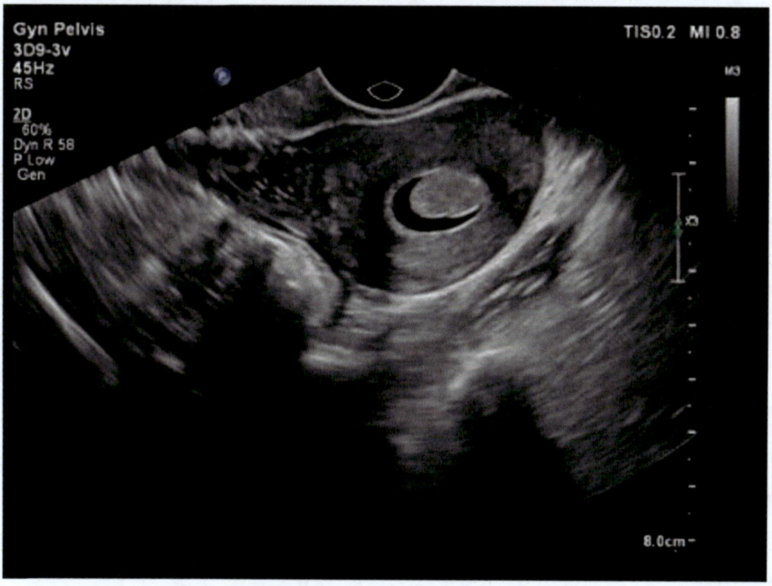

Figure 4. Saline-infused sonohysterography (SIS) image of an endometrial polyp, where the echogenic mass is clearly outlined by surrounding anechoic fluid.

Other imaging methods have notable drawbacks, such as ionizing radiation exposure, higher costs, and lower diagnostic accuracy. Hysterosalpingography (HSG) identifies polyps as filling defects within the endometrial cavity, but while its sensitivity is high (98%), specificity is limited (35%) [32]. Similarly, contrast-enhanced CT has a sensitivity of 53% and specificity of 94% [33]. Emerging methods like diffusion-weighted MRI may also play a role [34].

Diagnostic hysteroscopy enables direct visualization of intracavitary masses (Figure 5). However, without biopsies, its diagnostic accuracy varies, with sensitivity ranging from 58% to 99%, specificity from 87% to 100%, positive predictive value (PPV) of 21%–100%, and negative predictive value (NPV) of 66%–99% [27]. Blind sampling techniques, such as curettage, are less effective, with a sensitivity of only 8.4%–46% [35] (Table 1).

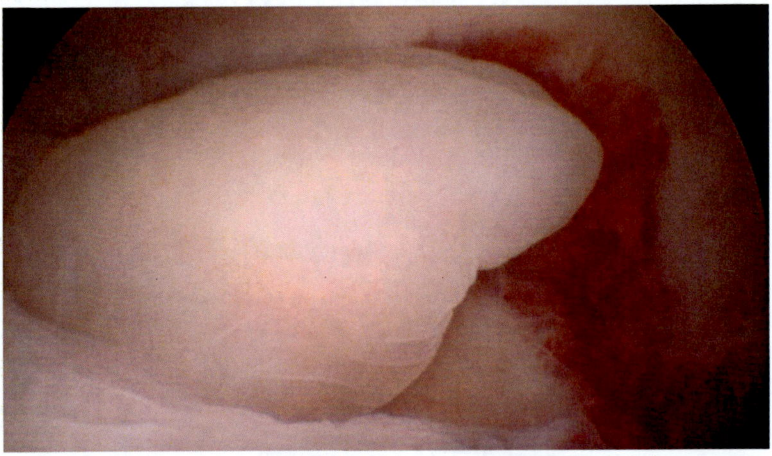

Figure 5. Hysteroscopic view of an endometrial polyp, showing the lesion within the uterine cavity under direct visualization.

The gold standard for diagnosis remains hysteroscopically guided biopsy, which offers the highest accuracy [36, 37]. Performing hysteroscopy in an outpatient setting can improve cost efficiency and feasibility [38–40]. Histopathological analysis of endometrial polyps typically reveals dense fibrous stroma, endometrial glands that are often dilated and closely spaced, and thick-walled stromal blood vessels [41].

Table 1. Sensitivity and specificity of different methods in diagnostics of endometrial polyps [27-35]

	Sensitivity	Specificity
2D	19% - 96%	53% - 100%
3D	65.6%	89%
Doppler	81.2% - 97%	88.2% - 100%
SIS	87% - 93%	81% - 91%
HSG	98%	35%
Contrast-enhanced CT	53%	94%
Diagnostic HSC	58% - 99%	87% - 100%
Blind procedure	8.4% - 46%	--

2.4. Classification

Endometrial polyps can be classified based on various criteria [42], including:

- Size: Less than or greater than 10 mm
- Number: Single or multiple
- Base: Pedunculated or sessile
- Menopausal status: Pre-menopausal or post-menopausal
- Histology: Benign, atypical, or malignant
- Type: Hyperplastic, atrophic, functional, adenomyomatous, or pseudopolyps.

2.5. Clinical Manifestations

Endometrial polyps can be asymptomatic or may cause abnormal uterine bleeding, post-coital spotting, and/or infertility [7, 43]. The majority (up to 40%) of premenopausal women with endometrial polyps complain of abnormal uterine bleeding, classified as "AUB-P" in the PALM COEIN classification [44]. The size, number or anatomical location of the polyp does not appear to correlate with the presence or severity of bleeding symptoms [44].

In case of malignancy, the most common histological subtypes are endometrioid adenocarcinoma and serous adenocarcinoma. The prevalence of premalignant and malignant lesions in patients with endometrial polyps is estimated to be 3.4%–4.9% in postmenopausal women and 1.1% in premenopausal women [45, 46]. Other studies report a broader prevalence range of 0%–12.9%, depending on the studied population [47]. Among patients diagnosed with uterine polyps, the malignancy rate rises to approximately 5% in symptomatic and postmenopausal groups [46].

The risk of malignancy in endometrial polyps increases with age, particularly in postmenopausal women experiencing vaginal bleeding [13, 48, 49].

This increased incidence in older women may be attributed to the absence of spontaneous regression mechanisms, which are characteristic of the cycling endometrium in younger, reproductive-age women [50–52].

Obesity is another risk factor for the malignant transformation of endometrial polyps due to the excess estrogen produced through aromatization of androgens in adipose tissue [53]. Hypertension has also been associated with an increased risk, although this may be an indirect correlation, as many hypertensive individuals also have a higher body mass index [54, 55].

Hormone replacement therapy (HRT) has not been definitively linked to an increased prevalence of endometrial polyps when balanced hormone regimens are used [56]. However, HRT is associated with a higher risk of malignant transformation, particularly in postmenopausal women [57]. Tamoxifen therapy for breast cancer has also been associated with malignancy in polyps, likely due to specific genetic mutations, such as mutations in codon 12 of the K-RAS gene (Kirsten Rat Sarcoma viral oncogene homolog) [58].

Genetic conditions such as Cowden syndrome and Lynch syndrome further increase the risk of endometrial cancer, with lifetime risks estimated at 5%–10% and 28%–60%, respectively [59, 60]. Postmenopausal bleeding remains a critical symptom that must be thoroughly investigated, as it is strongly associated with precancerous and malignant tissue changes. In these cases, histological evaluation is essential to exclude malignancy and ensure appropriate management [61].

2.6. Endometrial Polyps in Reproductive-Age Infertile Women

Endometrial polyps can negatively impact fertility by distorting the endometrial cavity, impairing endometrial receptivity, and increasing the risk of implantation failure [62]. One mechanism by which endometrial polyps contribute to infertility is through mechanical obstruction, which can hinder sperm transport by blocking the cervical canal or the entrance to the fallopian tubes [63, 64]. Another theory suggests that endometrial polyps exert their effects through biochemical mechanisms. Polyps have been shown to exhibit elevated levels of matrix metalloproteinases (MMPs) and cytokines, such as interferon-gamma and glycodelin (a molecule that interferes with sperm-oocyte interaction). Additionally, polyps have been associated with lower levels of placenta protein 14 compared to normal endometrial tissue, further supporting their potential role in infertility [65].

The reported prevalence of endometrial polyps in women with primary infertility ranges from 3.8% to 38.5%, while in women with secondary infertility, the range is 1.8% to 17% [66]. In infertile women with endometriosis, the prevalence of endometrial polyps diagnosed via hysteroscopy is approximately 46.7%. Furthermore, polyps are observed in 0.6% to 5% of women experiencing recurrent pregnancy loss [67, 68] (Table 2).

Table 2. Prevalence of endometrial polyps in different populations [66-68]

	Prevalence of polyps
Primary infertility	3.8% - 38.5%
Secondary infertility	1.8% - 17%
Infertility and Endometriosis	46.7%
Recurrent pregnancy loss	0.6% - 5%

Hysteroscopic resection of endometrial polyps has been shown to significantly improve pregnancy rates in infertile women with no other identifiable causes of infertility, regardless of the size or number of the polyps [69, 70]. Restoration of reproductive function after hysteroscopic polypectomy appears to enhance pregnancy outcomes consistently [71, 72]. In the context of assisted reproductive techniques (ART), polypectomy has been shown to improve outcomes for women undergoing intrauterine insemination (IUI) by increasing spontaneous pregnancy rates when performed prior to the first IUI cycle [73, 74]. Additionally, performing polypectomy prior to in vitro fertilization (IVF) or intracytoplasmic sperm injection (ICSI) may positively influence treatment outcomes when endometrial polyps are identified before the commencement of these procedures [75].

2.7. Hysteroscopic Management: When and How

Expectant management can be an option in cases where endometrial polyps are asymptomatic, as they may spontaneously regress in approximately 25% of cases. Smaller polyps are more likely to regress compared to those larger than 10 mm [7]. Medical treatment, including oral contraceptives, has shown a higher rate of regression for sessile polyps compared to pedunculated ones [76], and similar results have been observed with the use of the levonorgestrel intrauterine system (LNG-IUS) [77]. Additionally, the LNG-IUS may have a preventive role in polyp development [78]. For asymptomatic postmenopausal women, endometrial polyps are unlikely to be malignant, and observation can be considered following a detailed discussion with the patient [15].

Surgical removal of endometrial polyps is indicated in cases of symptoms such as abnormal uterine bleeding (AUB) or infertility, polyp recurrence, increased malignancy risk, or at the patient's request. For over 150 years, curettage has traditionally been the most commonly used method. However, as a blind procedure, curettage has proven to be ineffective and inaccurate, with limited success in achieving complete resection. Studies show that the area of the endometrial lining accessed by curettage represents less than half of the total endometrium, and the rate of incomplete polyp resection is significant [35]. In accordance with the FIGO-GCH ("Malaga") consensus, blind procedures should be avoided when appropriate hysteroscopic instrumentation is available [79].

Hysteroscopy is the preferred method for visualizing the uterine cavity and intracavitary lesions [80]. By inserting a scope connected to a camera and using fluid distension for enhanced visibility, the cervix and uterine cavity can be thoroughly assessed [81, 82] Procedures are best performed during the early proliferative phase when the endometrial thickness is minimal, ensuring optimal visualization [83–85]. Hysteroscopy enables not only visualization but also targeted removal of lesions using a "see-and-treat" approach, which allows for precise excision of the pathological mass while preserving the surrounding healthy endometrium [86–88] Thanks to the technical developments, the small diameter (4-5.5 mm) of the instruments and new techniques, hysteroscopy could be performed in an outpatient setting, without the need of operating room, anesthesia and high cost staff [89, 90]. The vaginoscopic technique further minimizes discomfort, often requiring only minimal pain management [91, 92].

The simplest and most straightforward method for endometrial polyp removal involves mechanical instruments. Hysteroscopic scissors or graspers, inserted through the working channel of the hysteroscope, allow for the precise mechanical resection of polyps at the level of the endometrium [93]. This technique is particularly effective for smaller, minimally vascularized polyps, as it minimizes bleeding. However, mechanical instruments are unable to address significant bleeding, and their use is limited in cases where vascularization or polyp size is substantial. When bleeding is encountered during mechanical resection, a bipolar electrosurgical electrode can be introduced through the working channel to coagulate bleeding vessels [94]. Bipolar electrodes also enable the slicing and resection of larger polyps while maintaining hemostasis [95]. Additionally, bipolar systems allow for the use of normal saline as a distension medium, which simplifies the procedure and makes office-based operative hysteroscopy more feasible [96].

For the resection of larger intrauterine lesions, the resectoscope represents a major advancement. This instrument, equipped with various types of electrodes, can manage a wide range of abnormalities using either monopolar or bipolar currents. Monopolar systems require non-conductive distension media, such as glycine or sorbitol, and are associated with higher rates of lateral electric and thermal spread, increasing the risk of complications. In recent years, the development of mini-resectoscopes with reduced diameters (5–6 mm) has enabled resectoscopy to be performed in outpatient settings [97]. These miniaturized instruments are predominantly designed for bipolar systems, allowing the use of saline as a distension medium, which further improves safety and practicality [98]. Resectoscopic polypectomy, whether performed in a traditional operating room or outpatient setting, is suitable for polyps of all sizes and numbers. Electrosurgical instruments provide simultaneous tissue cutting, slicing, and coagulation, ensuring complete resection while controlling bleeding [99] (Figure 6).

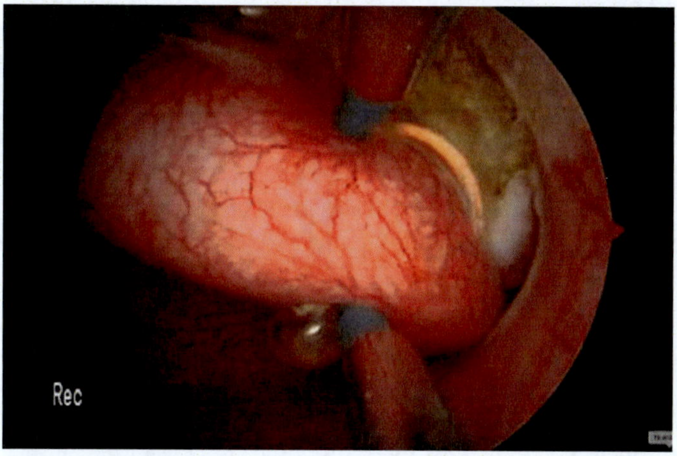

Figure 6. Resectoscopic polypectomy procedure, illustrating the use of electrosurgical instruments for precise resection of the polyp.

Laser technology (Light Amplification by Stimulated Emission of Radiation) was introduced to hysteroscopy in the 1970s and 1980s and has since become a valuable tool for polyp removal [100, 101]. Operating at wavelengths of 980 nm and 1470 nm, lasers enable precise cutting, coagulation, and hemostasis with minimal lateral thermal spread. This precision reduces pain during outpatient procedures and minimizes damage to surrounding healthy tissue, making lasers particularly suitable for delicate hysteroscopic interventions [102–104].

The Hysteroscopic Tissue Removal System (HTRS), first approved by the US Food and Drug Administration (FDA) in 2005, represents a significant innovation in polyp management. HTRS devices do not rely on electric energy; instead, they use a rotating or oscillating blade that "bites" pieces of the lesion while a suction system simultaneously removes the tissue from the uterine cavity. This continuous tissue removal ensures clear visualization by preventing floating tissue fragments from obstructing the operative field. HTRS also reduces the risk of uterine perforation, as the need for repeated instrument insertion and removal is minimized. Another key advantage of HTRS is its short learning curve compared to resectoscopes, as well as significantly shorter operative times. However, the system cannot coagulate bleeding vessels, necessitating the use of bipolar electrodes for hemostasis when bleeding occurs [105]. Comparative studies highlight that curettage, once widely practiced, is now considered outdated due to its low effectiveness and high rates of incomplete resection [106]. In contrast, hysteroscopically controlled polypectomy methods, particularly HTRS, offer superior outcomes. HTRS procedures are associated with lower rates of incomplete resection and shorter operative times compared to other techniques [107, 108]. Recurrence rates for endometrial polyps range between 5% and 15%, influenced by factors such as the surgical instrument used, the surgeon's expertise, and the size and location of the polyps. Although consensus on these relationships is lacking, studies suggest that laser technology may result in lower recurrence rates due to its superior ablation and vaporization effects. For instance, one study reported a recurrence rate of 32.6% with bipolar systems (Versapoint ™, Olympus America CORP. USA) compared to 2.2% with laser treatment at three months [109]. Additionally, complication rates, such as uterine perforation, are lower with mechanical instruments compared to electrosurgical devices. Postoperative adhesion formation is also rare with hysteroscopic techniques when compared to traditional dilatation and curettage (D&C) [74, 110].

Conclusion

Endometrial polyps are a common gynecological condition with significant implications for women's health, particularly in cases of abnormal uterine bleeding and infertility. Their pathogenesis is influenced by hormonal, genetic, and vascular factors, with estrogen overexpression playing a central role. While most polyps are benign, vigilance is required in high-risk populations due to the potential for malignancy. Advancements in diagnostic imaging and hysteroscopic techniques have revolutionized the management of endometrial polyps, enabling precise and minimally invasive interventions. Hysteroscopic polypectomy, in particular, has demonstrated efficacy in symptom relief and improved fertility outcomes. Future efforts should focus on reducing recurrence rates and further refining treatment options to ensure optimal patient care.

References

[1] Dreisler E, Stampe SS, Ibsen PH, Lose G. Prevalence of endometrial polyps and abnormal uterine bleeding in a Danish population aged 20–74 years. *Ultrasound Obs Gynecol.* 2009;33:102–8.

[2] Anastasiadis PG, Koutlaki NG, Skaphida PG, Galazios GC, Tsikouras PN, Liberis VA. Endometrial polyps: prevalence, detection, and malignant potential in women with abnormal uterine bleeding. *Eur J Gynaecol Oncol.* 2000;21:180–3.

[3] Clevenger-Hoeft M, Syrop CH, Stovall DW, Voorhis BJ. Sonohysterography in premenopausal women with and without abnormal bleeding. *Obs Gynecol.* 1999;94:516–20.

[4] Goldstein SR, Zeltser I, Horan CK, Snyder JR, Schwartz LB. Ultrasonography-based triage for perimenopausal patients with abnormal uterine bleeding. *Am J Obs Gynecol.* 1997;177:102–8.

[5] Nagele F, O'Connor H, Davies A, Badawy A, Mohamed H, Magos A. 2500 outpatient diagnostic hysteroscopies. *Obs Gynecol.* 1996;88:87–92.

[6] Van Bogaert L. Clinicopathologic ndings in endometrial polyps. *Obs Gynecol.* 1988;71:771–3.

[7] Lieng M, Istre O, Sandvik L, Prevalence QE. Prevalence, 1-year regression rate, and clinical signi cance of asymptomatic endometrial polyps: cross-sectional study. *J Minim Invasive Gynecol.* 2009;16:465–71.

[8] Hinckley MD, Milki AA. 1000 office-based hysteroscopies prior to in vitro fertilization: feasibility and ndings. *JSLS.* 2004;8:103–7.

[9] Frydman R, Eibschitz I, Fernandez H, Hamou J. Uterine evaluation by microhysteroscopy in IVF candidates. *Hum Reprod.* 1987;2:481–5.

[10] Seinera P, Maccario S, Visentin L, DiGregorio A. Hysteroscopy in an IVF-ER program. Clinical experience with 360 infertile patients. *Acta Obs Gynecol Scand.* 1988;67:135–7.

[11] Syrop CH, Sahakian V. Transvaginal sonographic detection of endometrial polyps with uid contrast augmentation. *Obs Gynecol.* 1992;79:1041–3.

[12] Ozelci R, Dilbaz B, Akpinar F. The significance of sonographically thickened endometrium in asymptomatic postmenopausal women. *Obs Gynecol Sci.* 2019;62:273–9.

[13] Lee SC, Kaunitz AM, Sanchez-Ramos L, Rhatigan RM. The oncogenic potential of endometrial polyps: a systematic review and meta-analysis. *Obs Gynecol.* 2010;116:1197–205.

[14] Sasaki LMP, Andrade KRC, Figueiredo A. Factors Associated with Malignancy in Hysteroscopically Resected Endometrial Polyps: A Systematic Review and Meta-Analysis. *J Minim Invasive Gynecol.* 2018;25:777–85.

[15] American Association Of Gynecologic Laparoscopists. AAGL practice report: practice guidelines for the diagnosis and management of endometrial polyps. *J Minim Invasive Gynecol.* 2012;19:3–10.

[16] King AE, Critchley HO. Oestrogen and progesterone regulation of inflammatory processes in the human endometrium. *J Steroid Biochem Mol Biol.* 2010;120:116.

[17] Critchley HOD, Kelly RW, Brenner RM, Baird DT. The endocrinology of menstruation-a role for the immune system." *Clin Endocrinol* (Oxf). 2001;55:701.

[18] Liu Z, Kuokkanen S, Pal L. Steroid hormone receptor profile of premenopausal endometrial polyps. *Reprod Sci.* 2010;17(377).

[19] Ye H, Xu X, Liu Y, Liu Z, Zhao A. Study on the relationship between estrogen receptor beta and etiology of human endometrial polyps. *Zhonghua Fu Chan Ke Za Zhi.* 2006;41(12):814.

[20] Pignata S, Ferrandina G, Scarfone G, Scollo P, Odicino F, Cormio G, Katsaros D, Frigerio L, Mereu L, Ghezzi F, Manzione L, Lauria R, Breda E, Alletti DG, Ballardini M, Vernaglia A, Sorio R, Tumolo S, Musso P, Magni G, Pisano C, Morabito A. Poor outcome of elderly patients with platinum-sensitive recurrent ovarian cancer: results from the SOCRATES retrospective study. *Crit Rev Oncol Hematol.* 2009;71(3):233–41.

[21] McGurgan P, Taylor LJ, Duffy SR, O.'Donovan PJ. Are endometrial polyps from pre-menopausal women similar to postmenopausal women? An immunohistochemical comparison of endometrial polyps from pre- and post-menopausal women. *Maturitas.* 2006;54:277.

[22] Indraccolo U, DiIorio R, Matteo M. The pathogenesis of endometrial polyps: a systematic semi-quantitative review. *Eur J Gynaecol Oncol.* 2013;34(1):5–22.

[23] Xuebing P, Tinchiu L, Enlan X, Jing L, Xiaowu H. Is endometrial polyp formation associated with increased expression of vascular endothelial growth factor and transforming growth factorbeta1? *Eur J Obs Gynecol Reprod Biol.* 2011;159:198–203.

[24] Taylor LJ, Jackson T, Reid J, Duffy SR. The difference expression of oestrogen receptors, progesterone receptors, Bcl-2 and Ki67 in endometrial polyps. *BJOG.* 2003;110:794.

[25] Meresman GF, Vighi S, Buquet RA, Contreras-Ortiz O, Tesone M, Rumi L. Apoptosis and expression of Bcl-2 and Bax in eutopic endometrium from women with endometriosis. *Fertil Steril.* 2000;74:760.

[26] Hague S, Manek S, Oehler M, MacKenzie I, Bicknell R, Rees M. Tamoxifen induction of angiogenic factor expression in endometrium. *Br J Cancer.* 2002;86:761.

[27] Vitale SG, Haimovich S, Laganà AS, Alonso L, Di Spiezio Sardo A, Carugno J. Endometrial polyps. An evidence-based diagnosis and management guide. *Eur J Obstet Gynecol Reprod Biol.* 2021;260:70–7.

[28] Fang L, Su Y, Guo Y, Sun Y. Value of 3-dimensional and power Doppler sonography for diagnosis of endometrial polyps. *J Ultrasound Med.* 2013;32:247–55.

[29] Jakab A, Ovari L, Juhasz B. Detection of feeding arteryimproves the ultrasound diagnosis of endometrial polyps in asymptomatic patients. *Eur J Obs Gynecol Reprod Biol.* 2005;119(1):103–107.

[30] Cil AP, Tulunay G, Kose MF, Haberal A. Power Doppler properties of endometrial polyps and submucosal fibroids: a preliminary observational study in women with known intracavitary lesions. *Ultrasound Obs Gynecol.* 2010;35:233–7.

[31] Vroom AJ, Timmermans A, Bongers MY. Diagnostic accuracy of saline contrast sonohysterography in detecting endometrial polyps in women with postmenopausal bleeding: systematic review and meta-analysis. *Ultrasound Obs Gynecol.* 54:28–34.

[32] Preutthipan S, Linasmita V. A prospective comparative study between hysterosalpingography and hysteroscopy in the detection of intrauterine pathology in patients with infertility. *J Obs Gynaecol Res.* 29:33–7.

[33] Grossman J, Ricci ZJ, Rozenblit A. Efficacy of contrast-enhanced CT in assessing the endometrium. *AJR Am J Roentgenol.* 2008;191:664–9.

[34] Grasel RP, Outwater EK, Siegelman ES, Capuzzi D, Parker L, Hussain SM. Endometrial polyps: MR imaging features and distinction from endometrial carcinoma. *Radiology.* 2000;214(1):47–52.

[35] Bettocchi S, Ceci O, Vicino M. Diagnostic inadequacy of dilatation and curettage. *Fertil Steril.* 2001;75:803–5.

[36] Fagioli R, Vitagliano A, Carugno J. Hysteroscopy in postmenopause: from diagnosis to the management of intrauterine pathologies. *Climacteric.* 23:360–8.

[37] Garuti G, Angioni S, Mereu L, Calzolari S, Mannini L, Scrimin F, Casadio P, Alberti DD, Nappi L, Busato E, Leone FPG, Perrini G, Cela V, Luerti M. Hysteroscopic view with targeted biopsy in the assessment of endometrial carcinoma. What is the rate of underestimatated diagnosis? The results of a multicenter Italian trial. *Gynecol Surg.* 2020;17(1).

[38] Di Spiezio Sardo A, Calagna G, Guida M, Perino A, Nappi C. Hysteroscopy and treatment of uterine polyps. *Best Pract Res Clin Obstet Gynaecol.* 2015;29(7):908–19.

[39] Vitale SG. The Biopsy Snake Grasper Sec. VITALE: A New Tool for Office Hysteroscopy. *J Minim Invasive Gynecol.* 2020;27(6):1414–6.

[40] Vitale SG, Laganà AS, Caruso S, Garzon S, Vecchio GM, La Rosa VL, Casarin J, Ghezzi F. Comparison of three biopsy forceps for hysteroscopic endometrial biopsy in postmenopausal patients (HYGREB-1): A multicenter, single-blind randomized clinical trial. *Int J Gynecol Obstet.* 2021;155(3):425–32.

[41] Kim KR, Peng R, Ro JY. A diagnostically useful histopathologic feature of endometrial polyp: the long axis of endometrial glands arranged parallel to surface epithelium. *Am J Surg Pathol.* 2004;28(8):1057–1062.

[42] Di Spiezio Sardo A, Di Carlo C, Minozzi S, Spinelli M, Pistotti V, Alviggi C, Placido G, Nappi C, Bifulco G. Efficacy of hysteroscopy in improving reproductive outcomes of infertile couples: a systematic review and metaanalysis. *Hum Reprod Updat.* 2016;22(4):479–496.

[43] Cai T, Mazzoli S, Migno S, Malossini G, Lanzafame P, Mereu L, Tateo S, Wagenlehner FM, Pickard RS, Bartoletti R. Development and validation of a nomogram predicting recurrence risk in women with symptomatic urinary tract infection. *Int J Urol.* 2014;21(9):929–34.

[44] Munro MG, Critchley H, Fraser IS. Research and clinical management for women with abnormal uterine bleeding in the reproductive years: more than PALM-COEIN. *BJOG.* 2017;124(2):185–9.

[45] Bel S, Billard C, Godet J, Viviani V, Akladios C, Host A. Risk of malignancy on suspicion of polyps in menopausal women. *Eur J Obs Gynecol Reprod Biol.* 2017;216:138–42.

[46] Uglietti A, Buggio L, Farella M, Chiaffarino F, Dridi D, Vercellini P. The risk of malignancy in uterine polyps: a systematic review and meta-analysis. *Eur J Obs Gynecol Reprod Biol.* 2019;237:48–56.

[47] Lieng M, Istre O, Qvigstad E. Treatment of endometrial polyps: a systematic review. *Acta Obs Gynecol Scand.* 2010;89(8):992–1002.

[48] Vitale SG, Riemma G, Haimovich S, Carugno J, Alonso Pacheco L, Perez-Medina T, Parry JP, Török P, Tesarik J, Della Corte L, Cobellis L, Di Spiezio Sardo A, De Franciscis P. Risk of endometrial cancer in asymptomatic postmenopausal women in relation to ultrasonographic endometrial thickness: systematic review and diagnostic test accuracy meta-analysis. *Am J Obstet Gynecol.* 2023;228(1):22-35.e2.

[49] Vitale SG, Angioni S, D'Alterio MN, Ronsini C, Saponara S, De Franciscis P, Riemma G. Risk of endometrial malignancy in women treated for breast cancer: the BLUSH prediction model–evidence from a comprehensive multicentric retrospective cohort study. *Climacteric.* 2024;27(5):482–8.

[50] Hileeto D, Fadare O, Martel M. Age dependent association of endometrial polyps with increased risk of cancer involvement. *World J Surg Oncol.* 2005;3(1):8.

[51] Prisco MG, Zannoni GF, De Stefano I, Vellone VG, Tortorella L, Fagotti A, Mereu L, Scambia G, Gallo D. Prognostic role of metastasis tumor antigen 1 in patients with ovarian cancer: a clinical study. *Hum Pathol.* 2012;43(2):282–8.

[52] Vitale SG, Caruso S, Rapisarda AMC, Valenti G, Rossetti D, Cianci S, Cianci A. Biocompatible porcine dermis graft to treat severe cystocele: impact on quality of life and sexuality. *Arch Gynecol Obstet.* 2016;293(1):125–31.

[53] Ali DES, Shah M, Ali A, Malik MO, Rehman F, Badshah H, Ehtesham E, Vitale SG. Treatment with Metformin and Combination of Metformin plus Pioglitazone on Serum Levels of IL-6 and IL-8 in Polycystic Ovary Syndrome: A Randomized Clinical Trial. *Horm Metab Res.* 2019;51(11):714–22.

[54] Gregoriou O, Konidaris S, Vrachnis N. Clinical parameters linked with malignancy in endometrial polyps. *Climacteric.* 12(5):454–458.

[55] Shi Y, Zhu Y, Fan S, Vitagliano A, Liu X, Liao Y, Liang Y, Vitale SG. Clinical Characteristics and Antifungal Susceptibility of Candida nivariensis from Vulvovaginal Candidiasis. *Gynecol Obstet Invest.* 2020;85(1):88–93.

[56] Oguz S, Sargin A, Kelekci S, H. A, O.L. T, L M. The role of hormone replacement therapy in endometrial polyp formation. *Maturitas.* 2005;50:231.

[57] Van Den Bosch T, Van Schoubroeck D, Ameye L. Ultrasound assessment of endometrial thickness and endometrial polyps in women on hormonal replacement therapy. *Am J Obs Gynecol.* 2003;188(5):1249–1253.

[58] Hachisuga T, Miyakawa T, Tsujioka H. K-ras mutation in tamoxifen-related endometrial polyps. *Cancer.* 2003;98(9):1890–1897.

[59] Kalin A, Merideth MA, Regier DS, Blumenthal GM, Dennis PA, Stratton P. Management of reproductive health in Cowden syndrome complicated by endometrial polyps and breast cancer. *Obs Gynecol.* 2013;121:461–4.

[60] Banno K, Kisu I, Yanokura M. Hereditary Endometrial Cancer: Lynch Syndrome. *Curr Obs Gynecol Rep.* 2013;2:11–18.

[61] American College of Obstetricians and Gynecologists. ACOG committee opinion no. 557: management of acute abnormal uterine bleeding in nonpregnant reproductive-aged women. *Obs Gynecol.* 2013;121(4):891–896.

[62] Alansari L, Wardle P. Endometrial polyps and subfertility. *Hum Fertil.* 2012;15(3):129–133.

[63] Salim S, Won H, Nesbitt-Hawes E, Campbell N, Abbott J. Diagnosis and management of endometrial polyps: a critical review of the literature. *J Minim Invasive Gynecol.* 2011;18(5):569–81.

[64] Vitale SG, De Angelis MC, Della Corte L, Saponara S, Carugno J, Laganà AS, Török P, Tinelli R, Pérez-Medina T, Ertas S, Urman B, Angioni S. Uterine cervical stenosis: from classification to advances in management. Overcoming the obstacles to access the uterine cavity. *Arch Gynecol Obstet.* 2024;309(3):755–64.

[65] Richlin SS, Ramachandran S, Shanti A. Glycodelin levels in uterine flushings and in plasma of patients with leiomyomas and polyps: implications for implantation. *Hum Reprod.* 2002;17(10):2742–2747.

[66] Shokeir TA, HM S, El-Shafei MM. Significance of endometrial polyps detected hysteroscopically in eumenorrheic infertile women. *J Obs Gynaecol Res.* 2004;30(2):84–89.

[67] Bosteels J, Weyers S, Puttemans P, Panayotidis C, Herendael B, Gomel V, Mol BW, Mathieu C, D'Hooghe T. The effectiveness of hysteroscopy in improving pregnancy rates in subfertile women without other gynaecological symptoms: a systematic review. *Hum Reprod Updat.* 2010;16(1):1–11.

[68] Ben-Nagi J, Miell J, Yazbek J, Holland T, Jurkovic D. The effect of hysteroscopic polypectomy on the concentrations of endometrial implantation factors in uterine flushings, Reprod. *Biomed Online.* 2009;19(5):737–744.

[69] Zhu H, Fu J, Lei H, Song Y, Shen L, Huang W. Evaluation of transvaginal sonography in detecting endometrial polyps and the pregnancy outcome following hysteroscopic polypectomy in infertile women. *Ther Med.* 2016;12(2):1196–1200.

[70] Vitale SG, Laganà AS, Török P, Lasmar RB, Carugno J, Palumbo M, Tesarik J. Virtual sonographic hysteroscopy in assisted reproduction: A retrospective cost-effectiveness analysis. *Int J Gynaecol Obstet.* 2022;156(1):112–8.

[71] Stamatellos I, Apostolides A, Stamatopoulos P, Bontis J. Pregnancy rates after hysteroscopic polypectomy depending on the size or number of the polyps. *Arch Gynecol Obstet.* 2008;277(5):395–9.

[72] Rackow BW, Jorgensen E, Taylor HS. Endometrial polyps affect uterine receptivity. *Fertil Steril.* 2011;95(8):2690–2692.

[73] Pérez-Medina T, Bajo-Arenas J, Salazar F, Redondo T, Sanfrutos L, Alvarez P, Engels V. Endometrial polyps and their implication in the pregnancy rates of patients undergoing intrauterine insemination: a prospective, randomized study. *Hum Reprod.* 2005;20(6):1632–5.

[74] Vitale SG, Riemma G, Carugno J, Perez-Medina T, Alonso Pacheco L, Haimovich S, Parry JP, Di Spiezio Sardo A, De Franciscis P. Postsurgical barrier strategies to avoid the recurrence of intrauterine adhesion formation after hysteroscopic adhesiolysis: a network meta-analysis of randomized controlled trials. *Am J Obstet Gynecol.* 2022;226(4):487-498.e8.

[75] Kodaman PH. Hysteroscopic polypectomy for women undergoing IVF treatment: when is it necessary? *Curr Opin Obstet Gynecol.* 2016;28(3):184–190.

[76] Fraser IS. The promise and reality of the intrauterine route for hormone delivery for prevention and therapy of gynecological disease. *Contraception.* 2007;75(6 Suppl):112– 117.

[77] Wada-Hiraike O, Osuga Y, Hiroi H. Sessile polyps and pedunculated polyps respond differently to oral contraceptives. *Gynecol Endocrinol.* 2011;27(5):351–355.

[78] Arnes M, Hvingel B, Orbo A. Levonorgestrel-impregnated intrauterine device reduces occurrence of hyperplastic polyps: a population-based follow-up cohort study. *Anticancer Res.* 2014;34(5):2319–2324.

[79] Villegas-Echeverri JD, Pope R, Robert M, Meinhold-Heerlein I, Haimovich S, Carugno J, Pacheco LA, Sardo ADS. FIGO-GCH joint consensus statement on the current status and recommendations for the use of blind intrauterine procedures in the evaluation and management of women with suspected intrauterine pathologies. *Int J Gynecol Obstet.* 2025;168(2):493–6.

[80] Vitale SG, Angioni S, Saponara S, Sicilia G, Mignacca A, Caiazzo A, De Franciscis P, Riemma G. Hysteroscopic metroplasty and its reproductive impact among the social networks: A cross-sectional analysis on video quality, reliability and creators' opinions on YouTube, TikTok and Instagram. *Int J Med Inform.* 2025;195:105776.

[81] Vitale SG, Angioni S, Saponara S, Sicilia G, Etrusco A, D'Alterio MN, Cobellis L, De Franciscis P, Riemma G. TikTok as a platform for hysteroscopy information: An analytical video-based cross-sectional study to assess quality, reliability, and accuracy. *Int J Gynecol Obstet.* 2025;168(1):353–61.

[82] Libretti A, Vitale SG, Saponara S, Corsini C, Aquino CI, Savasta F, Tizzoni E, Troìa L, Surico D, Angioni S, Remorgida V. Hysteroscopy in the new media: quality and reliability analysis of hysteroscopy procedures on YouTube™. *Arch Gynecol Obstet.* 2023;308(5):1515–24.

[83] Florio P, Filippeschi M, Imperatore A, Mereu L, Franchini M, Calzolari S, Mencaglia L, Litta P. The practicability and surgeons' subjective experiences with vaginal danazol before an operative hysteroscopy. *Steroids.* 2012;77:528–533.

[84] Mereu L, Giunta G, Carri C, Prasciolu C, Albis Florez ED, Mencaglia L. Nomegestrol acetate versus combined oral contraceptive as rapid endometrial preparation for operative hysteroscopy: a prospective randomised pilot study. *Gynecol Surg.* 2012;9:401–404.

[85] Saponara S, Angioni S, Parry JP, Pacheco LA, Carugno J, Moawad N, Haimovich S, Lasmar RB, Dealberti D, Aksakal E, Urman B, Nappi L, Vitale SG. The Pivotal role of hysteroscopy in diagnosing subtle uterine lesions in infertile patients: Seeing the unseen can make the difference. *Eur J Obstet Gynecol Reprod Biol.* 2025;305:132–41.

[86] Vitale SG, Di Spiezio Sardo A, Riemma G, De Franciscis P, Alonso Pacheco L, Carugno J. In-office hysteroscopic removal of retained or fragmented intrauterine device without anesthesia: a cross-sectional analysis of an international survey. *Updates Surg.* 2022;74(3):1079–85.

[87] Wortman M. "See-and-Treat" Hysteroscopy in the Management of Endometrial Polyps. *Surg Technol Int.* 2016;28:177–84.

[88] Chiofalo B, Palmara V, Vilos GA, Pacheco LA, Lasmar RB, Shawki O, Giacobbe V, Alibrandi A, Di Guardo F, Vitale SG. Reproductive outcomes of infertile women undergoing "see and treat" office hysteroscopy: a retrospective observational study. *Minim Invasive Ther Allied Technol.* 2021;30(3):147–53.

[89] Florio P, Puzzutiello R, Filippeschi M, D'Onofrio P, Mereu L, Morelli R, Marianello D, Litta P, Mencaglia L, Petraglia F. Low-dose spinal anesthesia with hyperbaric bupivacaine with intrathecal fentanyl for operative hysteroscopy: a case series study. *J Minim Invasive Gynecol.* 2012;19(1):107–12.

[90] Vitale SG, Carugno J, Saponara S, Mereu L, Haimovich S, Alonso Pacheco L, Giannini A, Chellani M, Urman B, De Angelis MC, Angioni S. What is the impact of simulation on the learning of hysteroscopic skills by residents and medical students? A systematic review. *Minim Invasive Ther Allied Technol.* 2024;33(6):373–86.

[91] Bettocchi S, Selvaggi L. A vaginoscopic approach to reduce the pain of office hysteroscopy. *J Am Assoc Gynecol Laparosc.* 1997;4(2):255–8.

[92] Török P, Molnár S, Herman T, Jashanjeet S, Lampé R, Riemma G, Vitale SG. Fallopian tubal obstruction is associated with increased pain experienced during office hysteroscopy: a retrospective study. *Updates Surg.* 2020;72(1):213–8.

[93] Vitale SG, Parry JP, Carugno J, Cholkeri-Singh A, Della Corte L, Cianci S, Schiattarella A, Riemma G, De Franciscis P. Surgical and Reproductive Outcomes after Hysteroscopic Removal of Retained Products of Conception: A Systematic Review and Meta-analysis. *J Minim Invasive Gynecol.* 2021;28(2):204–17.

[94] Golan A, Sagiv R, Berar M. Bipolar electrical energy in physiologic solution– a revolution in operative hysteroscopy. *J Am Assoc Gynecol Laparosc.* 2001;8:252–258.

[95] Mencaglia L, Carri G, Prasciolu C, Giunta G, Albis Florez ED, Cofelice V, Mereu L. Feasibility and complications in bipolar resectoscopy: preliminary experience. *Minim Invasive Ther Allied Technol.* 2013;22(1):50–5.

[96] Vilos GA. Intrauterine surgery using a new coaxial bipolar electrode in normal saline solution (Versapoint): a pilot study. *Fertil Steril.* 1999;72:740–743.

[97] Litta P, Cosmi E, Saccardi C. Outpatient operative polypectomy using a 5 mm-hysteroscope without anaesthesia and/or analgesia: advantages and limits. *Eur J Obs Gynecol Reprod Biol.* 2008;139:120–124.

[98] Papalampros P, Gambadauro P, Papadopoulos N, Polyzos D, Chapman L, Magos A. The mini-resectoscope: A new instrument for office hysteroscopic surgery. *Acta Obstet Gynecol Scand.* 2009;88(2):227–30.

[99] Deutsch A, Sasaki KJ, Cholkeri-Singh A. Resectoscopic surgery for polyps and myomas: a review of the literature. *J Minim Invasive Gynecol.* 2017;24:1104–1110.

[100] Vitale SG, Saponara S, Succu AG, Sicilia G, Martsidis K, D'Alterio MN, Angioni S. Efficacy and Safety of Non-Ablative Dual Wavelength Diode Laser Therapy for Genitourinary Syndrome of Menopause: A Single-Center Prospective Study. *Adv Ther.* 2024;41(12):4617–27.

[101] Etrusco A, Buzzaccarini G, Laganà AS, Chiantera V, Vitale SG, Angioni S, D'Alterio MN, Nappi L, Sorrentino F, Vitagliano A, Difonzo T, Riemma G, Mereu L, Favilli A, Peitsidis P, D'Amato A. Use of Diode Laser in Hysteroscopy for the Management of Intrauterine Pathology: A Systematic Review. *Diagnostics.* 2024;14(3):327.

[102] Vitale SG, Moore O, Riemma G, Carugno J, Yarto ML, Haimovich S. Hysteroscopic laser ablation of symptomatic uterine fibroids: insights from a prospective study. *Climacteric.* 2023;26(5):497–502.

[103] Donnez J, Polet R, Rabinovitz R. Endometrial laser intrauterine thermotherapy: the first series of 100 patients observed for 1 year. *Fertil Steril.* 2000;74:791–796.

[104] Vitale SG, Saponara S, Sicilia G, Klarić M, Sorrentino F, D'Alterio MN, Nappi L, Angioni S. Hysteroscopic diode laser myolysis: from a case series to literature review of incisionless myolysis techniques for managing heavy menstrual bleeding in premenopausal women. *Arch Gynecol Obstet.* 2024;309(3):949–59.

[105] Emanuel MH, Wamsteker K. The Intra Uterine Morcellator: a new hysteroscopic operating technique to remove intrauterine polyps and myomas. *J Minim Invasive Gynecol.* 2005;12(1):62–6.

[106] Annan JJ, Aquilina J, Ball E. The management of endometrial polyps in the 21st century. *Obs Gynaecol.* 2012;14:33–38.

[107] Raz N, Feinmesser L, Moore O, Haimovich S. Endometrial polyps: diagnosis and treatment options – a review of literature. *Minim Invasive Ther Allied Technol.* 2021;30(5):278–287.

[108] Smith P, Middleton L, Connor M. Hysteroscopic morcellation compared with electrical resection of endometrial polyps: a randomized controlled trial. *Obs Gynecol.* 2014;123:745–751.

[109] Al Hilli M, Nixon K, Hopkins M. Long-term outcomes after intrauterine morcellation vs hysteroscopic resection of endometrial polyps. *J Minim Invasive Gynecol.* 2013;20:215–221.

[110] Urman B, Yakin K, Ertas S, Alper E, Aksakal E, Riemma G, Angioni S, Vitale SG. Fertility and anatomical outcomes following hysteroscopic adhesiolysis: An 11-year retrospective cohort study to validate a new classification system for intrauterine adhesions (Urman-Vitale Classification System). *Int J Gynecol Obstet.* 2024;165(2):644–54.

Chapter 3

Uterine Fibroids and Endometrial Implications

Ricardo Bassil Lasmar[1,*], MD, PhD
Bernardo Portugal Lasmar[2], MD
Salvatore Giovanni Vitale[3], MD, PhD
Liliana Mereu[3], MD, PhD
and Vitor de Carvalho Banal Xavier[4], MD

[1]Department of Surgery and Specialized, Faculty of Medicine, Fluminense Federal University, UFF, Rio de Janeiro, Brazil
[2]Maternal-Infant Department, Faculty of Medicine, Fluminense Federal University, UFF, Rio de Janeiro, Brazil
[3]Obstetrics and Gynecology Unit, "*Gaspare Rodolico*" University Hospital, Department of General Surgery and Medical Surgical Specialties, University of Catania, Catania, Italy
[4]Crispi Institute of Minimally Invasive Surgery, Department of Gynecology, Rio de Janeiro, Brazil

Abstract

Uterine fibroids are benign tumors that can cause a variety of symptoms, including heavy menstrual bleeding, pelvic pain, and infertility. Although fibroids are common, they are directly responsible for infertility in only a small percentage of cases (3–5%), particularly those located submucosally. These fibroids can distort the uterine cavity, impair sperm transport, and interfere with embryo implantation, leading to reduced fertility and lower success rates in assisted reproductive technologies. Fibroids can also cause chronic pelvic pain, urinary and bowel issues, and other gynecological complaints, especially when

---

[*] Corresponding Author's Email: ricardo@lasmar.com.br

In: Endometrium and Related Endouterine Pathologies
Editors: Liliana Mereu and Salvatore Giovanni Vitale
ISBN: 979-8-89530-818-9

associated with conditions like adenomyosis or pelvic inflammatory disease.
Medical treatments for fibroids, including hormonal therapies (combined oral contraceptives, levonorgestrel-releasing IUD, GnRH agonists, and progesterone receptor modulators), offer symptomatic relief but have limited long-term efficacy. Surgical options such as myomectomy, performed via hysteroscopic, laparoscopic, or laparotomic approaches, are effective for symptom control and fertility preservation. Minimally invasive techniques, particularly hysteroscopic myomectomy, offer advantages like reduced blood loss, shorter recovery times, and better reproductive outcomes. However, further research is needed to elucidate the precise mechanisms through which fibroids affect fertility and to optimize treatment strategies.
This review highlights the complexities of fibroid-related infertility, the role of medical and surgical interventions, and the need for individualized treatment plans to improve patient outcomes.

Keywords: uterine fibroids, infertility, submucosal fibroids, hysteroscopy, myomectomy, reproductive outcomes, fibroid management, fibroid-related symptoms

Introduction

Uterine leiomyomatosis, also known as uterine fibroids or fibromyomas, is the most common benign neoplasm of the female reproductive tract. These tumors, predominantly composed of smooth muscle cells and extracellular matrix, can reach significant sizes and, in many cases, cause symptoms that significantly affect women's quality of life. Clinical manifestations include abnormal menstrual bleeding, pelvic pain, compressive symptoms (such as increased urinary frequency and constipation), and, in some cases, infertility or pregnancy complications. Although most fibroids are asymptomatic, the condition affects millions of women of reproductive age worldwide, with prevalence rates ranging from 20% to 80%, depending on the population studied and diagnostic methods employed [1, 2].

Due to its high prevalence, uterine leiomyomatosis represents a significant public health concern, especially when considering the economic costs associated with its treatment, both in terms of surgical procedures such as myomectomy or hysterectomy and in terms of productivity loss related to its symptoms [3]. Furthermore, fibroids can profoundly impact the physical and mental health of women, exacerbating conditions like anemia due to excessive bleeding and leading to psychological disorders as a result of chronic pain or infertility.

3.1. Epidemiology and Risk Factors

3.1.1. Epidemiology of Uterine Leiomyomatosis

The prevalence of uterine fibroids varies widely depending on factors such as age, race, reproductive status, and others. Several epidemiological studies indicate that Black women have a significantly higher risk of developing fibroids compared to White women. In a study conducted by Baird et al., substantial cumulative incidence of fibroids was observed in Black and White women, showing that by the age of 50, approximately 80% of Black women and about 70% of White women will have developed some degree of uterine leiomyomatosis [1].

The risk of developing fibroids increases with age, peaking between the ages of 30 and 50. After menopause, the incidence of new fibroids tends to decrease significantly, suggesting a direct relationship with levels of sex hormones such as estrogen and progesterone, which drop drastically during this phase of life [4]. The use of ultrasound as a diagnostic method, in addition to clinical exams, has revealed an even higher prevalence of asymptomatic fibroids than previously reported. In a study by Laughlin-Tommaso et al., the use of ultrasonography as a screening tool in a cohort of women identified a considerable prevalence of fibroids that would otherwise go unnoticed [2].

3.1.2. Risk Factors Associated with Uterine Leiomyomatosis

3.1.2.1. Age

Age is undoubtedly one of the most strongly associated risk factors for the development of uterine fibroids. Women of reproductive age, particularly between 30 and 50 years old, are the most affected by the condition. The incidence of fibroids steadily increases with age, peaking during the perimenopausal period when hormonal fluctuations are more pronounced. The development of fibroids in young women, under the age of 20, is rare, and after menopause, fibroids tend to shrink or stop growing due to the decrease in estrogen and progesterone levels [5].

Longitudinal epidemiological studies, such as those by Laughlin et al. [5], show that the incidence of fibroids is directly proportional to the aging process in women up to menopause, when the prevalence decreases. This is due to the fact that fibroids are highly dependent on sex hormones, especially estrogen, for their growth and development [6].

3.1.2.2. Race

Race is another important and well-documented risk factor for the development of uterine leiomyomatosis. Black women have a significantly higher risk of developing fibroids compared to White women. According to Marshall et al. [3], black women not only have a higher prevalence of fibroids but also tend to develop the disease earlier, with a greater number of tumors and more severe symptoms. In some populations, the relative risk of fibroid development in Black women is up to three times higher than that of White women.

This racial disparity may be related to a combination of genetic, hormonal, and environmental factors. For example, Black women are more likely to have higher levels of estrogen and other hormones related to fibroid growth, which may partially explain this difference. Additionally, factors such as disparities in access to healthcare and differences in living conditions may exacerbate this vulnerability [7].

3.1.2.3. Parity and Reproductive Factors

The relationship between parity and the risk of uterine leiomyomatosis has been extensively studied. Women who have never had children (nulliparous) have a significantly higher risk of developing fibroids compared to those who have had one or more pregnancies. Pregnancy appears to offer a protective effect against the development of fibroids, possibly due to the high levels of progesterone and other reproductive hormones maintained during gestation. These hormones may inhibit fibroid growth or induce their regression [8].

Studies such as that by Schulze-Rath et al. [7] confirm this association, demonstrating that women with a greater number of pregnancies have a reduced risk of developing fibroids. These findings are consistent with the theory that elevated hormone levels during pregnancy, particularly progesterone, play a crucial role in inhibiting fibroid growth.

3.1.2.4. Hormonal Factors

Sex hormones, particularly estrogen and progesterone, are widely recognized as key players in the development and growth of uterine fibroids. These hormones stimulate cellular proliferation in the myometrium, as well as the production of extracellular matrix, both of which are essential for fibroid formation. Women who use hormonal contraceptives or are on hormone replacement therapy may have a higher risk of developing fibroids, although data on the magnitude of this risk are inconsistent [9].

Studies such as those by Flake et al. [9] explore the role of these hormones in fibroid development, highlighting that estrogen, in particular, promotes cellular proliferation in fibroids. However, it is important to note that the use of hormonal contraceptives, depending on dosage and type of hormone, may have variable effects on fibroid risk.

3.1.2.5. Obesity

Obesity is another well-established risk factor for the development of uterine fibroids. Overweight or obese women have an increased risk of developing fibroids compared to women with normal weight. Adipose tissue is a significant source of estrogen production, especially in postmenopausal women, which may partially explain the increased risk in women with higher body mass index (BMI) [10, 11].

Studies such as that by Wise et al. [8] show that obesity is associated with an increased risk of fibroid development, particularly in women with elevated BMI before menopause. This finding suggests that the excess estrogen produced by adipose tissue may act as a growth factor for fibroids.

3.1.2.6. Smoking and Alcohol Consumption

Smoking and alcohol consumption have also been studied as possible risk factors for uterine leiomyomatosis, with variable results. Some studies suggest that smoking may have a protective effect due to nicotine's ability to lower estrogen levels in the body. However, this effect is still controversial, and other studies indicate that smoking may be associated with an increased risk of other gynecological complications [12].

On the other hand, alcohol consumption, particularly frequent beer drinking, has been associated with an increased risk of fibroid development, as highlighted by Radin et al. [13]. The mechanism behind this association may be related to the impact of alcohol on estrogen metabolism, although further studies are needed to fully understand this relationship.

3.1.2.7. Stress and Mental Health

The impact of psychological stress and other mental health factors on the development of fibroids has been increasingly recognized. Recent epidemiological studies suggest that women experiencing high levels of stress, anxiety, or depression may have an increased risk of developing fibroids [10].

The theory is that chronic stress can trigger an inflammatory response in the body, exacerbating fibroid growth through activation of the hypothalamic-pituitary-adrenal axis.

Studies like those by Vitonis et al. [10] explore this relationship, suggesting that psychological stress may be associated with an increased incidence of uterine fibroids. The connection between mental and reproductive health is complex, and stress, in particular, has been implicated in a variety of health conditions. In the case of uterine leiomyomatosis, chronic stress may result in hormonal changes, such as elevated cortisol levels and other substances related to the body's inflammatory response. These changes, in turn, may stimulate fibroid growth or influence the severity of symptoms related to the condition [10].

Vitonis et al. [10] conducted an extensive investigation to determine the relationship between stress and fibroid presence. Their results indicate that women reporting high levels of anxiety and depression had an increased risk of developing fibroids compared to those reporting lower psychological stress levels. Although the exact mechanisms by which stress affects fibroid growth are not yet fully understood, this relationship underscores the importance of a more holistic approach to the treatment and management of patients with Leiomyomas, considering not only the physical factors but also the psychological ones.

3.2. Diagnosis and Classification

Abnormal uterine bleeding is the most common symptom associated with fibroids, while other complaints include infertility and findings from imaging studies. For diagnosis, ultrasound is the initial and sufficient examination to identify measure, locate, and count the fibroids. In specific cases, usually involving multiple fibroids in patients indicated for surgery, magnetic resonance imaging (MRI) may provide more detailed information.

Submucosal fibroids are classified by their location in the uterine wall, being submucosal when part of it is within the uterine cavity; intramural when it is in the myometrium; and subserosal when part of it extends beyond the serosa. In 2018, Munro et al. published a new classification ranging from 0 to 8, with 0 being completely submucosal; 1 having the largest submucosal portion; 2 having the largest intramural portion; 3 being intramural in contact with the cavity; and up to 8 for cervical fibroids [14] (Figure 1).

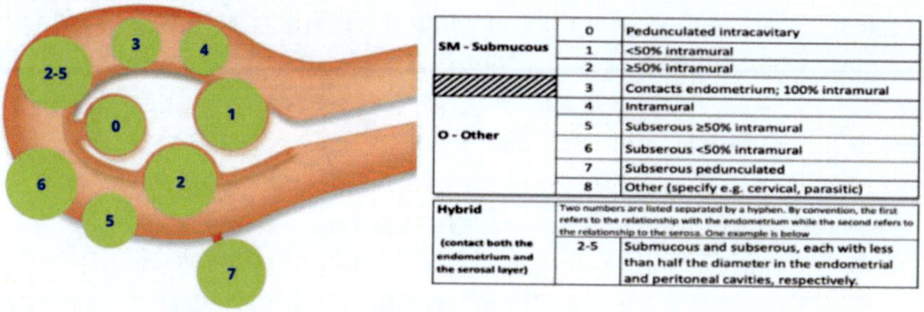

Figure 1. FIGO classification of fibroids [14].

In 2005, Lasmar et al. published a classification for submucosal fibroids, correlating the degree of surgical complexity based on five parameters: size, location, penetration into the myometrium, base, and wall [15] (Table 1).

Table 1. Lasmar submucous myoma classification [15]

Score	Size	Topography	Base	Penetration	Lateral Wall	Total
0	≤ 2 cm	Inferior	≤ 1/3	0		
1	> 2 to 5 cm	Middle	>1/3 to 2/3	≥ 50%		
2	> 5cm	Upper	> 2/3	< 50%	+ 1	
	+	+	+	+	=	

Score	Group	Indication
0 to 4	I	Low complexity hysteroscopic myomectomy.
5 to 6	II	High complexity hysteroscopic myomectomy. GnRH? Two-step hysteroscopic myomectomy.
7 to 9	III	Hysteroscopic myomectomy is contraindicated.

3.3. Clinical Manifestations

Among the various complaints associated with uterine fibroids, abnormal uterine bleeding (AUB) is the most frequent, affecting up to 30% of patients. Bleeding caused by uterine fibroids tends to occur during the menstrual period, increasing flow or prolonging the menstrual duration. Intermenstrual bleeding and postmenopausal bleeding are more related to other types of uterine diseases, and appropriate investigation should be conducted [16–18].

In 1956, Jacobson and Enzer [19] described the correlation between submucosal fibroids and AUB, demonstrating that submucosal fibroids were found in 57% of AUB cases. The number and size of these fibroids, as well as their location, can interfere with symptoms. AUB related to uterine fibroids can be associated with several factors [20]:

- Increased endometrial surface area
- Increased uterine vascularization
- Changes in uterine contractility patterns
- Exposure and ulceration of the submucosal fibroid surface
- Degeneration of the fibroid nodule
- Venous ectasia due to compression of the venous plexus by the nodules.

With fibroids inside the uterus, the endometrial surface area increases, leading to a larger area for shedding and bleeding. On the other hand, fibroids are poorly vascularized, with peripheral vascularization, which can lead to bleeding from the rupture of a vessel on their surface in some cases.

Yang et al. [21] compared hemoglobin levels in patients with single submucosal fibroids in the absence of other pathologies associated with menorrhagia and concluded that the size of the fibroid is the main factor associated with anemia. Additionally, the degree of protrusion of the nodule into the uterine cavity also showed a relationship with hemoglobin levels. Patients with fibroids smaller than 2 cm exhibited similar hematimetric levels regardless of the degree of protrusion of the fibroid into the cavity. Fibroids measuring 2 to 3.9 cm had an inverse association of hemoglobin values with the degree of protrusion. Fibroids with less than 50% protrusion into the cavity had similar hemoglobin levels regardless of nodule size. In cases of fibroids with 50 to 79% protrusion and those equal to or greater than 80%, hemoglobin levels were lower as the diameter of the nodule increased.

Korompelis et al. [22] conducted a case-control study to compare the expression of MMP-2, MMP-9, their tissue inhibitor (TIMP-1), and VEGF in patients with and without fibroids. TIMP-1 promotes the inactivation of MMPs when bound. MMPs play a crucial role in the extracellular matrix remodeling process, acting in its degradation. In this work by Korompelis et al., higher serum levels of VEGF were demonstrated in patients with fibroids, as well as higher levels of VEGF in fibroid tissue versus normal myometrium. This difference in VEGF concentration in tissues may confirm the importance of local angiogenesis as a growth and development factor for fibroids. Regarding MMPs, the researchers identified an increase in MMP-2 concentration in fibroid tissue compared to normal myometrium. MMP-2 mediates the cleavage of type IV collagen, leading to extracellular matrix instability and cell-to-cell and cell-to-matrix interactions, interfering with cell proliferation and differentiation [22].

The fibroid, especially the submucosal type, alters uterine contractility, interrupting normal peristaltic movement, which is important for sperm transport during fertilization. This interference in uterine contractility may be associated with increased AUB, as it prevents adequate hemostasis of the myometrial vessels.

In 2014, Kido et al. [23] compared uterine peristalsis in patients with and without fibroids using 3 Tesla magnetic resonance imaging (MRI). The direction of peristalsis was towards the cervix-fundus in most patients, regardless of the presence of a nodule. However, patients with myomatosis exhibited a significant reduction in uterine peristalsis, supporting the theory that fibroids would impede the transmission of the contraction wave from normal myometrium [23, 24]. In this study, the reduction of uterine peristalsis had no relation to the size or location of the nodules, as only symptomatic patients were included.

The vascularization of fibroids is usually peripheral, and when their growth exceeds the blood supply, degeneration and necrosis occur. This process is more frequent during pregnancy, when accelerated growth of the fibroid can occur. In some cases, degeneration of the fibroid may expose the vascularization of the nodule, leading to abundant transvaginal bleeding [25, 26].

3.3.1. Fibroids and Other Gynecological Complaints

Some gynecological complaints may be reported by patients with fibroids, even if infrequently [27]. Chronic pelvic pain, whether dyspareunia or dysmenorrhea, may be present. Fibroid nodules are not usually associated with pain; however, pain can occur in cases of pedunculated fibroids with torsion of the pedicle or degeneration of the nodule (when growth exceeds vascular supply), leading to ischemia, pain, and sometimes fever.

It is crucial to rule out common causes of pelvic pain in patients with myomatosis, as these conditions often overlap [28]. There is a common association with adenomyosis, which can be better differentiated by MRI and satisfactorily managed with hormonal treatment. Pelvic inflammatory disease may also be present, causing chronic pelvic pain, and thus should be excluded.

Urinary and intestinal complaints may also be present [29–31]. Large subserosal nodules can lead to bladder compression (when on the anterior wall) and intestinal compression (when on the posterior wall). The patient may report difficulty retaining urine (decreased total bladder capacity) due to direct compression from the nodule, as well as difficulty with bowel movements.

3.4. Fibroids and Infertility: What's There, What's New?

3.4.1. Fibroids and Infertility

Uterine fibroids, despite being very prevalent, are directly related to infertility in only 3 to 5% of cases. The relationship between fibroids and infertility is intricate and multifactorial, with fibroid size, location, and number playing critical roles in reproductive outcomes. The nodules that most hinder pregnancy or are associated with miscarriages are those located submucosally [32]. This is because their proximity to the endometrium, the inner lining of the uterus where embryo implantation occurs, can distort the uterine cavity, interfere with sperm transport, and impair embryo implantation. Studies suggest that women with submucosal fibroids may experience reduced fertility and lower success rates with assisted reproductive technologies (ART) like in vitro fertilization (IVF) [33–38].

Intramural fibroids, especially those larger than 3 cm, may also negatively impact fertility by altering the uterine architecture and disrupting blood flow to the endometrium [39]. Although the effect of subserosal fibroids on fertility is less clear, large subserosal fibroids can cause mechanical interference with the fallopian tubes, impairing the passage of sperm or eggs [40, 41].

Fibroids can affect fertility through several mechanisms, including:

1) Distortion of the uterine cavity: Submucosal fibroids can distort the uterine cavity, leading to difficulties in embryo implantation. Even small fibroids can have this effect when located near the endometrium.
2) Altered blood flow: Large intramural fibroids can compress blood vessels in the uterus, reducing blood flow to the endometrium, which is critical for embryo implantation and pregnancy maintenance.
3) Endometrial changes: Fibroids can alter the structure and function of the endometrium, leading to an inflammatory environment, impaired cell signaling, and changes in cytokine levels, all of which may hinder embryo implantation. Hoxa 10 (an important gene regulating endometrial receptivity) is globally decreased in submucosal myomas. Intramural fibroids also seem to reduce Hoxa10 levels,

though likely to a lesser extent [42]. This mechanism may explain the impact of type 3 fibroids on fertility.

4) Tubal blockage: Subserosal fibroids, especially when large, may cause mechanical compression or distortion of the fallopian tubes, preventing the normal passage of sperm and eggs.
5) Cervical and uterine contractions: Fibroids can also affect the normal contractility of the uterus and cervix, potentially interfering with sperm migration and embryo transport [43].

New prospective controlled studies should be conducted in order to establish the precise relationship between fibroids and infertility.

3.5. Medical Treatment: Indications and Options

Pharmacological treatment of fibroids is associated with a 75% remission/control rate of symptoms within one year. However, its long-term efficacy is low [44]. There is a higher cure rate in women when abnormal bleeding is an isolated symptom. In a population receiving drug treatment, 60% of cases underwent surgery within two years [45]. The frequent association of fibroids with adenomyosis may resolve symptoms with the use of hormonal medications when adenomyosis is the cause.

3.5.1. Hormonal Therapy

3.5.1.1. Combined Oral Contraceptives

They are administered as therapy in cases of menorrhagia/heavy menstrual bleeding associated with fibroids, as a result of endometrial atrophy [46]. Their use is limited in women with contraindications to combined hormonal therapy or in those experiencing side effects that hinder treatment adherence [47]. In general, combined oral contraceptives are not able to control uterine bleeding caused by fibroids, but there is no evidence that they can cause the growth of the fibroid.

3.5.1.2. Levonorgestrel-Releasing Intrauterine Device (IUD) and Progestogens

Progestogens can act ambiguously concerning fibroids, by promoting the increase of epidermal growth factor, which stimulates fibroid growth, while inhibiting IGF-1, which can suppress growth. Moreover, progestogens promote downregulation of estrogen and progesterone receptors in fibroids, potentially modulating their growth. The medicated IUD releases 20 μg of levonorgestrel daily, and its use is associated with a reduction in uterine and menstrual volumes, as well as an increase in hematocrit/hemoglobin levels, with an effect superior to combined oral contraceptives [48, 49]. Submucosal fibroids contraindicate the use of medicated IUDs. One study showed that the medicated IUD significantly reduced menstrual flow and uterine volume in patients with menorrhagia, with or without fibroids, but without a significant reduction in fibroid size [50].

3.5.1.3. GnRH Agonists

This class of drugs initially stimulates pituitary receptors, causing an increase in gonadotropins, followed by desensitization and inhibition of follicle-stimulating hormone (FSH) and luteinizing hormone (LH) production, leading to hypogonadotropic hypogonadism. This initial elevation of gonadotropins is responsible for the "flare-up" effect, characterized by bleeding 7 to 10 days after the first dose of the agonist. GnRH analogs cause amenorrhea, improve anemia, and reduce uterine size by up to 50% in three months [51, 52]. However, they are associated with side effects from hypoestrogenism, such as vaginal dryness, hot flashes, sleep disturbances, and bone loss. Significant bone mineral loss is the main barrier to long-term therapy. The use of certain agents can reduce this bone loss, requiring "add-back" therapy with tibolone or even some progestogens. The reduction in volume and resolution of abnormal uterine bleeding (AUB) is temporary, with symptoms returning a few months after medication discontinuation. Some studies have shown a residual effect for a prolonged period, such as decreased menstrual flow after discontinuation of the analog, but there is no scientific basis to support this finding.

The primary indication for GnRH analogs is preoperative, for a period of 3 to 6 months, to facilitate surgical procedures and improve preoperative hematological levels, preferably with associated iron supplementation [53]. This allows for a more conservative and minimally invasive approach. They are also prescribed short-term for women nearing menopause who have contraindications to surgery. To minimize side effects, they can be combined with low-dose estrogen and progestogen therapy, the same as used in HRT [54].

3.5.1.4. GnRH Antagonists

GnRH antagonists, including elagolix and relugolix, provide a targeted approach in the management of uterine fibroids by directly inhibiting the action of endogenous GnRH at pituitary receptors [55]. Unlike GnRH agonists, which initially induce a surge in gonadotropin levels (flare-up effect) before achieving downregulation, antagonists immediately suppress gonadotropin secretion, leading to a rapid reduction in circulating estrogen levels [56]. This mechanism minimizes the risk of symptom exacerbation at treatment initiation and achieves therapeutic effects more quickly. The efficacy of GnRH antagonists is dose-dependent, and their side effects—predominantly related to hypoestrogenism—are generally similar to those seen with GnRH agonists [55, 56].

A significant advancement in this therapeutic class is the introduction of a fixed-dose combination therapy containing relugolix (40 mg), estradiol (1 mg), and norethisterone acetate (0.5 mg) [57]. Approved in Europe in 2021, marketed under the brand name Ryeqo, this formulation is specifically indicated for the management of heavy menstrual bleeding associated with uterine fibroids [57]. The inclusion of estradiol and norethisterone acetate in the formulation provides "add-back therapy," effectively countering the hypoestrogenic side effects such as bone density loss and vasomotor symptoms, which are common with GnRH antagonist monotherapy [58].

3.5.1.5. Progesterone Receptor Modulators

Compared to normal myometrium, fibroids have a greater expression of estrogen and progesterone receptors. Some studies have shown that fibroid growth occurs during the secretory phase, directly influenced by progesterone. With this in mind, progesterone receptor modulators were developed to control fibroid growth. Their advantages include oral administration and fewer side effects, though the long-term endometrial effects are not well known, and high doses may lead to elevated liver enzymes [59–61].

3.5.1.6. Mifepristone

Mifepristone is a progesterone receptor modulator with pure antagonist properties, directly reducing the expression of progesterone receptors in the myometrium and fibroid. It has the same limitation as ulipristal acetate concerning high doses and inappropriate market availability for treating uterine fibroids. It is prescribed at a dose of 5 mg/day, with an average 50% fibroid volume reduction and few side effects. Some cases of endometrial hyperplasia have been reported with the use of mifepristone, but this adverse effect is rare at the 5 mg/day dose.

A Cochrane review showed improvement in the quality of life for mifepristone users but did not show significant fibroid volume reduction [62].

3.5.1.7. Aromatase Inhibitors (Letrozole)
Myometrial cell cultures have shown overexpression of aromatase P450 and synthesized high levels of estradiol to accelerate their cellular growth. Aromatase inhibitors block the conversion of androgens into estrogens. Studies with small sample sizes have described symptom reduction in women during the climacteric transition [63–65]. These inhibitors cause up to a 50% reduction in fibroid volume, an effect comparable to or even superior to that of GnRH analogs, as they do not cause vasomotor symptoms. However, further investigation on this topic is still necessary.

3.6. Surgical and Endoscopic Approaches

Myomectomy can be performed via vaginal, hysteroscopic, laparotomic, laparoscopic/robotic, or a combination of these approaches. The minimally invasive approach tends to reduce blood loss, estimated at 200 to 800 ml for laparotomic myomectomy, compared to 80 to 250 ml for laparoscopic myomectomy.

3.6.1. Vaginal Myomectomy
This approach is associated with submucosal fibroids during childbirth, characterized by a mass at the external os, which may present as friable and with abundant bleeding, leading to hypovolemic shock. This nodule is associated with sinusorrhea and metrorrhagia, and it can easily be confused with cervical tumors. Treatment consists of resecting its base, preferably in a surgical center, which can be done through suturing and sectioning or sectioning with energy instruments. If available, hysteroscopy can adequately resect this lesion, allowing for investigation of the uterine cavity and complete resection of the entire vascular pedicle [66].

There are also reports in the literature of vaginal myomectomy for nodules affecting the lower uterine region, accessed through the opening of the vaginal pouch, allowing access to the nodule, resection, and suturing of the uterine wall [66].

3.6.2. Hysteroscopic Myomectomy

Symptomatic submucosal nodules or those associated with infertility should preferably be addressed via hysteroscopy [67, 68]. In patients desiring to maintain fertility, if laparotomic or laparoscopic myomectomy is indicated and a submucosal fibroid is present, the hysteroscopic approach should be combined for its removal, yielding better reproductive outcomes [69].

Hysteroscopic myomectomy can be classified as outpatient or inpatient. The outpatient procedure, performed without sedation, is limited to fibroids up to 3 cm with minimal penetration into the myometrium (level 0 or 1) [70]. Outpatient hysteroscopic surgery, like myomectomy, has advantages: immediate treatment of the lesion at the time of diagnosis, reduced patient anxiety (along with complaints), lower costs compared to inpatient surgery, and the satisfaction of performing the best art of hysteroscopy [71, 72] (Figure 2).

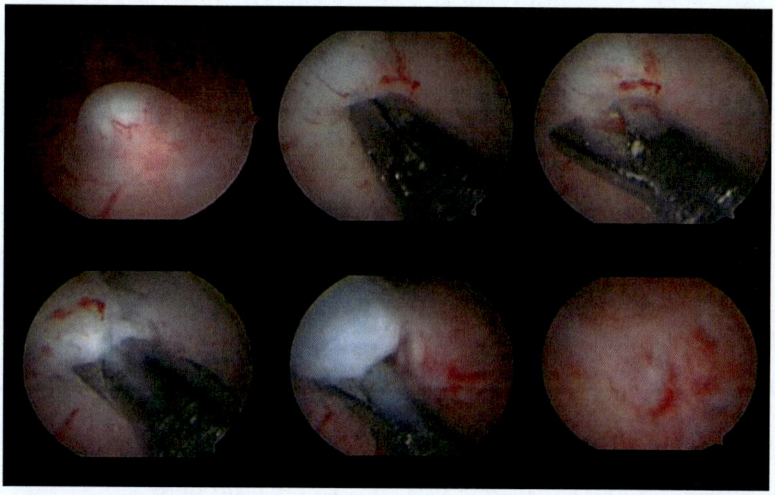

Figure 2. Office Myomectomy.

A grasping forceps or scissors are used to access the pseudocapsule plane, and with the hysteroscopic setup, the nodule is protruded and dissected [73]. At the end, the nodule is left free in the cavity and can be fragmented or removed entirely with grasping forceps [74]. In cases where the free nodule is difficult to remove from the cavity, the patient can be advised to return in 7 to 10 days, during which the nodule may either be expelled spontaneously (the patient should be informed about this possibility) or drastically reduced in size, facilitating its removal. Currently, the mini-resectoscope is available, allowing the use of monopolar or bipolar energy, in a final diameter instrument of 16 fr (5.3 mm). This instrument permits the resection of larger polyps and fibroids without the need for analgesia in an outpatient setting, as it enables the fragmentation of large nodules and complete removal of the lesion with associated hemostasis.

Another technology applied to fibroids is laser [75, 76]. Under hysteroscopic vision, it is possible to "vaporize" the nodule using a laser fiber with a special tip, showing excellent results in preliminary studies for submucosal nodules and even for large intramural components [77, 78].

Inpatient myomectomy is reserved for larger or deeper nodules or in patients with low tolerance for outpatient procedures. The analgesia of choice for the procedure is spinal or epidural block, often requiring cervical dilation for the introduction of a resectoscope [79].

The resectoscope, whether bipolar or monopolar, requires dexterity and skill from the surgeon [80]. The electrode movements must be planned, and the angulation of the resectoscope during the activation of the cutting pedal defines the depth of resection. The electrode movement should always be directed towards the uterine fundus (cervix, and never the opposite), to avoid uterine perforation and the need for laparoscopic or laparotomic conversion. Cornual regions are thinner and require extreme caution for resections in these areas. Uterine perforation using current requires evaluation of the abdominal cavity for associated intestinal loop injuries [81].

Lasmar et al. developed a preoperative classification to predict the complexity of hysteroscopic myomectomy [15]. The Lasmar Classification or STEPW allows the surgeon to stratify the difficulty of hysteroscopic myomectomy, anticipating whether it will be a low-complexity, medium-complexity, or non-recommended procedure. Various parameters are considered, and with this information, it is possible to predict the expected surgery time and the degree of difficulty of the procedure.

The technique used for hysteroscopic myomectomy was described by Ricardo Lasmar in 2002 [82], involving direct mobilization of the nodule from the development of the pseudocapsule plane. For this, a knife electrode or Collins electrode is used to circumscribe the fibroid and reach the pseudocapsule. From this point, the fibroid is mobilized, and the fibrous bundles are individualized and sectioned using energy [83-84]. This technique enables myomectomies in nodules with extremely thin myometrial mantles (3 mm), with a low risk of uterine perforation and intravasation syndrome [69, 70]. The vessels are cauterized punctually, under direct vision, preserving the adjacent endometrium and myometrium, thus improving reproductive outcomes (Figure 3).

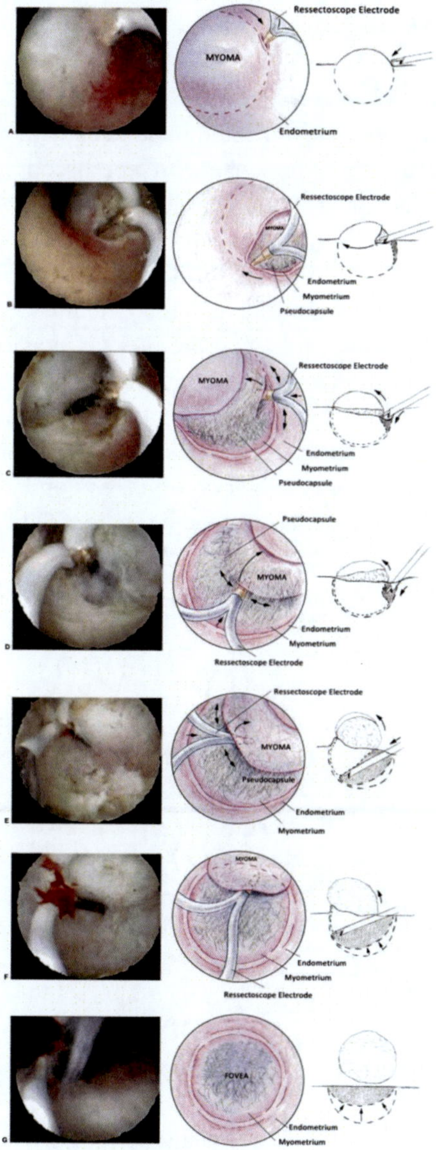

Figure 3. Enucleation with Collins knife.

After hysteroscopic myomectomy, it is advisable to perform an outpatient hysteroscopy for review in 45 to 60 days. Any scar adhesions that may arise after the procedure can often be easily undone during this period, sometimes even with the simple passage of the hysteroscope [85–87].

3.6.3. Laparotomic Myomectomy

Laparotomic myomectomy is indicated in patients with multiple fibroids or in cases where the team lacks experience with laparoscopy. There is no record of a maximum number of fibroids that can be removed laparoscopically; however, multiple nodules (more than six) tend to increase the laparoscopic suturing time and make it difficult to locate intramural nodules, as laparoscopy prevents the tactile sensation of the nodule in the myometrium [88].

The technique involves planning the uterine incisions to minimize their number to avoid postoperative adhesions. Posterior incisions are more associated with adhesions. Whenever possible, the incision should be used to remove the maximum number of nodules. Opening the uterine cavity should always be avoided to minimize the risk of adhesions and infertility. After the uterine incision, the nodule is grasped with toothed forceps, and a Kelly forceps or scissors are used to dissect the pseudocapsule. Sometimes, the index finger can be used for this purpose [88] (Figure 4).

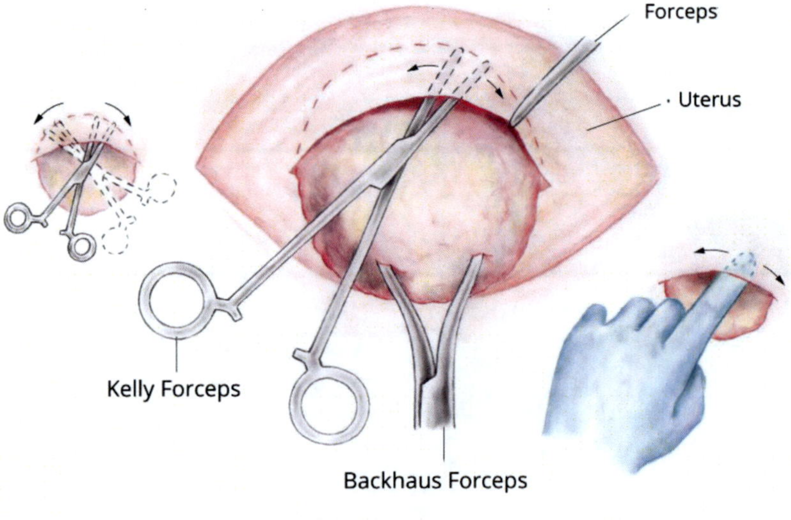

Figure 4. Pseudocapsule plane at laparotomy.

After the removal of the nodules, the uterine wall should be closed while respecting the layers. Absorbable polyglycatin 3-0 suture can be used for the endometrial mucosa/submucosa, polyglycatin 0 for the myometrium with separate "X" stitches (avoiding the formation of myometrial pockets that can accumulate blood and compromise healing), and polyglycatin 2-0 for the uterine serosa. Depending on the surgeon's experience and speed, the suturing of the incisions can be done at the end of the nodule removal or after each one is removed. Estimated blood loss for this procedure varies according to the number and location of the nodules and can exceed 1 liter, with a transfusion rate of up to 20%. In some cases, ligation of the uterine or hypogastric arteries must be performed for effective control of bleeding [88].

3.6.4. Laparoscopic Myomectomy

The laparoscopic approach to fibroids combines the challenges of laparotomic myomectomy (bleeding, the need to reduce the number of incisions, proper suturing) with the necessity to master laparoscopic suturing techniques, the difficulty in removing/morcellating large nodules, and the loss of tactile sensation of the myometrium [89]. It is the laparoscopic surgery with the highest conversion rate to laparotomy, ranging from 0 to 41%. However, it is associated with shorter hospitalization time, lower incidence of adhesions, faster recovery, and reduced blood loss. The pregnancy outcomes after the procedure in patients operated on by experienced surgeons are similar to those of laparotomic myomectomy [90, 91].

The technique involves making an incision at the area of greatest protrusion of the fibroid in the serosa of the uterus, always respecting the uterine tension lines whenever possible, using a monopolar hook or ultrasonic energy forceps to section serosa and muscle until reaching the fibroid's pseudocapsule (Figure 5). The nodule is grasped with toothed forceps, and dissection is initiated within the pseudocapsule with scissors or blunt forceps. Then, through traction movements, while rotating the fibroid and contracting the myometrium, gradual release of the fibroid from its bed is performed, followed by point coagulation of the bleeding vessels. Subserosal fibroids are resected by sectioning their pedicle after cauterization [92].

To reduce intraoperative bleeding or as an adjunctive action for small fibroids that are not removed, ligation of the uterine arteries may be helpful, as well as the infusion of vasopressin before each incision. Myometrial suturing requires extreme skill and an experienced team and should be performed layer by layer, ensuring that the edges are adequately coapted and that hemostasis is achieved without causing ischemia of the myometrium, as in laparotomy [93]. Currently, barbed sutures are available, which eliminate the need to tie knots, providing time savings and reduced blood loss.

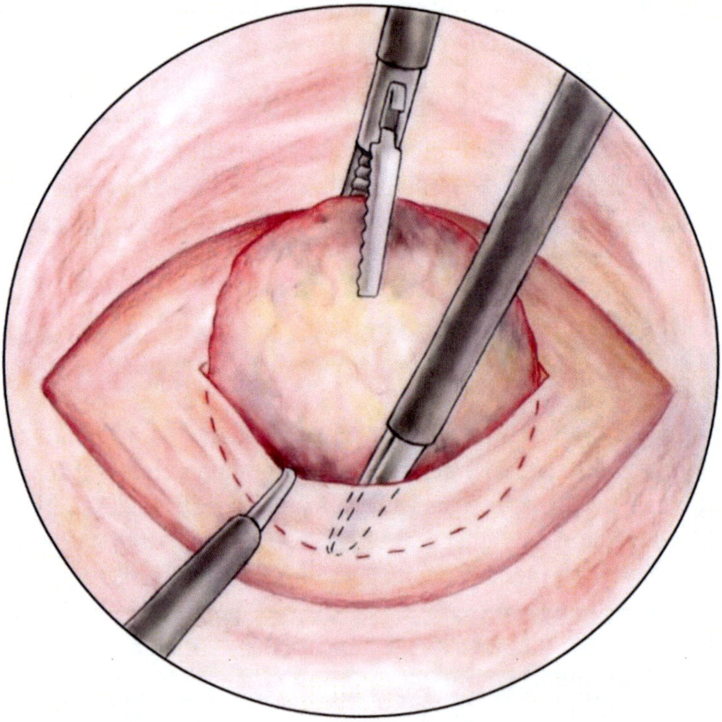

Figure 5. Pseudocapsule plane at laparoscopy.

In laparoscopic myomectomy, the removal of the specimen from the cavity can be more challenging than the rest of the surgery. During mini laparotomy for uterine repair, the same incision can be used for specimen removal from the cavity. Fibroids smaller than 10 mm can exit through trocars of that same diameter. Larger ones must be fragmented using mechanical or electrical morcellators. Fibroids can also be removed via posterior colpotomy.

There is currently a constant concern about the dissemination of malignant disease from the use of morcellators in the cavity [94]. Undiagnosed sarcomas in the preoperative period could have fragments disseminated throughout the abdominal cavity during morcellation [95]. Therefore, the use of morcellators has been banned in some countries. To avoid this problem, a technique for morcellation within bags has been developed, where a resistant plastic bag is inflated with CO2 inside the abdominal cavity, covering the entire cavity, making it possible to morcellate the fibroid within it without the risk of dissemination or injury to organs or vessels.

At the end of the surgery, hemostasis should be reviewed, and all clots and debris should be removed from the cavity through thorough irrigation and aspiration. One option is to leave a volume of 1,000 to 1,500 ml of heated lactated Ringer's solution in the abdominal cavity at the end of the surgery to provide a heat buffer for the patient and completely remove the CO2 from the cavity, preventing the formation of carbonic acid and subsequent phrenic irritation that causes shoulder pain.

Conclusion

Uterine fibroids are a prevalent and complex condition with significant clinical and reproductive implications. Their impact extends from symptomatic burdens like abnormal bleeding and pelvic pain to challenges in fertility, particularly in cases involving submucosal fibroids. While advances in medical therapies, including hormonal treatments and novel pharmacological agents, provide symptom relief, their long-term efficacy remains limited, underscoring the need for continued innovation.

Minimally invasive surgical techniques, such as hysteroscopic and laparoscopic myomectomy, have revolutionized fibroid management, offering improved recovery times and better reproductive outcomes. However, the variability in fibroid size, location, and number necessitates personalized treatment strategies tailored to individual patient needs.

Further research into the molecular and physiological mechanisms of fibroid growth and their interaction with the endometrium is essential. This knowledge will guide the development of more effective and targeted therapies, addressing both symptomatic relief and fertility preservation. By combining technological advancements with a patient-centered approach, the management of uterine fibroids can continue to evolve, improving outcomes and quality of life for affected women.

References

[1] Baird DD, Dunson DB, Hill MC, Cousins D, Schectman JM. High cumulative incidence of uterine leiomyoma in black and white women: Ultrasound evidence. *Am J Obstet Gynecol.* 2003;188(1):100–7.

[2] Wise LA, Laughlin-Tommaso SK. Epidemiology of uterine fibroids: from menarche to. *Clin Obs Gynecol.* 2016;59(1):2–24.

[3] Marshall LM, Spiegelman D, Barbieri RL, Goldman MB, Manson JE, Colditz GA, et. Variation in the incidence of uterine leiomyoma among premenopausal women by age and race. *Obs Gynaecol.* 1997;90(6):967–73.

[4] Bulun SE. Uterine Fibroids. Longo DL, editor. *N Engl J Med.* 2010;369(14):1344–55.

[5] Laughlin SK, Schroeder JC, Baird DD. New directions in the epidemiology of uterine. *Semin Reprod Med.* 2010;28(3):204–17.

[6] Stewart EA. Uterine fibroids. Lancet. 2015;379(9822):1235–45.

[7] Schulze-Rath R, Shapiro S, Jick SS. Uterine fibroids and reproductive factors: a case-control study. *Am J Obs Gynecol.* 2005;193(1):161–7.

[8] Wise LA, Palmer JR, Harlow B, Spiegelman D, EA S. Risk of uterine leiomyomata in relation to tobacco, alcohol and caffeine consumption in the Black Women's Health Study. *Hum Reprod.* 2004;19(8):1746–54.

[9] Flake GP, Andersen J, Dixon D. Etiology and pathogenesis of uterine leiomyomas: a review. *Env Heal Perspect.* 2003;111(8):1037–54.

[10] Vitonis AF, Vincent K, Kawachi I, Cramer DW, Missmer SA. Stress, anxiety, and depression and risk of uterine leiomyomata. *Am J Obs Gynecol.* 2014;210(3):244.e1-244.e8.

[11] Giannini A, D'Oria O, Vizza E, Congiu MA, Cuccu I, Golia D'Augè T, Saponara S, Capalbo G, Di Donato V, Raspagliesi F, Bogani G. Robotic-assisted, laparoscopic, and vaginal hysterectomy in morbidly obese patients with endometrial hyperplasia and endometrial cancer. *Minim Invasive Ther Allied Technol.* 2024;33(6):358–64.

[12] Aloiso AA, Baird DD, DeRoo LA, Sandler DP. Early-life exposures and early-onset uterine leiomyomata in black women in the Sister Study. *Env Heal Perspect.* 2012;120(3):406–12.

[13] Radin RG, Rosenberg L, Palmer JR W, L.A. Drug use and risk of uterine leiomyomata in African-American women. *Am J Epidemiol.* 2010;171(2):218–28.

[14] Munro MG, Critchley HOD, Fraser IS. The two FIGO systems for normal and abnormal uterine bleeding symptoms and classification of causes of abnormal uterine bleeding in the reproductive years: 2018 revisions. *Int J Gynecol Obstet.* 2018;143(3):393–408.

[15] Lasmar RB, Barrozo PR, Dias R, Oliveira MA. Submucous myomas: a new presurgical classification to evaluate the viability of hysteroscopic surgical treatment preliminary report. *J Minim Invasive Gynecol.* 2005;12(4):308–11.

[16] Vitale SG, Riemma G, Haimovich S, Carugno J, Alonso Pacheco L, Perez-Medina T, Parry JP, Török P, Tesarik J, Della Corte L, Cobellis L, Di Spiezio Sardo A, De Franciscis P. Risk of endometrial cancer in asymptomatic postmenopausal women in relation to ultrasonographic endometrial thickness: systematic review and diagnostic test accuracy meta-analysis. *Am J Obstet Gynecol.* 2023;228(1):22-35.e2.

[17] Vitale SG, Angioni S, D'Alterio MN, Ronsini C, Saponara S, De Franciscis P, Riemma G. Risk of endometrial malignancy in women treated for breast cancer: the

BLUSH prediction model–evidence from a comprehensive multicentric retrospective cohort study. *Climacteric.* 2024;27(5):482–8.

[18] Garuti G, Angioni S, Mereu L, Calzolari S, Mannini L, Scrimin F, Casadio P, Alberti D De, Nappi L, Busato E, Leone FPG, Perrini G, Cela V, Luerti M. Hysteroscopic view with targeted biopsy in the assessment of endometrial carcinoma. What is the rate of underestimatated diagnosis? The results of a multicenter Italian trial. *Gynecol Surg.* 2020;17(1).

[19] Jacobson FJ, Enzer N. Uterine myomas and the endometrium; study of the mechanism of bleeding. *Obs Gynaecol.* 1956;7(2):206–10.

[20] Lasmar RB, Lasmar BP. The role of leiomyomas in the genesis of abnormal uterine bleeding (AUB). *Best Pr Res Clin Obs Gynaecol.* 2017;40:82–8.

[21] Yang JH, Chen MJ, Chen CD. Impact of submucousmyoma on the severity of anemia. *Fertil Steril.* 2011;95(5):1769–72.

[22] Korompelis P, Piperi C, Adamopoulos C, Dalagiorgou G. Expression of vascular endothelial factor-A, gelatinases (MMP-2, MMP-9) and TIMP-1 in uterine leiomyomas. *Clin Chem Lab Med.* 2015;53(9):1415–24.

[23] Kido A, Ascher SM, Hahn W, Kishimoto K, Kashitani N, Jha RC, Togashi K, Spies. 3 T MRI uterine peristalsis: comparison of symptomatic fibroid patients versus controls. *Clin Radiol.* 2014;69(5):468–72.

[24] Nishino M, Togashi K, A N. Uterine contractions evaluated oncine MR imaging in patients with uterine leiomyomas. *Eur J Radiol.* 2005;53(1):142–6.

[25] Buhimschi CS, Marvel RP. Degenerated uterine leiomyoma mimicking a hematoma associated with gas formation. *Int J Gynaecol Obs.* 2001;73(3):271–3.

[26] Sim CH, Lee JH, Kwak JS, Song SH. Necrotizing ruptured vaginal leiomyoma mimicking a malignant neoplasm. *Obstet Gynecol Sci.* 2014;57(6):560.

[27] Shi Y, Zhu Y, Fan S, Vitagliano A, Liu X, Liao Y, Liang Y, Vitale SG. Clinical Characteristics and Antifungal Susceptibility of Candida nivariensis from Vulvovaginal Candidiasis. *Gynecol Obstet Invest.* 2020;85(1):88–93.

[28] Saponara S, Angioni S, Parry JP, Pacheco LA, Carugno J, Moawad N, Haimovich S, Lasmar RB, Dealberti D, Aksakal E, Urman B, Nappi L, Vitale SG. The Pivotal role of hysteroscopy in diagnosing subtle uterine lesions in infertile patients: Seeing the unseen can make the difference. *Eur J Obstet Gynecol Reprod Biol.* 2025;305:132–41.

[29] Vitale SG, Caruso S, Rapisarda AMC, Valenti G, Rossetti D, Cianci S, Cianci A. Biocompatible porcine dermis graft to treat severe cystocele: impact on quality of life and sexuality. *Arch Gynecol Obstet.* 2016;293(1):125–31.

[30] Cai T, Mazzoli S, Migno S, Malossini G, Lanzafame P, Mereu L, Tateo S, Wagenlehner FM, Pickard RS, Bartoletti R. Development and validation of a nomogram predicting recurrence risk in women with symptomatic urinary tract infection. *Int J Urol.* 2014;21(9):929–34.

[31] Vitale SG, Laganà AS, Noventa M, Giampaolino P, Zizolfi B, Butticè S, La Rosa VL, Gullo G, Rossetti D. Transvaginal bilateral sacrospinous fixation after second recurrence of vaginal vault prolapse: Efficacy and impact on quality of life and sexuality. *Biomed Res Int.* 2018;2018:5727165.

[32] Donnez J, Taylor HS, Marcellin L, Dolmans MM. Uterine fibroid-related infertility: mechanisms and management. *Fertil Steril.* 2024;122(1):31–9.

[33] Don EE, Mijatovic V, van Eekelen R, Huirne JAF. The effect of myomectomy on reproductive outcomes in patients with uterine fibroids: a retrospective cohort study. *Reprod Biomed Online.* 2022;45(5):970–8.

[34] Donnez J. Intramural myomas-related infertility: should the myomas be removed? Fertil Steril. 2021;116(943–944).

[35] Dolmans MM, Isaacson K, Zhang W, Gordts S. Intramural myomas more than 3-4 centimeters should be surgically removed before in vitro fertilization. *Fertil Steril.* 2021;116(4):945–58.

[36] Pritts EA. Fibroids and infertility: a systematic review of the evidence. *Obstet Gynecol Surv.* 2001;56(8):483–91.

[37] Vitale SG, Laganà AS, Török P, Lasmar RB, Carugno J, Palumbo M, Tesarik J. Virtual sonographic hysteroscopy in assisted reproduction: A retrospective cost-effectiveness analysis. *Int J Gynaecol Obstet.* 2022;156(1):112–8.

[38] Vitale SG, Parry JP, Carugno J, Cholkeri-Singh A, Della Corte L, Cianci S, Schiattarella A, Riemma G, De Franciscis P. Surgical and Reproductive Outcomes after Hysteroscopic Removal of Retained Products of Conception: A Systematic Review and Meta-analysis. *J Minim Invasive Gynecol.* 2021;28(2):204–17.

[39] Yan L, Ding L, Li C, Wang Y, Tang R, Chen Z. Effect of fibroids not distorting the endometrial cavity on the outcome of in vitro fertilization treatment: a retrospective cohort study. *Fertil Steril.* 2014;101(3):716–21.

[40] Vitale SG, Di Spiezio Sardo A, Riemma G, De Franciscis P, Alonso Pacheco L, Carugno J. In-office hysteroscopic removal of retained or fragmented intrauterine device without anesthesia: a cross-sectional analysis of an international survey. *Updates Surg.* 2022;74(3):1079–85.

[41] Chiofalo B, Palmara V, Vilos GA, Pacheco LA, Lasmar RB, Shawki O, Giacobbe V, Alibrandi A, Di Guardo F, Vitale SG. Reproductive outcomes of infertile women undergoing "see and treat" office hysteroscopy: a retrospective observational study. *Minim Invasive Ther Allied Technol.* 2021;30(3):147–53.

[42] Taylor HS. Fibroids: when should they be removed to improve in vitro fertilization success? *Fertil Steril.* 2018;109:784–5.

[43] Orisaka M, Kurokawa T, Shukunami KI, Orisaka S, Fukuda MT, Shinagawa A, Fukuda S, Ihara N, Yamada H, Itoh H, Kotsuji F. A comparison of uterine peristalsis in women with normal uteri and uterine leiomyoma by cine magnetic resonance imaging. *Eur J Obstet Gynecol Reprod Biol.* 2007;135(1):111–5.

[44] Pritts EA, Parker WH, Olive DL. Fibroids and infertility: an updated systematic review of the evidence. *Fertil Steril.* 2009;91(4):1215–23.

[45] Lee DW, Gibson TB, Carls GS, Ozminkowski RJ, Wang S, Stewart EA. Uterine fibroid treatment patterns in a population of insured women. *Fertil Steril.* 2009;91(2):566–74.

[46] Mereu L, Giunta G, Carri C, Prasciolu C, Albis Florez ED, Mencaglia L. Nomegestrol acetate versus combined oral contraceptive as rapid endometrial preparation for operative hysteroscopy: a prospective randomised pilot study. *Gynecol Surg.* 2012;9:401–404.

[47] Ali DES, Shah M, Ali A, Malik MO, Rehman F, Badshah H, Ehtesham E, Vitale SG. Treatment with Metformin and Combination of Metformin plus Pioglitazone on Serum Levels of IL-6 and IL-8 in Polycystic Ovary Syndrome: A Randomized Clinical Trial. *Horm Metab Res.* 2019;51(11):714–22.

[48] Grigorieva V, Chen-Mok M, Tarasova M, Mikhailov A. Use of a levonorgestrel-releasing intrauterine system to treat bleeding related to uterine leiomyomas. *Fertil Steril.* 2003;79(5):1194–8.

[49] Senol T, Kahramanoglu I, Dogan Y, Baktiroglu M, Karateke A, Suer N. Levonorgestrel-releasing intrauterine device use as an alternative to surgical therapy for uterine leiomyoma. *Clin Exp Obstet Gynecol.* 2015;42(2):224–7.

[50] Magalhães J, Aldrighi JM, de Lima GR. Uterine volume and menstrual patterns in users of the levonorgestrel-releasing intrauterine system with idiopathic menorrhagia or menorrhagia due to leiomyomas. *Contraception.* 2007;75(3):193–8.

[51] Friedman AJ, Barbieri RL, Doubilet PM, Fine C, Schiff I. A randomized, double-blind trial of a gonadotropin releasing-hormone agonist (leuprolide) with or without medroxyprogesterone acetate in the treatment of leiomyomata uteri. *Fertil Steril.* 1988;49(3):404–9.

[52] Minaguchi H, Wong JM, Snabes MC. Clinical use of nafarelin in the treatment of leiomyomas: a review of the literature. *J Reprod Med Obstet Gynecol.* 2000;45(6):481–9.

[53] Lethaby A, Vollenhoven B, Sowter M. Efficacy of pre-operative gonadotrophin hormone releasing analogues for women with uterine fibroids undergoing hysterectomy or myomectomy: a systematic review. *BJOG.* 2002;109(10):1097–108.

[54] Thomas EJ. Add-back therapy for long-term use in dysfunctional uterine bleeding and uterine fibroids. *Br J Obstet Gynaecol.* 1996;103 Suppl:18–21.

[55] Ciebiera M, Madueke-Laveaux OS, Feduniw S, Ulin M, Spaczyński R, Zgliczyńska M, Bączkowska M, Zarychta E, Łoziński T, Ali M, Al-Hendy A. GnRH agonists and antagonists in therapy of symptomatic uterine fibroids - current roles and future perspectives. *Expert Opin Pharmacother.* 2023;24(16):1799–809.

[56] Niaz R, Saeed M, Khan H, Ali MA, Irshad A, Faiz M, Irshad A, Fatima F, Tunio SA, Aiman W. Efficacy and Safety of Oral GnRh Antagonists in Patients With Uterine Fibroids: A Systematic Review. *J Obstet Gynaecol Can.* 2022;44(12):1279–88.

[57] Al-Hendy A, Lukes AS, Poindexter AN, Venturella R, Villarroel C, Critchley HOD, Li Y, McKain L, Arjona Ferreira JC, Langenberg AGM, Wagman RB, Stewart EA. Treatment of Uterine Fibroid Symptoms with Relugolix Combination Therapy. *N Engl J Med.* 2021;384(7):630–42.

[58] Arjona Ferreira JC, Migoya E. Development of relugolix combination therapy as a medical treatment option for women with uterine fibroids or endometriosis. *F&S reports.* 2022;4(2 Suppl):73–82.

[59] Mutter GL, Bergeron C, Deligdisch L, Ferenczy A, Glant M, Merino M, Williams ARW, Blithe DL. The spectrum of endometrial pathology induced by progesterone receptor modulators. *Mod Pathol.* 2008;21(5):591–8.

[60] Wilkens J, Williams ARW, Chwalisz K, Han C, Cameron IT, Critchley HOD. Effect of asoprisnil on uterine proliferation markers and endometrial expression of the tumour suppressor gene, PTEN. *Hum Reprod.* 2009;24(5):1036–44.

[61] Steinauer J, Pritts EA, Jackson R, Jacoby AF. Systematic review of mifepristone for the treatment of uterine leiomyomata. Obstet Gynecol. 2004;103(6):1331–6.

[62] Tristan M, Orozco LJ, Steed A, Ramirez-Morera A, Stone P. Mifepristone for uterine fibroids. *Cochrane database Syst Rev.* 2012;2012(8).

[63] Varelas FK, Papanicolaou AN, Vavatsi-Christaki N, Makedos GA, Vlassis GD. The effect of anastrazole on symptomatic uterine leiomyomata. *Obstet Gynecol.* 2007;110(3):643–9.

[64] Hilário SG, Bozzini N, Borsari R, Baracat EC. Action of aromatase inhibitor for treatment of uterine leiomyoma in perimenopausal patients. *Fertil Steril.* 2009;91(1):240–3.

[65] Parsanezhad ME, Azmoon M, Alborzi S, Rajaeefard A, Zarei A, Kazerooni T, Frank V, Schmidt EH. A randomized, controlled clinical trial comparing the effects of aromatase inhibitor (letrozole) and gonadotropin-releasing hormone agonist (triptorelin) on uterine leiomyoma volume and hormonal status. *Fertil Steril.* 2010;93(1):192–8.

[66] Faivre E, Surroca MM, Deffieux X, Pages F, Gervaise A, Fernandez H. Vaginal myomectomy: literature review. *J Minim Invasive Gynecol.* 2010;17(2):154–60.

[67] Vitale SG, Angioni S, Saponara S, Sicilia G, Etrusco A, D'Alterio MN, Cobellis L, De Franciscis P, Riemma G. TikTok as a platform for hysteroscopy information: An analytical video-based cross-sectional study to assess quality, reliability, and accuracy. *Int J Gynecol Obstet.* 2025;168(1):353–61.

[68] Libretti A, Vitale SG, Saponara S, Corsini C, Aquino CI, Savasta F, Tizzoni E, Troìa L, Surico D, Angioni S, Remorgida V. Hysteroscopy in the new media: quality and reliability analysis of hysteroscopy procedures on YouTube™. *Arch Gynecol Obstet.* 2023;308(5):1515–24.

[69] Vitale SG, Angioni S, Saponara S, Sicilia G, Mignacca A, Caiazzo A, De Franciscis P, Riemma G. Hysteroscopic metroplasty and its reproductive impact among the social networks: A cross-sectional analysis on video quality, reliability and creators' opinions on YouTube, TikTok and Instagram. *Int J Med Inform.* 2025;195:105776.

[70] Riemma G, Vitale SG, Lipták MG, Ciebiera M, Boldogh BZ, Mereu L, Kovács KS, Török P. Surgical parameters affecting procedure duration of hysteroscopic fibroid resection: results of a retrospective longitudinal study. *Arch Gynecol Obstet.* 2024;311(1):91–8.

[71] Török P, Molnár S, Herman T, Jashanjeet S, Lampé R, Riemma G, Vitale SG. Fallopian tubal obstruction is associated with increased pain experienced during office hysteroscopy: a retrospective study. *Updates Surg.* 2020;72(1):213–8.

[72] Florio P, Filippeschi M, Imperatore A, Mereu L, Franchini M, Calzolari S, Mencaglia L, Litta P. The practicability and surgeons' subjective experiences with vaginal danazol before an operative hysteroscopy. *Steroids.* 2012;77:528–533.

[73] Vitale SG, Laganà AS, Caruso S, Garzon S, Vecchio GM, La Rosa VL, Casarin J, Ghezzi F. Comparison of three biopsy forceps for hysteroscopic endometrial biopsy

in postmenopausal patients (HYGREB-1): A multicenter, single-blind randomized clinical trial. *Int J Gynecol Obstet.* 2021;155(3):425–32.

[74] Vitale SG. The Biopsy Snake Grasper Sec. VITALE: A New Tool for Office Hysteroscopy. *J Minim Invasive Gynecol.* 2020;27(6):1414–6.

[75] Vitale SG, Saponara S, Succu AG, Sicilia G, Martsidis K, D'Alterio MN, Angioni S. Efficacy and Safety of Non-Ablative Dual Wavelength Diode Laser Therapy for Genitourinary Syndrome of Menopause: A Single-Center Prospective Study. *Adv Ther.* 2024;41(12):4617–27.

[76] Etrusco A, Buzzaccarini G, Laganà AS, Chiantera V, Vitale SG, Angioni S, D'Alterio MN, Nappi L, Sorrentino F, Vitagliano A, Difonzo T, Riemma G, Mereu L, Favilli A, Peitsidis P, D'Amato A. Use of Diode Laser in Hysteroscopy for the Management of Intrauterine Pathology: A Systematic Review. *Diagnostics.* 2024;14(3):327.

[77] Vitale SG, Moore O, Riemma G, Carugno J, Yarto ML, Haimovich S. Hysteroscopic laser ablation of symptomatic uterine fibroids: insights from a prospective study. *Climacteric.* 2023;26(5):497–502.

[78] Vitale SG, Saponara S, Sicilia G, Klarić M, Sorrentino F, D'Alterio MN, Nappi L, Angioni S. Hysteroscopic diode laser myolysis: from a case series to literature review of incisionless myolysis techniques for managing heavy menstrual bleeding in premenopausal women. *Arch Gynecol Obstet.* 2024;309(3):949–59.

[79] Florio P, Puzzutiello R, Filippeschi M, D'Onofrio P, Mereu L, Morelli R, Marianello D, Litta P, Mencaglia L, Petraglia F. Low-dose spinal anesthesia with hyperbaric bupivacaine with intrathecal fentanyl for operative hysteroscopy: a case series study. *J Minim Invasive Gynecol*. 2012;19(1):107–12.

[80] Vitale SG, Carugno J, Saponara S, Mereu L, Haimovich S, Alonso Pacheco L, Giannini A, Chellani M, Urman B, De Angelis MC, Angioni S. What is the impact of simulation on the learning of hysteroscopic skills by residents and medical students? A systematic review. *Minim Invasive Ther Allied Technol.* 2024;33(6):373–86.

[81] Mencaglia L, Carri G, Prasciolu C, Giunta G, Albis Florez ED, Cofelice V, Mereu L. Feasibility and complications in bipolar resectoscopy: preliminary experience. *Minim Invasive Ther Allied Technol.* 2013;22(1):50–5.

[82] Lasmar RB, Barozzo P. Histeroscopia: uma abordagem prática. 1a Ed. Rio de Janeiro: MEDSI; 2002.

[83] Lasmar RB, Barrozo PRM, Da Rosa DB, Lasmar BP, Modotte WP, Dias R. Hysteroscopic myomectomy in a submucous fibroid near from tubal ostia and 5 mm from the serosa: A case report from the Endoscopy Service of Ginendo-RJ. *Gynecol Surg.* 2009;6(3):283–6.

[84] Lasmar RB, Barrozo PRM, Da Rosa DB, Dias R. Hysteroscopic myomectomy in a submucous fibroid 3 mm from the serosa: A case report - Case report from the endoscopy service of Ginendo-RJ. *Gynecol Surg.* 2007;4(2):149–52.

[85] Vitale SG, Riemma G, Carugno J, Perez-Medina T, Alonso Pacheco L, Haimovich S, Parry JP, Di Spiezio Sardo A, De Franciscis P. Postsurgical barrier strategies to avoid the recurrence of intrauterine adhesion formation after hysteroscopic

adhesiolysis: a network meta-analysis of randomized controlled trials. *Am J Obstet Gynecol.* 2022;226(4):487-498.e8.

[86] Urman B, Yakin K, Ertas S, Alper E, Aksakal E, Riemma G, Angioni S, Vitale SG. Fertility and anatomical outcomes following hysteroscopic adhesiolysis: An 11-year retrospective cohort study to validate a new classification system for intrauterine adhesions (Urman-Vitale Classification System). *Int J Gynecol Obstet.* 2024;165(2):644–54.

[87] Vitale SG, De Angelis MC, Della Corte L, Saponara S, Carugno J, Laganà AS, Török P, Tinelli R, Pérez-Medina T, Ertas S, Urman B, Angioni S. Uterine cervical stenosis: from classification to advances in management. Overcoming the obstacles to access the uterine cavity. *Arch Gynecol Obstet.* 2024;309(3):755–64.

[88] Giannini A, Cuccu I, D'Auge TG, De Angelis E, Laganà AS, Chiantera V, Caserta D, Vitale SG, Muzii L, D'Oria O, Perniola G, Bogani G, Di Donato V. The great debate: Surgical outcomes of laparoscopic versus laparotomic myomectomy. A meta-analysis to critically evaluate current evidence and look over the horizon. *Eur J Obstet Gynecol Reprod Biol.* 2024;297:50–8.

[89] Angioni S, Saponara S, D'Ancona G, Sicilia G, D'Alterio MN, Vitale SG. Safety, Efficacy, and Cost-effectiveness of Organ Suspension in Laparoscopic Gynecologic Surgery: A Retrospective Cohort Study to Validate an Innovative Technique: Laparoscopic Organ Suspension sec. Angioni. *Gynecol Obstet Invest.* 2024;89(6):445–52.

[90] Dubuisson JB, O'Leary T, Feki A, Bouquet De Jolinière J, Dubuisson J. Laparoscopic myomectomy: the current status. *Curr Opin Obstet Gynecol.* 2003;15(4):345–51.

[91] Sizzi O, Rossetti A, Malzoni M, Minelli L, La Grotta F, Soranna L, Panunzi S, Spagnolo R, Imperato F, Landi S, Fiaccamento A, Stola E. Italian multicenter study on complications of laparoscopic myomectomy. *J Minim Invasive Gynecol.* 2007;14(4):453–62.

[92] Pontis A, Sedda F, Mereu L, Podda M, Melis GB, Pisanu A, Angioni S. Review and meta-analysis of prospective randomized controlled trials (RCTs) comparing laparo-endoscopic single site and multiport laparoscopy in gynecologic operative procedures. *Arch Gynecol Obstet.* 2016;294(3):567–77.

[93] Angioni S, Pontis A, Pisanu A, Mereu L, Roman H. Single-port access subtotal laparoscopic hysterectomy: A prospective case-control study. *J Minim Invasive Gynecol.* 2015;22(5):807–12.

[94] Prisco MG, Zannoni GF, De Stefano I, Vellone VG, Tortorella L, Fagotti A, Mereu L, Scambia G, Gallo D. Prognostic role of metastasis tumor antigen 1 in patients with ovarian cancer: a clinical study. *Hum Pathol.* 2012;43(2):282–8.

[95] Pignata S, Ferrandina G, Scarfone G, Scollo P, Odicino F, Cormio G, Katsaros D, Frigerio L, Mereu L, Ghezzi F, Manzione L, Lauria R, Breda E, Alletti DG, Ballardini M, Vernaglia A, Sorio R, Tumolo S, Musso P, Magni G, Pisano C, Morabito A. Poor outcome of elderly patients with platinum-sensitive recurrent ovarian cancer: results from the SOCRATES retrospective study. *Crit Rev Oncol Hematol.* 2009;71(3):233–41.

Chapter 4

Adenomyosis

Liliana Mereu[1,*], MD, PhD
Basilio Pecorino[2], MD
Saverio Tateo[3], MD, PhD
Stefania Saponara[4], MD
Giuseppe Scibilia[5], MD
and Salvatore Giovanni Vitale[1], MD, PhD
[1]Obstetrics and Gynecology Unit, "*Gaspare Rodolico*" University Hospital, Department of General Surgery and Medical Surgical Specialties, University of Catania, Catania, Italy
[2]Gynecology and Obstetrics, "*Umberto I*" Hospital Enna, Kore University of Enna, Enna, Italy
[3]Department of Obstetrics and Gynecology, Centre Hospitalier de Troyes, Troyes, France
[4]Division of Gynecology and Obstetrics, Department of Surgical Sciences, University of Cagliari, Cagliari, Italy
[5]Gynecology and Obstetrics "*Giovanni Paolo II*" Hospital, Ragusa, Kore University of Enna, Enna, Italy

Abstract

Adenomyosis is a gynecological disease characterized by endometrial tissue within the muscular wall of the uterus. This disorder, which can cause a range of disabling symptoms, including chronic pelvic pain, heavy and irregular menstruation, and dysmenorrhea, is often diagnosed in women of childbearing age but may persist even during menopause. The precise cause of adenomyosis is not fully understood, although

---

* Corresponding Author's Email: liliana.mereu@unict.it

In: Endometrium and Related Endouterine Pathologies
Editors: Liliana Mereu and Salvatore Giovanni Vitale
ISBN: 979-8-89530-818-9

genetic, hormonal and inflammatory factors seem to play an important role in the development of the condition. Diagnosis is mainly based on transvaginal ultrasound and MRI, while therapeutic management can range from drugs to control pain and blood loss to surgical treatments such as hysterectomy in severe cases. Despite its incidence, adenomyosis remains a relatively little known and often underdiagnosed disease, which makes increased awareness and research essential to improve diagnostic and therapeutic pathways.

Keywords: adenomyosis, pelvic pain, abnormal uterine bleeding.

Introduction

Adenomyosis is histologically characterized by the presence of ectopic endometrial tissue, including glands and stroma, within the myometrium, often accompanied by hyperplasia of the surrounding smooth muscle cells. The condition is particularly prevalent in women aged 40–49 years, with reported rates ranging from 20% to 32%, and its prevalence increases significantly in patients undergoing hysterectomy for benign gynecological conditions, reaching as high as 62% in this population [1, 2]. Although adenomyosis is frequently associated with abnormal uterine bleeding (AUB) and chronic pelvic pain, its diagnosis can be challenging due to the absence of highly sensitive and specific diagnostic tools and the presence of asymptomatic cases. Notably, asymptomatic adenomyosis is often linked to infertility, further complicating its recognition. Historically, the diagnosis has often been incidental, identified only after hysterectomy, particularly in multiparous women between the ages of 40 and 50 [3, 4]. Over the past 15 years, advancements in imaging techniques, particularly transvaginal ultrasound and magnetic resonance imaging (MRI), have significantly improved the ability to diagnose adenomyosis non-invasively. These developments have facilitated earlier detection, allowing diagnosis in younger patients and enabling clinicians to address critical issues such as infertility, recurrent spontaneous abortions, and obstetric complications more effectively [5, 6]. Early and accurate diagnosis through these modern imaging modalities has expanded therapeutic opportunities and underscored the importance of tailored management strategies for this complex condition.

4.1. Definition, Etiology and Classification

The definition of adenomyosis has evolved significantly over time due to ongoing debates about its etiology. Carl von Rokitansky described it in 1860 as "adenoid cystosarcoma of the uterus," identifying endometrial glands within the myometrium [7]. In 1921 and later in 1925, Frankl proposed a theory of diffuse endometrial invasion into the myometrium. By 1927, Sampson introduced the peritoneal invasion hypothesis, initially associating adenomyosis with endometriosis but eventually distinguishing the two conditions. That same year, Bird provided the modern definition of adenomyosis as a benign invasion of endometrial tissue into the myometrium, resulting in a diffusely enlarged uterus [7]. Microscopically, this condition is characterized by ectopic, non-neoplastic endometrial glands and stroma surrounded by hypertrophic and hyperplastic myometrium [8].

Despite extensive study, the exact etiology of adenomyosis remains unclear. Two predominant theories—*invagination* and *metaplasia*—have been proposed, but neither fully satisfies the criteria of falsifiability, explanatory capacity, and predictive capability. Leyendecker, in 2009 and later in 2015, introduced the "tissue injury and repair" (TIAR) hypothesis [9, 10]. According to this model, the myocytes and fibroblasts of the junctional zone (JZ), visualized on MRI as the endometrial-myometrial interface (EMI), are damaged by abnormal myometrial hyperperistalsis of unknown origin. This damage activates the TIAR system, leading to an increase in inflammatory mediators and estrogen. Through feedback mechanisms, such as estrogen receptor α (ERα)-induced oxytocin/oxytocin receptor expression, hyperperistalsis is further exacerbated, causing chronic microtrauma [11].

The metaplasia theory suggests that pluripotent Müllerian cells, acting as endometrial progenitors or niche cells, migrate into the myometrium instead of residing within the junctional zone. This migration is thought to be driven by yet unrecognized mechanisms [12]. Risk factors for adenomyosis include early menarche, frequent menstrual cycles, and late menopause, which increase estrogenic exposure. Additionally, trauma to the junctional zone, often resulting from uterine revisions after abortions, cesarean sections, or myomectomies, may contribute to endometrial-myometrial disruption (EMID) [13].

Current diagnostic imaging has facilitated the classification of adenomyosis into four distinct types based on ultrasound findings [14]:

1) *Focal adenomyosis*: The lesion involves less than 25% of the myometrium, with more than 25% of the lesion surrounded by normal myometrium.
2) *Diffuse adenomyosis*: The lesion affects more than 25% of the myometrium, with less than 25% of the lesion surrounded by normal myometrium.
3) *Adenomyoma*: A localized lesion characterized by hypertrophy of the surrounding myometrial cells.
4) *Mixed adenomyosis*: A combination of both diffuse and focal adenomyosis.

Magnetic resonance imaging (MRI) has further refined the classification of adenomyosis into *internal* and *external* subtypes, often associated with different clinical presentations [15]. Internal adenomyosis is commonly observed in women aged 40–50 years and is frequently linked to menometrorrhagia and a history of uterine surgeries, such as uterine revisions or cesarean sections. This type typically presents without concurrent endometriosis. In contrast, external adenomyosis is more prevalent in younger, nulliparous patients and is often associated with deep infiltrating endometriosis [15].

Despite these advances, no universally accepted classification system exists to integrate ultrasound and MRI findings, highlighting the need for standardization in diagnostic criteria.

4.2. Histopathological Characteristics

Adenomyosis is characterized by distinct macroscopic and microscopic features. Macroscopically, it manifests as a globular and cystic enlargement of the myometrium. The cysts are often filled with red blood, usually hemolyzed, and contain siderophages, reflecting repeated hemorrhage and iron deposition episodes.

Microscopically, adenomyosis is defined by the presence of ectopic endometrial glands and stroma located beyond the last basal glands of the endometrium, arranged in a disordered manner within the myometrium. These glands are surrounded by a collar of hypertrophic smooth muscle cells [16]. The endometrial glands and stroma within adenomyotic lesions typically exhibit a proliferative appearance, although they can also mirror various phases of the menstrual cycle depending on hormonal influences. In approximately 5% of cases, the glands become cystic, containing cellular debris and iron-laden macrophages, indicative of chronic hemorrhagic activity [16] (Figure 1).

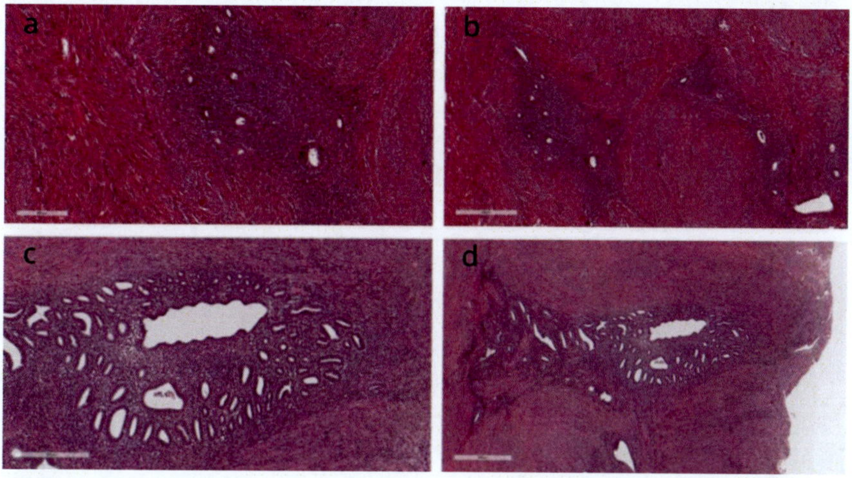

Figure 1. Histological images of uterine tissue with adenomyosis, stained with hematoxylin and eosin (H&E). (a) Myometrial section with ectopic endometrial glands surrounded by fibrous stroma and hypertrophic muscle; (b) Myometrium showing scattered glands within areas of disorganized tissue and fibrosis; (c) Ectopic glands of various shapes and sizes within the myometrium, surrounded by proliferative stroma and hyperplastic muscle; (d) Adenomyotic lesion with disorganized glandular patterns embedded in thickened fibrous and muscular tissue.

Rarely, epithelial metaplasia is observed, predominantly of the ciliated or tubal type. In the gland-poor variant, which is more commonly found in postmenopausal women, the endometrioid glands are sparse, appearing only in isolated adenomyotic foci [17]. Stromal decidualization, either focal or extensive, may occur during pregnancy or with progestin treatment, while atrophic changes in the stroma are more common during menopause or following certain hormonal therapies. Additionally, adenomyotic lesions show an increase in microvascular density, supported by the expression of vascular endothelial growth factor (VEGF) and hypoxia-inducible factor-1 alpha (HIFα), which are key mediators of angiogenesis in response to tissue hypoxia [18].

The topographic distribution of adenomyotic lesions varies. Most lesions are thought to originate at the endometrial–myometrial interface (the junctional zone), with a centrifugal pattern of extension into the outer myometrium [19]. This pattern highlights the progressive nature of the disease and its tendency to invade deeper myometrial layers over time.

Differential diagnosis is critical when evaluating adenomyosis. It must be distinguished from *endometriosis*, in which the ectopic glands and stroma are typically confined to the outer layers of the myometrium and do not affect at least 90% of the myometrium. Additionally, differentiation from *adenomyoma* is important. Adenomyoma presents as a well-circumscribed lesion within the myometrium and may protrude into the uterine cavity, in which case it is referred to as an adenomatous polyp [20].

4.3. Clinical Appearance

Adenomyosis manifests through a variety of symptoms, including gynecological pain, abnormal uterine bleeding (AUB), dysmenorrhea, dyspareunia, and is frequently associated with infertility and adverse obstetric outcomes. The clinical presentation often overlaps with other gynecological conditions, particularly uterine fibroids, complicating the attribution of specific symptoms solely to adenomyosis [21].

Abnormal uterine bleeding (AUB) is one of the hallmark symptoms of adenomyosis and encompasses heavy menstrual bleeding (HMB), prolonged or irregular menstrual cycles, intermenstrual bleeding, and pre- or post-menstrual spotting. The pathophysiology underlying AUB in adenomyosis includes increased uterine volume, enhanced vascularization, improper uterine contractions, and elevated levels of estrogen and prostaglandins [22]. However, the high prevalence of comorbidities, especially uterine fibroids, in 60-80% of adenomyosis cases has led to debates about whether these symptoms are attributable to adenomyosis itself or its coexisting pathologies [23].

Chronic pelvic pain (CPP) and dysmenorrhea are also common clinical features. Chronic pelvic pain has been found to persist even after surgical removal of endometriotic lesions when preoperative MRI reveals a junctional zone (JZ) thickness exceeding 11 mm, suggesting a link between adenomyosis and sustained pain [24]. Dysmenorrhea severity correlates with the depth and degree of adenomyotic invasion into the myometrium, with more extensive infiltration leading to more severe symptoms [25]. Moreover, patients with both uterine fibroids and adenomyosis report a broader range of pain types compared to those with fibroids alone. In addition to pain, the increased uterine size associated with adenomyosis can lead to a sensation of pelvic heaviness or weight and in some cases, dysuria.

Adenomyosis is also associated with adverse obstetric outcomes, including recurrent miscarriages, fetal malpositions, uterine rupture, haemoperitoneum [26, 27] and an increased likelihood of cesarean sections [28]. These outcomes are often attributed to reduced elasticity of the myometrium, explaining the uterine rupture also in non-pregnant uterus [29, 30], abnormal placental localization or invasion, and reduced uterine cavity size. These structural abnormalities arise partly from the disrupted architecture of the myometrium due to adenomyosis and partly from coexisting leiomyomas.

During pregnancy, adenomyosis is linked to a higher risk of preeclampsia, fetal intrauterine growth restriction (IUGR), and preterm delivery. While the precise mechanisms remain unclear, these complications are thought to result from spiral artery dysfunction, oxidative stress, and diminished placental perfusion [31]. Additionally, placental anomalies related to location and invasion exacerbate the risk of pre-, peri-, and postpartum hemorrhage. Fragile neoangiogenesis, coupled with the abnormal myometrial architecture in adenomyosis, contributes to metrorrhagia during pregnancy and postpartum hemorrhages [32].

4.4. Adenomyosis and Infertility

The association between adenomyosis and infertility has become increasingly evident over the years. However, a direct causal relationship remains unproven due to the lack of randomized controlled trials, limitations in diagnostic tools, and the heterogeneity of the disease itself [33, 34]. Current estimates suggest that the prevalence of adenomyosis among infertile women ranges from 7% to 27% [8]. While the exact pathological mechanisms remain poorly understood, several contributing factors have been identified.

One major factor is altered tubal uterine migration of gametes and embryos, which likely explains the increased incidence of ectopic pregnancies in patients with adenomyosis [35]. Additionally, the distortion of the uterine cavity caused by adenomyotic lesions disrupts the structural and functional environment necessary for successful implantation [36]. More importantly, there is evidence of altered endometrial receptivity, characterized by the dysregulation of implantation-associated factors such as HOXA10, LIF, MMP2, IL-6, cytochrome P450, and RCAS1 in the eutopic endometrium [37].

These abnormalities impair the ability of the endometrium to support implantation and early pregnancy. Furthermore, inflammation plays a critical role, with increased expression of IL-1β and CRH observed in patients with adenomyosis, suggesting that inflammatory pathways within the endometrium contribute significantly to infertility [22].

In addition to endometrial abnormalities, the architecture of the normal myometrium is disrupted in adenomyosis. The typical arrangement of smooth muscle fibers is replaced by hyperplastic muscle tissue with an irregular distribution. This leads to dysfunctional uterine peristalsis, which is highly sensitive to endocrine and paracrine stimuli, resulting in elevated intrauterine pressure [38, 39]. These abnormalities further compromise the migration of gametes and embryos within the reproductive tract, reducing the likelihood of successful fertilization and implantation.

Another proposed mechanism involves the alteration of ovarian function. Emerging evidence suggests that adenomyosis may negatively impact ovarian reserve, granulosa cell function, and oocyte quality. Preliminary studies have even linked the depth of adenomyotic invasion to the degree of oocyte immaturity, underscoring the potential impact of the disease on ovarian health [40, 41].

Infertility associated with adenomyosis is also characterized by higher rates of miscarriage and failures in assisted reproductive technologies (ART) [42]. This highlights the complexity of the condition and the challenges it poses in achieving successful pregnancies. Despite advances in treatment, there is insufficient evidence to definitively recommend one approach over another for managing infertility in adenomyosis patients.[43]. Medical therapy, surgical intervention, ART, and expectant management all play roles, but their relative efficacy depends on individual patient characteristics [44].

Medical therapy is currently considered the first-line treatment for infertility associated with adenomyosis. Among available options, GnRH analogues have shown promise [45]. These agents improve endometrial receptivity by reducing nitric oxide synthetase activity, thereby decreasing free radical levels in the glandular epithelium. Additionally, GnRH analogues suppress aromatase P450 expression, further optimizing the endometrial environment without impairing the decidualization process or blastocyst invasion [46]. This treatment strategy has been shown to enhance implantation and pregnancy rates, particularly in ART cycles.

The role of surgery in treating infertility caused by adenomyosis remains controversial [47]. Surgical intervention may be beneficial in select cases, particularly for patients with focal adenomyosis, as it may improve uterine anatomy and function. However, the risks associated with surgery, including uterine trauma, must be carefully weighed against the potential benefits, particularly in women with diffuse adenomyosis [48].

When considering assisted reproductive techniques, there is no consensus on whether ART should be prioritized over surgical or medical treatment, or whether it should follow an expectant management approach [48]. Decisions should be guided by individual patient characteristics, including the extent of the disease, the patient's age, and their reproductive goals.

4.5. Diagnosis

The advent of increasingly sophisticated imaging techniques has significantly improved the ability to diagnose adenomyosis, often before obtaining histological confirmation. Early detection is critical given the condition's strong association with infertility and its potential to impair reproductive outcomes. A combination of imaging modalities, alongside adjunctive diagnostic tools such as hysteroscopy, provides a comprehensive framework for evaluating adenomyosis.

Transvaginal ultrasound (TVUS) is the first-line diagnostic tool for adenomyosis due to its accessibility, non-invasiveness, and cost-effectiveness. TVUS offers a sensitivity of 74% and a specificity of 76% [49]. When enhanced with three-dimensional (3D) imaging, diagnostic performance improves to 84% for both sensitivity and specificity, making it a reliable initial screening method [49]. The diagnostic approach is guided by the Morphological Uterus Sonographic Assessment (MUSA) criteria, which have been revised to define both direct and indirect signs of adenomyosis [50].

Direct signs visible on TVUS include *myometrial cysts*, *hyperechogenic islands*, and *echogenic subendometrial lines or buds*, indicating ectopic endometrial tissue within the myometrium. These findings are often accompanied by indirect signs, such as *a globular uterus*, a*symmetrical myometrial thickening, fan-shaped shadowing, translesional vascularity,* and abnormalities in the *junctional zone (JZ),* such as irregularities or interruptions. The junctional zone, which represents the interface between the endometrium and myometrium, is a critical diagnostic parameter. Regularity and lack of interruptions should exclude adenomyosis only after a 3D evaluation by an experienced gynecologist (Figure 2).

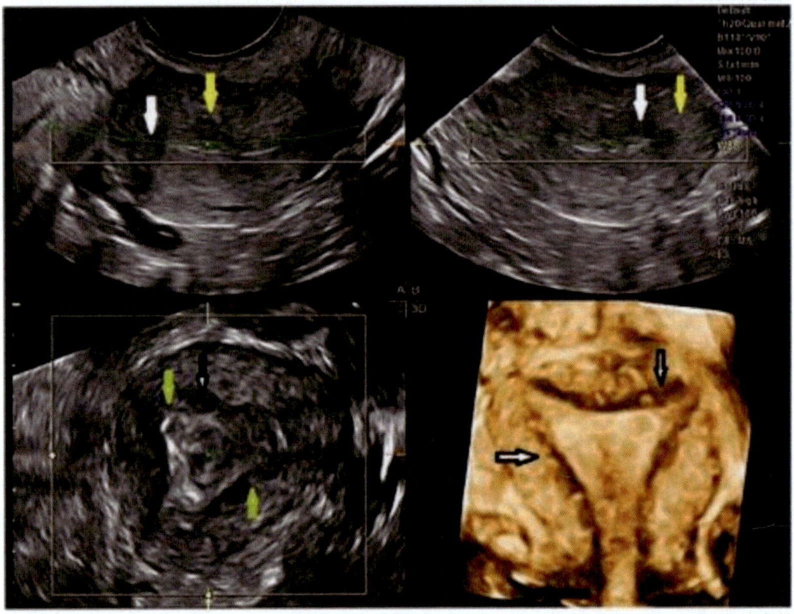

Figure 2. Severe adenomyosis with multiple sonographic signs: multiplanar and 3D rendering of an anteverted uterus with multiple sonographic signs: myometrial cysts (white arrow), hyperechoic islands (yellow arrow), linear striations (green arrow), and irregular EMJ (black arrow). *(©2017 From Eisenberg VH et al.* Sonographic Signs of Adenomyosis Are Prevalent in Women Undergoing Surgery for Endometriosis and May Suggest a Higher Risk of Infertility. *Licensed under the Attribution 4.0 International*).

Magnetic resonance imaging (MRI) is the second-line diagnostic method, typically reserved for cases with inconclusive TVUS results. It is particularly valuable in patients with infertility or abnormal uterine bleeding (e.g., menorrhagia) who are of reproductive age. MRI is recommended by the European Society of Urogenital Radiology (ESUR 2017) due to its superior specificity of 89% compared to TVUS, alongside a sensitivity of 77% and an exceptionally high positive predictive value of 92.3% [51–53].

MRI enables detailed visualization of the uterus, distinguishing adenomyosis from other uterine pathologies such as leiomyomas. Similar to ultrasound, MRI findings are categorized as direct and indirect signs. *Direct signs* include cystic components within the myometrium, which represent glandular foci trapped in ectopic locations. *Indirect signs* primarily involve abnormalities of the junctional zone, such as focal or diffuse thickening exceeding 12 mm, poorly defined low-signal margins in T2-weighted sequences, and subendometrial cysts or glandular foci with hyperintensity in T1 fat-suppressed and T2-weighted images. The combined observation of these features—particularly when junctional zone thickening is associated with cystic glandular foci—provides highly specific evidence of adenomyosis. MRI's ability to detect subclinical disease and its high anatomical resolution make it indispensable for complex or ambiguous cases, particularly in infertility evaluations [54] (Figure 3).

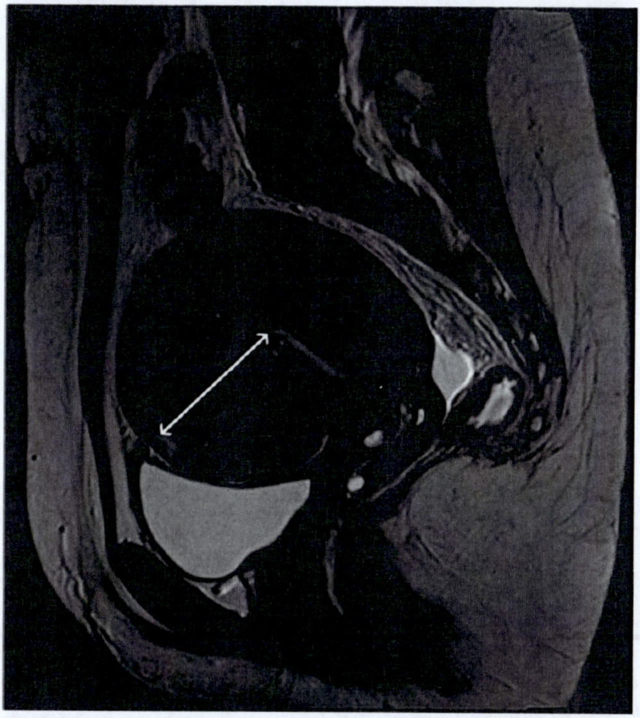

Figure 3. Diffuse adenomyosis: Sagittal T2-weighed image; thickening of the junctional zone forming an ill-defined area of low signal intensity, with punctate high-intensity myometrial foci (white arrow) *(©2017 From Agostinho L et al. MRI for adenomyosis: a pictorial review. Licensed under the Attribution 4.0 International).*

Hysteroscopy is a valuable adjunctive diagnostic tool for adenomyosis, providing direct visualization of the uterine cavity and enabling targeted biopsies [55, 56]. Although hysteroscopy is limited in its ability to visualize pathology beyond the endometrial surface, it can provide suggestive evidence of adenomyosis through characteristic findings [57, 58]. These include an irregular endometrium with *small openings, pronounced hypervascularization,* and a *"strawberry-like" appearance* of the endometrium (Figure 4). Hemorrhagic cystic lesions, appearing dark blue or chocolate brown, may also be observed, representing ectopic endometrial tissue that has undergone repeated intra-myometrial hemorrhage (Figure 5). Fibrous cystic lesions can develop following multiple episodes of bleeding within the myometrium [59].

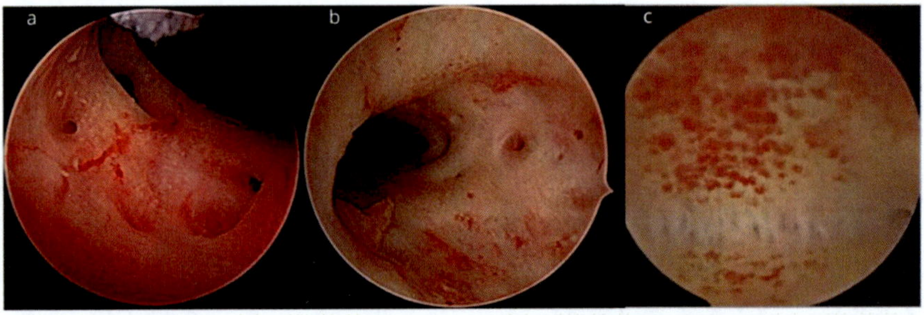

Figure 4. Hysteroscopic view of adenomyosis: (a-b) Tiny adenomyotic openings scattered across an irregular endometrial surface; (c) Typical 'strawberry' pattern of the endometrium, characterized by hyperemia with bright red areas surrounding white central dots. (*©2024 Modified from Saponara S et al. The Pivotal role of hysteroscopy in diagnosing subtle uterine lesions in infertile patients: Seeing the unseen can make the difference. Licensed under the Creative Commons Attribution 4.0).*

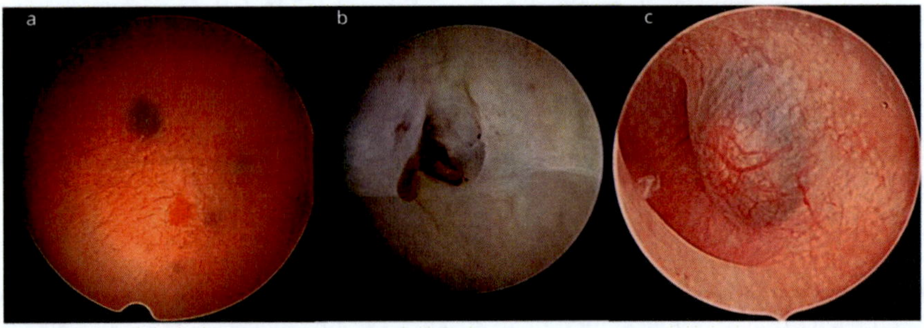

Figure 5. Hysteroscopic view of adenomyosis: (a-b-c) Hemorrhagic cystic lesions exhibiting a dark blue to chocolate brown appearance (*©2024 Modified from Saponara S et al. The Pivotal role of hysteroscopy in diagnosing subtle uterine lesions in infertile patients: Seeing the unseen can make the difference. Licensed under the Creative Commons Attribution 4.0).*

The timing of the procedure influences the accuracy of hysteroscopy in diagnosing adenomyosis. The early post-menstrual phase is considered optimal, as adenomyotic lesions are more likely to impact the uterine cavity and can be better visualized during this time [59]. Additionally, reducing intracavitary pressure during the procedure enhances the ability to evaluate superficial vascular abnormalities, improving diagnostic accuracy. Hysteroscopy also facilitates biopsy collection from both the endometrium and sub-endometrial myometrium [60, 61]. Biopsy instruments such as grasping forceps, scissors, or bipolar electrodes allow precise sampling, while advanced tools like the Spirotome (Bioncise NV, Wellen, Belgium) can obtain samples from deeper sub-endometrial layers, providing critical insights into the depth of adenomyotic penetration [62, 63].

4.6. Treatment

Adenomyosis significantly impacts the quality of life in approximately two-thirds of affected individuals, primarily due to symptoms such as heavy menstrual bleeding (HMB), chronic pelvic pain, dysmenorrhea, and dyspareunia [64, 65]. Management involves both medical and surgical approaches, with medical therapy preferred for patients wishing to conceive, those aiming to preserve their uterus, or in cases where surgery is contraindicated.

4.6.1. Medical Treatment

Medical therapy is the first-line approach for managing adenomyosis in many patients, especially those seeking to preserve fertility or avoid surgical interventions. The primary aim of medical treatment is to alleviate symptoms, including reducing HMB, pelvic pain, and uterine volume. Hormonal treatments form the backbone of this approach, often supplemented with analgesic or anti-hemorrhagic agents to address specific symptoms.

Nonsteroidal anti-inflammatory drugs (NSAIDs) are frequently employed for symptomatic relief, particularly for dysmenorrhea and pelvic pain. By inhibiting cyclooxygenase (COX) enzymes, NSAIDs reduce prostaglandin production, thereby mitigating inflammation and pain. While effective for mild cases or as an adjunct to hormonal therapy, their efficacy is limited in severe cases, as approximately 20% of women with adenomyosis experience dysmenorrhea that does not respond to NSAID treatment [66]. Moreover, NSAIDs are less effective than hormonal options for managing heavy menstrual bleeding, making them a supportive rather than primary therapy [67].

Progestins play a central role in the hormonal management of adenomyosis due to their diverse mechanisms of action. These include the induction of negative feedback pathways that suppress follicle-stimulating hormone (FSH) and luteinizing hormone (LH), the inhibition of endometrial proliferation, and the promotion of decidualization and atrophy of adenomyotic tissue. However, studies have revealed a decreased expression of progesterone receptors (PR) A and B in adenomyotic tissue, which is similar to the changes observed in endometriosis [68]. Progesterone exerts its antiproliferative effects primarily through binding to these receptors. The observed reduction in PR expression may partially explain both the pathogenesis of adenomyosis and the reduced responsiveness to progestin-based therapies in some patients [69]. Progestins are available in various formulations, including oral, injectable, and intrauterine delivery systems, each offering distinct advantages tailored to the specific clinical needs and preferences of patients.

Dienogest (DNG) is the preferred first-line treatment for adenomyosis. DNG is a 19-norsteroid progestin that selectively binds to progesterone receptors, exerting a potent antiproliferative effect on endometrial tissue [70]. This action reduces the hyperplasia and inflammation characteristic of adenomyosis. DNG is effective in managing dysmenorrhea, heavy menstrual bleeding, and chronic pelvic pain, as well as in reducing uterine volume. Its hypoestrogenic and mild anti-ovulatory properties further contribute to its efficacy. Multiple studies have demonstrated the effectiveness of DNG, showing marked improvements in pain scores and reductions in bleeding volume [71]. However, irregular bleeding and spotting are common side effects that can impact patient adherence, particularly during long-term use. These adverse effects must be carefully discussed with patients during treatment planning.

The *levonorgestrel-releasing intrauterine system (LNG-IUS)* is another cornerstone of medical treatment for adenomyosis. The LNG-IUS delivers high concentrations of levonorgestrel directly to the uterine cavity, inducing endometrial atrophy and suppressing local inflammation. This localized action minimizes systemic side effects, making LNG-IUS a well-tolerated option [72]. It effectively reduces heavy menstrual bleeding, pelvic pain, and dysmenorrhea, with studies showing long-term symptom control comparable to surgical interventions like hysterectomy. Additionally, LNG-IUS has been associated with fewer adverse events than systemic hormonal therapies, enhancing patient compliance. However, its efficacy diminishes in cases of significantly enlarged uteri (>200 ml), where the risk of spontaneous expulsion increases [73]. In such cases, pre-treatment with a GnRH analog to reduce uterine size can improve outcomes.

Combined Oral Contraceptives (COCs) offer another hormonal option for managing adenomyosis, particularly in younger patients or those with mild symptoms. By inducing a pseudo-pregnancy state, COCs suppress ovulation, induce endometrial atrophy, and reduce menstrual volume and pelvic pain. COCs also inhibit aromatase activity within adenomyotic lesions, decreasing local estrogen production. While effective for controlling symptoms, studies suggest that COCs are less effective than DNG or LNG-IUS for long-term symptom management [71]. Therefore, they are generally considered a secondary option for adenomyosis treatment.

Gonadotropin-Releasing Hormone (GnRH) Analogs are among the most effective drugs for symptom control, particularly in patients with severe or refractory symptoms. These agents suppress gonadotropin release, leading to systemic and local hypoestrogenism, which directly inhibits the growth of adenomyotic tissue. GnRH analogs reduce uterine volume more effectively than progestins, making them particularly valuable for patients with bulky uteri (>200 ml) or as pre-treatment before LNG-IUS insertion [74]. However, the hypoestrogenic state induced by GnRH analogs is associated with significant adverse effects, including vasomotor symptoms, bone mineral density loss, genital atrophy, and mood instability [75, 76]. For this reason, treatment is generally limited to six months, followed by progestin maintenance therapy to sustain symptom control. In refractory cases, longer durations with "add-back therapy" (low-dose estrogen and progestin supplementation) are employed to mitigate hypoestrogenic side effects. Emerging approaches, such as "draw-back therapy," use lower doses of GnRH analogs combined with progestins, offering effective symptom relief with fewer adverse effects [75, 76]. However, no specific progestin has proven superior in this combination.

Emerging Treatments for adenomyosis include newer hormonal therapies that target specific molecular pathways involved in the disease. *GnRH antagonists*, such as relugolix, elagolix and linzagolix, directly suppress gonadotropin release without the initial flare effect seen with GnRH analogs. These agents show promise in managing adenomyosis-related pain and bleeding, but long-term data on safety and efficacy are still limited [77]. Similarly, *Selective Progesterone Receptor Modulators (SPRMs)*, such as ulipristal acetate, have demonstrated efficacy in reducing dysmenorrhea and heavy menstrual bleeding. However, the potential for liver toxicity associated with SPRMs necessitates careful patient monitoring and further research [78].

*Aromatase Inhibitors***,** which suppress local estrogen production within adenomyotic tissue, are another emerging option. While early studies show promise, their safety profile and long-term efficacy remain to be fully established [79].

Despite the availability of these treatments, medical therapy for adenomyosis remains a challenge due to the heterogeneity of clinical presentations and individual responses (Table 1). No single treatment is universally effective, and therapy must be carefully tailored to each patient based on their symptom severity, fertility goals, and preferences. The variability in clinical outcomes underscores the need for further research to refine treatment protocols and establish evidence-based guidelines for managing this complex condition.

Table 1. Medical treatment of adenomyosis

Intervention	Mechanism of Action	Adverse Effects
Nonsteroidal anti-inflammatory drugs	Decreased pain and abnormal bleeding from decreasing circulating prostaglandin	Potential for renal toxicity and gastrointestinal irritation
Combined oral contraceptives	Atrophy of endometrial tissue causing decreased menstrual bleeding	Contraception, irregular bleeding, thromboembolism
Progestins	Atrophy of endometrium	Irregular bleeding, weight gain
Progestin-releasing intrauterine device	Atrophy of endometrium from local progestin	Irregular bleeding, contraception
Gonadotropin-releasing hormone analogues	Hypoestrogenism, endometrial atrophy	Vasomotor symptoms, risk of osteoporosis
Gonadotropin-releasing hormone antagonists	Endometrial atrophy, mild hypoestrogenism	Vasomotor symptoms

4.6.2. Surgical Treatment

Surgical intervention is a key option for managing adenomyosis when medical therapy fails to control symptoms adequately [80]. Although no universal guidelines exist, treatment strategies are tailored to the patient's specific needs, whether symptom relief or fertility preservation. Surgical options range from definitive hysterectomy to fertility-preserving procedures, including excisional and non-excisional techniques [81], as well as hysteroscopic and ablative methods (Table 2).

Table 2. Surgical treatment of adenomyosis

Preoperative Evaluation	Surgical Options	Details
Fertility Sparing	Excisional Techniques	1. Classic Adenomyomectomy 2. Triple-flap method 3. Transverse H incision 4. Wedge resection 5. Asymmetric dissection of the uterus 6. PUSH technique
	Non-excisional Techniques	1. HIFU (High-Intensity Focused Ultrasound 2. Uterine Artery Embolization (UAE) 3. Radiofrequency Ablation (RFA) 4. Percutaneous Microwave Ablation (PMWA)
	Hysteroscopic procedures	1. Hemorrhagic cystic lesions evacuation 2. Endometrial ablation 3. Endomyometrial ablation
No Fertility-Sparing Needs	Hysterectomy	1. Vaginal Hysterectomy 2. Laparoscopically Assisted Vaginal Hysterectomy (LAVH) 3. Total Laparoscopic Hysterectomy (TLH) 4. Laparotomic Hysterectomy

4.6.2.1. Hysterectomy: The Definitive Option

Hysterectomy remains the gold-standard treatment for adenomyosis, particularly for patients who no longer wish to preserve fertility. By removing the uterus, hysterectomy ensures complete symptom resolution and eliminates the risk of recurrence [82, 83]. Total hysterectomy is often preferred over subtotal to prevent recurrence in the cervical stump or rectovaginal septum. This approach is especially effective for diffuse adenomyosis, where the disease extensively affects the uterine wall.

The choice of surgical technique depends on patient factors and disease complexity. Vaginal hysterectomy is often preferred due to its lower morbidity, shorter hospital stay, and faster recovery. However, it carries a higher risk of bladder injury, attributed to the difficulty in identifying critical anatomical planes, such as the vesicovaginal and vesicocervical septa [84]. Laparoscopically assisted vaginal hysterectomy (LAVH) offers improved visualization of these planes but is associated with a higher risk of ureteral injury due to the complexity of the dissection [85–87]. Laparotomy, while more invasive, allows better visualization of adhesions and deeply infiltrated adenomyotic tissue, making it a useful option for complex cases. Nevertheless, it comes with longer recovery times and greater postoperative pain. Laparoscopic hysterectomy is considered the optimal method for many patients, combining excellent visualization, lower surgical risks, and quicker recovery [88–91].

4.6.2.2. Fertility-Preserving Techniques

For women seeking to preserve fertility, conservative surgical techniques aim to alleviate symptoms while maintaining uterine functionality [92]. These approaches are broadly categorized into *excisional techniques* and *non-excisional techniques.*

4.6.2.3. Excisional Techniques

Excisional techniques involve the targeted removal of adenomyotic tissue, followed by meticulous uterine reconstruction to restore its structural and functional integrity. The most commonly performed procedure is *adenomyomectomy*, which can be tailored to the extent and location of the disease.

1. *Classic Adenomyomectomy*
   This technique involves a longitudinal incision along the adenomyotic region, allowing sharp and blunt dissection of the lesion using scissors, diathermy, or graspers. The uterine wall is reconstructed in multiple layers with absorbable sutures, restoring the endometrial cavity and seromuscular wall properly. This approach is particularly suited for focal adenomyosis [93].
2. *Triple-Flap Method*
   Designed for diffuse adenomyosis, this technique involves midline bisection of the uterus to open the endometrial cavity. Diseased tissue is excised with a 1 cm margin of healthy myometrium to minimize recurrence. Reconstruction is performed using overlapping flaps, which provide robust structural support and reduce the risk of uterine rupture during pregnancy [94].
3. *Transverse H Incision*
   The transverse H incision technique is particularly effective for diffuse adenomyosis of the anterior wall. A vertical midline incision is made, complemented by two transverse incisions at the upper and lower edges of the uterus. This allows wide exposure for precise excision of adenomyotic tissue while preserving healthy myometrium. The uterus is then reconstructed in multiple layers [95].

4. *Wedge Resection*
   Wedge resection targets localized adenomyosis by excising a cone-shaped section of the uterine wall, including both the serosal and adenomyotic layers. Layered suturing is performed to restore uterine integrity and functionality [93].
5. *Asymmetric Dissection*
   Asymmetric dissection involves diagonally hollowing out the uterus to remove deep adenomyotic tissue while preserving the uterine arteries and cavity. Reconstruction focuses on restoring the uterine wall with attention to its structural stability [96].
6. *PUSH (Protection of Uterine Structure for Healing)*
   The PUSH technique emphasizes optimal uterine reconstruction after excision. Submucosal and subserosal muscle flaps are overlapped and secured with vertical mattress sutures, ensuring robust healing and uterine integrity [97].

Outcomes from excisional techniques are promising, with pregnancy rates reaching 60-65% in women under 40 years of age. However, these procedures are complex and carry risks such as uterine rupture during pregnancy, necessitating cesarean delivery, as well as intrauterine adhesions [88].

4.6.2.4. Non-Excisional Techniques
Non-excisional approaches reduce symptoms by ablating or altering adenomyotic tissue without removing it. These minimally invasive methods are particularly useful for patients with smaller or localized lesions.

- *High-Intensity Focused Ultrasound (HIFU)*
  HIFU uses focused ultrasound energy to thermally ablate adenomyotic tissue under MRI or ultrasound guidance. It achieves significant symptom control, with over 80% of patients experiencing improvement in pain and bleeding [98]. In addition to improving symptoms, HIFU reduces uterine volume by an average of 33.6%, making it particularly effective for focal adenomyosis or lesions with reduced vascularity [99]. However, HIFU's efficacy decreases in cases of diffuse adenomyosis or highly vascularized lesions, where the non-perfused volume ratio (NPVr) is reduced [100]. Patients with isointense or hypointense lesions on T2-weighted MRI tend to show better outcomes, as these lesions absorb thermal energy more effectively than hyperintense, vascular lesions [100]. HIFU is non-

invasive and preserves ovarian function, as demonstrated by stable anti-Müllerian hormone (AMH) levels post-procedure [101]. Nevertheless, procedural times can be lengthy (92–115 minutes), and while complications are rare, they can include superficial burns, vaginal discharge, and, in rare cases, bowel injury [99, 101].

- *Uterine Artery Embolization (UAE)*
  UAE involves the injection of synthetic particles into the uterine arteries to induce ischemia and necrosis of adenomyotic tissue. This approach achieves symptom improvement in 74-90% of patients, with uterine volume reductions up to 51% [102]. UAE is particularly effective in patients with hypervascular lesions, as its mechanism relies on reducing blood flow to the affected tissue [103]. However, recurrence rates are higher than excisional methods, ranging from 10-29%, and UAE is less effective for diffuse adenomyosis [102]. Complications include post-procedural pain, premature ovarian failure, amenorrhea, and rare occurrences of intrauterine adhesions or pseudoaneurysms [103].
- *Radiofrequency Ablation (RFA)*
  RFA applies high-frequency electrical currents to coagulate adenomyotic tissue. It effectively reduces menstrual bleeding, dysmenorrhea, and uterine size [99]. Symptom control rates are reported between 59% and 89%, with long-term studies showing uterine volume reductions of 33–64 [99, 104, 105] RFA is associated with high patient satisfaction, with up to 78% of patients recommending the procedure to others [104, 105] Additionally, RFA has a low complication profile and shorter recovery times compared to hysterectomy [99, 104]. However, reintervention rates range from 18.5–39.5%, with hysterectomy being the most common subsequent procedure in some cases [104, 105].
- *Percutaneous Microwave Ablation (PMWA)*
  PMWA delivers microwave energy through a percutaneous needle to create large ablation zones. It achieves symptom control rates exceeding 85%, with shorter procedural times. [98, 99]. Studies demonstrate sustained improvements in dysmenorrhea, menorrhagia, and uterine volume over 12 months, with reductions in uterine size ranging from 33% to 46% [105]. PMWA has a minimal impact on ovarian function, making it an attractive option for younger patients seeking fertility preservation. Minor complications, including abdominal pain and vaginal discharge, are common but self-limiting,

typically resolving within 6–8 weeks [105, 106]. While long-term data is limited, preliminary studies suggest durable symptom control and low recurrence rates [105, 107].

4.6.2.5. Hysteroscopic Treatment and Endometrial Ablation

Hysteroscopic treatment and endometrial ablation are minimally invasive options for managing superficial adenomyosis or small lesions near the endometrium [108]. These techniques are particularly useful in cases where the disease is localized and accessible, offering an alternative for patients who wish to avoid more invasive surgeries [57, 109]. Hysteroscopy effectively treats focal adenomyosis by evacuating hemorrhagic cystic lesions or enucleating adenomyomas smaller than 1.5 cm in diameter [59, 110]. The procedure uses mechanical instruments, 5-Fr bipolar electrodes, or resectoscopes to precisely remove diseased tissue while preserving the surrounding healthy myometrium [111]. The success of hysteroscopic treatment depends heavily on accurate preoperative imaging, typically with transvaginal ultrasound or MRI, to determine lesion size, location, and depth [59, 110, 112].

Endometrial ablation and resection are also commonly employed to manage abnormal uterine bleeding, including cases associated with adenomyosis [113]. Techniques vary widely, ranging from first-generation methods using lasers and rollerballs to third-generation approaches such as thermal balloons and radiofrequency devices [114–116] These techniques aim to destroy the endometrium and superficial myometrium, reducing symptoms like heavy bleeding and pain. However, traditional endometrial ablation has limitations in treating adenomyosis, particularly in cases involving diffuse or deeply infiltrating disease. Clinical failure rates remain high, and hysterectomy may still be required in a significant proportion of cases [117].

For superficial diffuse adenomyosis, endomyometrial ablation (or endomyometrectomy) offers a more targeted approach. This technique involves removing the endometrium along with superficial layers of the myometrium until healthy tissue is exposed. Coagulation of residual endometrial tissue is then performed to minimize recurrence. Specialized tools, such as 3-mm or 5-mm straight loops and classic cutting loops, are used to target specific areas, including the uterine fundus, cornual recesses, and lateral walls [59]. The procedure's success depends on the extent of intramyometrial infiltration, with extensive disease posing greater challenges. Complications such as uterine perforation, intraoperative hemorrhage, fluid intravasation, and incomplete removal of adenomyotic tissue are more likely in advanced cases. In some instances, persistent or recurrent disease may necessitate a second surgical procedure. Preoperative imaging is critical for evaluating the thickness of the myometrium between the adenomyosis and the uterine serosa to guide surgical planning and minimize complications [118, 119].

Despite its potential benefits, endomyometrectomy carries certain risks, including the dissemination and proliferation of ectopic endometrial cells, which could worsen the condition or promote new adenomyosis development [59, 113].

4.6.2.6. Combination Therapies

Combining conservative surgery or non-excisional methods with hormonal treatments, such as GnRH analogs or levonorgestrel-releasing IUDs, improves long-term outcomes [120]. These therapies reduce recurrence rates and enhance symptom control, particularly when paired with techniques like adenomyomectomy, HIFU, or RFA [120].

Surgical treatment of adenomyosis encompasses a wide array of options tailored to disease severity and patient needs. While hysterectomy provides definitive symptom relief, fertility-preserving approaches, minimally invasive techniques, and hysteroscopic treatments offer alternatives for managing symptoms and preserving uterine function. Advances in surgical methods continue to improve outcomes, offering hope to patients with this challenging condition.

Conclusion

Adenomyosis is a challenging gynecological condition due to its complex nature and varied presentations. While diagnostic tools like transvaginal ultrasound and MRI have improved early detection, the clinical diversity complicates management. Advances in understanding its pathogenesis, including hormonal and inflammatory factors, have informed new therapeutic strategies.

Management must be tailored to symptoms, disease severity, and reproductive goals. Options range from symptom control and fertility-preserving treatments to hysterectomy in severe cases. Despite progress, optimal care remains debated and requires individualized assessment.

Further research is vital to standardize diagnostic criteria and refine treatments, ultimately improving patient outcomes and addressing the impact of this underdiagnosed condition.

References

[1] Vercellini P, Viganò P, Somigliana E, Daguati R, Abbiati A, Fedele L. Adenomyosis: epidemiological factors. *Best Pr Res Clin Obs Gynaecol.* 2006;20(4):465–77.

[2] Naftalin J, Hoo W, Pateman K, Mavrelos D, Holland T, Jurkovic D. How common is adenomyosis? A prospective study of prevalence using transvaginal ultrasound in a gynaecology clinic. *Hum Reprod.* 2012;27(12):3432–9.

[3] Hamouda S Ben, Ouerdiane N, Zina H Ben, Abdelwaheb, Masmoudi Ines Ennine Bouguerra B, Sfar R. [Adenomyosis at hysterectomy]. *Tunis Med.* 2007;85(7):559–62.

[4] Parazzini F, Mais V, Cipriani S, Busacca M, Venturini P, G.I.S.E. Determinants of adenomyosis in women who underwent hysterectomy for benign gynecological conditions: results from a prospective multicentric study in Italy. *Eur J Obs Gynecol Reprod Biol.* 2009;143(2):103–6.

[5] Vannuccini S, Petraglia F. Recent advances in understanding and managing adenomyosis. *F1000Research.* 2019;8:F1000 Faculty Rev-283.

[6] Cai T, Mazzoli S, Migno S, Malossini G, Lanzafame P, Mereu L, Tateo S, Wagenlehner FM, Pickard RS, Bartoletti R. Development and validation of a nomogram predicting recurrence risk in women with symptomatic urinary tract infection. *Int J Urol.* 2014;21(9):929–34.

[7] Benagiano G, Brosens I. History of adenomyosis. *Best Pr Res Clin Obs Gynaecol.* 2006;20(4):1–8.

[8] Bergeron C, Amant F, Ferenczy A. Pathology and physiopathology of adenomyosis. *Best Pract Res Clin Obstet Gynaecol.* 2006;20(4):511–21.

[9] Leyendecker G, Wildt L, Mall G. The pathophysiology of endometriosis and adenomyosis: tissue injury and repair. *Arch Gynecol Obs.* 2009;280(4):529–38.

[10] Leyendecker G, Bilgicyildirim A, Inacker M, Stalf T, Huppert P, Mall G, Böttcher B, Wildt L. Adenomyosis and endometriosis. Re-visiting their association and further insights into the mechanisms of auto-traumatisation. *An MRI study. Arch Gynecol Obstet.* 2015;291(4):917–32.

[11] Leyendecker G, Wildt L, Leyendecker G. A new concept of endometriosis and adenomyosis: Tissue injury and repair (TIAR). *Horm Mol Biol Clin Investig.* 2011;5(2):125–42.

[12] Gargett CE. Uterine stem cells: What is the evidence? *Hum Reprod Update.* 2007;13(1):87–101.

[13] Guo SW. The Pathogenesis of Adenomyosis vis-à-vis Endometriosis. *J Clin Med.* 2020;9(2).

[14] Van den Bosch T, de Bruijn AM, de Leeuw RA, Dueholm M, Exacoustos C, Valentin L, Bourne T, Timmerman D, Huirne JAF. Sonographic classification and reporting system for diagnosing adenomyosis. *Ultrasound Obstet Gynecol.* 2019;53(5):576–82.

[15] Kishi Y, Suginami H, Kuramori R, Yabuta M, Suginami R, Taniguchi F. Four subtypes of adenomyosis assessed by magnetic resonance imaging and their specification. *Am J Obstet Gynecol.* 2012;207(2):114.e1-114.e7.

[16] Liu Z, Guo Y, Pan X, Liu G, Yang X. Histopathological characteristics of adenomyosis: structure and microstructure. *Histol Histopathol.* 2023;38(10):1099–107.

[17] Goldblum JR, Clement PB, Hart WR. Adenomyosis with sparse glands: A potential mimic of low-grade endometrial stromal sarcoma. *Am J Clin Pathol.* 1995;103(2):218–23.

[18] Goteri G, Lucarini G, Montik N, Zizzi A, Stramazzotti D, Fabris G, Tranquilli AL, Ciavattini A. Expression of vascular endothelial growth factor (VEGF), hypoxia inducible factor-1alpha (HIF-1alpha), and microvessel density in endometrial tissue in women with adenomyosis. *Int J Gynecol Pathol.* 2009;28(2):157–163.

[19] Benagiano G, Brosens I, Habiba M. Adenomyosis: a life-cycle approach. *Reprod Biomed Online.* 2015;30:220–232.

[20] Bergeron C, Amant F, Ferenczy A. Pathology and physiopathology of adenomyosis. *Best Pr Res Clin Obs Gynaecol.* 20(4):511–21.

[21] Ali DES, Shah M, Ali A, Malik MO, Rehman F, Badshah H, Ehtesham E, Vitale SG. Treatment with Metformin and Combination of Metformin plus Pioglitazone on Serum Levels of IL-6 and IL-8 in Polycystic Ovary Syndrome: A Randomized Clinical Trial. *Horm Metab Res.* 2019;51(11):714–22.

[22] Vannuccini S, Tosti C, Carmona F, Huang SJ, Chapron C, S-W G. Pathogenesis of adenomyosis: an update on molecular mechanisms. *Reprod Biomed Online.* 2017;35:592–601.

[23] Gracia M, Carmona F. Uterine Fibroids and Adenomyosis. In: *Endocrinology* (Switzerland). Springer, Cham; 2020. p. 173–92.

[24] Parker JD, Leondires M, Sinaii N, Premkumar A, Nieman LK, Stratton P. Persistence of dysmenorrhea and nonmenstrual pain after optimal endometriosis surgery may indicate adenomyosis. *Fertil Steril.* 2006;86:711–715.

[25] Sammour A, Pirwany I, Usubutun A. Correlations between extent and spread of adenomyosis and clinical symptoms. *Gynecol Obs Invest.* 2002;54(4):213e216.

[26] Krajec M, Lebar V, Cerar LK, Lukanovic D, Meglic L. Spontaneous Haemoperitoneum in the Third Trimester of Pregnancy Due to Adenomyosis: A Case Report. *Cureus.* 2024;16(7):e63718.

[27] Phillips L, Brown H, Williams A. Uterine rupture of an unscarred gravid uterus at term attributed to adenomyosis. *BMJ Case Rep.* 2023;16(12):e257145.

[28] Tower AM, Frishman GN. Cesarean scar defects: an underrecognized cause of abnormal uterine bleeding and other gynecologic complications. *J Minim Invasive Gynecol.* 2013;20(5):562–72.

[29] Kim NI, Lee JS, Nam JH. Uterine rupture due to adenomyosis in an adolescent: A case report and review of literature. *World J Clin Cases.* 2023;11(32):7888.

[30] Liu Y, Hu X, Lv W, Xu Y. A case report of adenomyosis-induced spontaneous rupture in an unscarred and unpregnant uterus. *Medicine* (Baltimore). 2024;103(51):e41037.
[31] Upson K, Missmer SA. Epidemiology of Adenomyosis. *Semin Reprod Med.* 2020;38(2–3):089–107.
[32] Guo SW. Cracking the enigma of adenomyosis: an update on its pathogenesis and pathophysiology. *Reproduction.* 2022;164(5):R101–21.
[33] Sunkara SK, Khan KS. Adenomyosis and female fertility: A critical review of the evidence. *J Obstet Gynaecol* (Lahore). 2012;32(2):113–6.
[34] Sharma S, Bathwal S, Agarwal N, Chattopadhyay R, Saha I, Chakravarty B. Does presence of adenomyosis affect reproductive outcome in IVF cycles? A retrospective analysis of 973 patients. *Reprod Biomed Online*. 2019;38(1):13–21.
[35] Török P, Molnár S, Herman T, Jashanjeet S, Lampé R, Riemma G, Vitale SG. Fallopian tubal obstruction is associated with increased pain experienced during office hysteroscopy: a retrospective study. *Updates Surg.* 2020;72(1):213–8.
[36] Cao Y, Yang D, Cai S, Yang L, Yu S, Geng Q, Mo M, Li W, Wei Y, Li Y, Yin T, Diao L. Adenomyosis associated infertility: an update on immunological perspective. *Reprod Biomed Online.* 2024;0(0):104703.
[37] Fischer CP, Kayisili U, Taylor HS. HOXA10 expression is decreased in endometrium of women with adenomyosis. *Fertil Steril*. 2011;95(3):1133–6.
[38] Leyendecker G, Herbertz M, Kunz G, Mall G. Endometriosis results from the dislocation of basal endometrium. *Hum Reprod.* 2002;17(10):2725–36.
[39] Bulletti C, Ziegler D De, Polli V, Del Ferro E, Palini S, Flamigni C. Characteristics of uterine contractility during menses in women with mild to moderate endometriosis. *Fertil Steril.* 2002;77(6):1156–61.
[40] Kunz G, Leyendecker G. Uterine peristaltic activity during the menstrual cycle: characterization, regulation, function and dysfunction. *Reprod Biomed Online.* 2002;4 Suppl 3:5–9.
[41] Furuhashi M, Miyabe Y, Katsumata Y. Comparison of complications of vaginal hysterectomy in patients with leiomyomas and in patients with adenomyosis. *Arch Gynecol Obs.* 1998;262:69–73.
[42] Pados G, Gordts S, Sorrentino F, Nisolle M, Nappi L, Daniilidis A. Adenomyosis and Infertility: A Literature Review [Internet]. Vol. 59, *Medicina* (Kaunas). Multidisciplinary Digital Publishing Institute (MDPI); 2023 [cited 2024 Aug 8]available from. p. 1551.
[43] Urman B, Yakin K, Ertas S, Alper E, Aksakal E, Riemma G, Angioni S, Vitale SG. Fertility and anatomical outcomes following hysteroscopic adhesiolysis: An 11-year retrospective cohort study to validate a new classification system for intrauterine adhesions (Urman-Vitale Classification System). *Int J Gynecol Obstet.* 2024;165(2):644–54.
[44] Vitale SG, Laganà AS, Török P, Lasmar RB, Carugno J, Palumbo M, Tesarik J. Virtual sonographic hysteroscopy in assisted reproduction: A retrospective cost-effectiveness analysis. *Int J Gynaecol Obstet*. 2022;156(1):112–8.
[45] Lan J, Wu Y, Wu Z, Wu Y, Yang R, Liu Y, Lin H, Jiao X, Zhang Q. Ultra-Long GnRH Agonist Protocol During IVF/ICSI Improves Pregnancy Outcomes in

Women With Adenomyosis: A Retrospective Cohort Study. *Front Endocrinol* (Lausanne). 2021;12:609771.

[46] Kamada Y, Nakatsuka M, Asagiri K, Noguchi S, Habara T, Takata M, Kudo T. GnRH agonist-suppressed expression of nitric oxide synthases and generation of peroxynitrite in adenomyosis. *Hum Reprod.* 2000;15(12):2512–9.

[47] Chiofalo B, Palmara V, Vilos GA, Pacheco LA, Lasmar RB, Shawki O, Giacobbe V, Alibrandi A, Di Guardo F, Vitale SG. Reproductive outcomes of infertile women undergoing “see and treat” office hysteroscopy: a retrospective observational study. *Minim Invasive Ther Allied Technol.* 2021;30(3):147–53.

[48] Szubert M, Koziróg E, Olszak O, Krygier-Kurz K, Kazmierczak J, Wilczynski J. Adenomyosis and infertility—review of medical and surgical approaches. *Int J Environ Res Public Health.* 2021;18(3):1–12.

[49] Tellum T, Nygaard S, Lieng M. Noninvasive Diagnosis of Adenomyosis: A Structured Review and Meta-analysis of Diagnostic Accuracy in Imaging. *J Minim Invasive Gynecol.* 2020;27:408–418.

[50] Harmsen MJ, Van den Bosch T, de Leeuw RA, Dueholm M, Exacoustos C, Valentin L, Hehenkamp WJK, Groenman F, De Bruyn C, Rasmussen C, Lazzeri L, Jokubkiene L, Jurkovic D, Naftalin J, Tellum T, Bourne T, Timmerman D, Huirne JAF. Consensus on revised definitions of Morphological Uterus Sonographic Assessment (MUSA) features of adenomyosis: results of modified Delphi procedure. *Ultrasound Obstet Gynecol.* 2022;60(1):118–31.

[51] Bazot M, Bharwani N, Huchon C, Kinkel K, Cunha TM, Guerra A, Manganaro L, Buñesch L, Kido A, Togashi K. European Society of Urogenital Radiology (ESUR) Guidelines: MR Imaging of Pelvic Endometriosis. *Eur Radiol.* 2017;27(7):2765–2775.

[52] Guerriero S, Saba L, Pascual MA, Ajossa S, Rodriguez I, Mais V, Alcazar JL. Transvaginal ultrasound versus magnetic resonance imaging for diagnosing adenomyosis. A systematic review and head-to-head meta-analysis. *Ultrasound Obs Gynecol.* 2018;51(5):586–95.

[53] Champaneria R, Abedin P, Daniels J, Balogun M, Khan KS. Ultrasound scan and magnetic resonance imaging for the diagnosis of adenomyosis: systematic review comparing test accuracy. *Acta Obs Gynecol Scand.* 2010;89:1374–84.

[54] Celli V, Dolciami M, Ninkova R, Ercolani G, Rizzo S, Porpora MG, Catalano C, Manganaro L. MRI and Adenomyosis: What Can Radiologists Evaluate? *Int J Environ Res Public Heal* 2022, Vol 19, Page 5840. 2022;19(10):5840.

[55] Vitale SG, Angioni S, Saponara S, Sicilia G, Mignacca A, Caiazzo A, De Franciscis P, Riemma G. Hysteroscopic metroplasty and its reproductive impact among the social networks: A cross-sectional analysis on video quality, reliability and creators' opinions on YouTube, TikTok and Instagram. *Int J Med Inform.* 2025;195:105776.

[56] Vitale SG, Di Spiezio Sardo A, Riemma G, De Franciscis P, Alonso Pacheco L, Carugno J. In-office hysteroscopic removal of retained or fragmented intrauterine device without anesthesia: a cross-sectional analysis of an international survey. *Updates Surg.* 2022;74(3):1079–85.

[57] Saponara S, Angioni S, Parry JP, Pacheco LA, Carugno J, Moawad N, Haimovich S, Lasmar RB, Dealberti D, Aksakal E, Urman B, Nappi L, Vitale SG. The Pivotal role of hysteroscopy in diagnosing subtle uterine lesions in infertile patients: Seeing the unseen can make the difference. *Eur J Obstet Gynecol Reprod Biol.* 2025;305:132–41.

[58] Vitale SG, Angioni S, Saponara S, Sicilia G, Etrusco A, D'Alterio MN, Cobellis L, De Franciscis P, Riemma G. TikTok as a platform for hysteroscopy information: An analytical video-based cross-sectional study to assess quality, reliability, and accuracy. *Int J Gynecol Obstet.* 2025;168(1):353–61.

[59] Di Spiezio Sardo A, Calagna G, Santangelo F, Zizolfi B, Tanos V, Perino A, De Wilde RL. The Role of Hysteroscopy in the Diagnosis and Treatment of Adenomyosis. *Biomed Res Int.* 2017;2017:2518396.

[60] Vitale SG, Laganà AS, Caruso S, Garzon S, Vecchio GM, La Rosa VL, Casarin J, Ghezzi F. Comparison of three biopsy forceps for hysteroscopic endometrial biopsy in postmenopausal patients (HYGREB-1): A multicenter, single-blind randomized clinical trial. *Int J Gynecol Obstet.* 2021;155(3):425–32.

[61] Vitale SG. The Biopsy Snake Grasper Sec. VITALE: A New Tool for Office Hysteroscopy. *J Minim Invasive Gynecol*. 2020;27(6):1414–6.

[62] Gordts S, Campo R, Brosens I. Hysteroscopic diagnosis and excision of myometrial cystic adenomyosis. *Gynecol Surg.* 2014;11(4):273.

[63] Vitale SG, Angioni S, D'Alterio MN, Ronsini C, Saponara S, De Franciscis P, Riemma G. Risk of endometrial malignancy in women treated for breast cancer: the BLUSH prediction model–evidence from a comprehensive multicentric retrospective cohort study. *Climacteric.* 2024;27(5):482–8.

[64] Vitale SG, Caruso S, Rapisarda AMC, Valenti G, Rossetti D, Cianci S, Cianci A. Biocompatible porcine dermis graft to treat severe cystocele: impact on quality of life and sexuality. *Arch Gynecol Obstet.* 2016;293(1):125–31.

[65] Shi Y, Zhu Y, Fan S, Vitagliano A, Liu X, Liao Y, Liang Y, Vitale SG. Clinical Characteristics and Antifungal Susceptibility of Candida nivariensis from Vulvovaginal Candidiasis. *Gynecol Obstet Invest.* 2020;85(1):88–93.

[66] Oladosu FA, Tu FF, Hellman KM. Nonsteroidal antiinflammatory drug resistance in dysmenorrhea: epidemiology, causes, and treatment. *Am J Obstet Gynecol.* 2018;218(4):390–400.

[67] Marjoribanks J, Ayeleke RO, Farquhar C, Proctor M. Nonsteroidal anti-inflammatory drugs for dysmenorrhoea. *Cochrane Database Syst Rev.* 2015;2015(7):CD001751.

[68] Szegeczki V, Fazekas L, Kulcsár M, Reglodi D, Török P, Orlik B, Laganà AS, Jakab A, Juhasz T. Endometrium as Control of Endometriosis in Experimental Research: Assessment of Sample Suitability. *Diagnostics.* 2022;12(4).

[69] Mehasseb MK, Panchal R, Taylor AH, Brown L, Bell SC, Habiba M. Estrogen and progesterone receptor isoform distribution through the menstrual cycle in uteri with and without adenomyosis. *Fertil Steril.* 2011;95(7):2228–35.

[70] Sasagawa S, Shimizu Y, Kami H, Takeuchi T, Mita S, Imada K. Dienogest is a selective progesterone receptor agonist in transactivation analysis with potent oral

endometrial activity due to its efficient pharmacokinetic profile. *Steroids.* 2008;73:222–31.

[71] Kobayashi H. Efficacy, Adverse Events, and Challenges of Dienogest in the Management of Symptomatic Adenomyosis: A Comparison with Different Hormonal Treatments. *Gynecol Obstet Invest.* 2023;88(2):71–80.

[72] Ikomi A, Pepra EF. Efficacy of the levonorgestrel intrauterine system in treating menorrhagia: Actualities and ambiguities. *BMJ Sex Reprod Heal.* 2002;28(2):99–100.

[73] Magalhaes J, Ferreira-Filho ES, Soares-Junior JM, Baracat EC. Uterine volume, menstrual patterns, and contraceptive outcomes in users of the levonorgestrel-releasing intrauterine system: A cohort study with a five-year follow-up. *Eur J Obstet Gynecol Reprod Biol.* 2022;276:56–62.

[74] Vannuccini S, Luisi S, Tosti C, Sorbi F, Petraglia F. Role of medical therapy in the management of uterine adenomyosis. *Fertil Steril.* 2018;109(3):398–405.

[75] Streuli I, Dubuisson J, Santulli P, Ziegler D, Batteux F, Chapron C. An update on the pharmacological management of adenomyosis. *Expert Opin Pharmacother.* 2014;15(16):2347–60.

[76] Akira S, Mine K, Kuwabara Y, Takeshita T. Efficacy of long-term, low-dose gonadotropin-releasing hormone agonist therapy (draw-back therapy) for adenomyosis. *Med Sci Monit.* 2009;15(1):CR1-4.

[77] Donnez O, Donnez J. Gonadotropin-releasing hormone antagonist (linzagolix): a new therapy for uterine adenomyosis. *Fertil Steril.* 2020;114(3):640–5.

[78] Kim ES, Nie T. Consider fertility-preserving medications when treating adenomyosis. *Drugs Ther Perspect.* 2024;40(9):357–62.

[79] Farquhar C, Brosens I. Medical and surgical management of adenomyosis. *Best Pract Res Clin Obstet Gynaecol.* 2006;20(4):603–16.

[80] Mereu L, Florio P, Carri G, Pontis A, Petraglia F, Mencaglia L. Clinical outcomes associated with surgical treatment of endometrioma coupled with resection of the posterior broad ligament. *Int J Gynaecol Obstet.* 2012;116(1):57–60.

[81] Vitale SG, Laganà AS, Noventa M, Giampaolino P, Zizolfi B, Butticè S, La Rosa VL, Gullo G, Rossetti D. Transvaginal Bilateral Sacrospinous Fixation after Second Recurrence of Vaginal Vault Prolapse: Efficacy and Impact on Quality of Life and Sexuality. *Biomed Res Int.* 2018;2018:5727165.

[82] Prisco MG, Zannoni GF, De Stefano I, Vellone VG, Tortorella L, Fagotti A, Mereu L, Scambia G, Gallo D. Prognostic role of metastasis tumor antigen 1 in patients with ovarian cancer: a clinical study. *Hum Pathol.* 2012;43(2):282–8.

[83] Pignata S, Ferrandina G, Scarfone G, Scollo P, Odicino F, Cormio G, Katsaros D, Frigerio L, Mereu L, Ghezzi F, Manzione L, Lauria R, Breda E, Alletti DG, Ballardini M, Vernaglia A, Sorio R, Tumolo S, Musso P, Magni G, Pisano C, Morabito A. Poor outcome of elderly patients with platinum-sensitive recurrent ovarian cancer: results from the SOCRATES retrospective study. *Crit Rev Oncol Hematol.* 2009;71(3):233–41.

[84] Landi S, Mereu L, Pontrelli G, Stepniewska A, Romano L, Tateo S, Dorizzi C, Minelli L. The influence of adenomyosis in patients laparoscopically treated for deep endometriosis. *J Minim Invasive Gynecol.* 2008;15(5):566–70.

[85] Restaino S, Mereu L, Finelli A, Spina MR, Marini G, Catena U, Turco LC, Moroni R, Milani M, Cela V, Scambia G, Fanfani F. Robotic surgery vs laparoscopic surgery in patients with diagnosis of endometriosis: a systematic review and meta-analysis. *J Robot Surg.* 2020;14(5):687–94.

[86] Minelli L, Fanfam F, Fagotti A, Ruffo G, Ceccaroni M, Mereu L, Landi S, Pomini P, Scambia G. Laparoscopic colorectal resection for bowel endometriosis: feasibility, complications, and clinical outcome. *Arch Surg.* 2009;144(3):234–9.

[87] Mereu L, Ruffo G, Landi S, Barbieri F, Zaccoletti R, Fiaccavento A, Stepniewska A, Pontrelli G, Minelli L. Laparoscopic treatment of deep endometriosis with segmental colorectal resection: short-term morbidity. *J Minim Invasive Gynecol.* 2007;14(4):463–9.

[88] Oliveira MAP, Crispi CP, Brollo LC, De Wilde RL. Surgery in adenomyosis. *Arch Gynecol Obstet.* 2018;297(3):581–9.

[89] Angioni S, Pontis A, Pisanu A, Mereu L, Roman H. Single-port access subtotal laparoscopic hysterectomy: A prospective case-control study. *J Minim Invasive Gynecol.* 2015;22(5):807–12.

[90] Mereu L, Gagliardi ML, Clarizia R, Mainardi P, Landi S, Minelli L. Laparoscopic management of ureteral endometriosis in case of moderate-severe hydroureteronephrosis. *Fertil Steril.* 2010;93(1):46–51.

[91] Landi S, Pontrelli G, Surico D, Ruffo G, Benini M, Soriano D, Mereu L, Minelli L. Laparoscopic disk resection for bowel endometriosis using a circular stapler and a new endoscopic method to control postoperative bleeding from the stapler line. *J Am Coll Surg.* 2008;207(2):205–9.

[92] Stepniewska A, Pomini P, Scioscia M, Mereu L, Ruffo G, Minelli L. Fertility and clinical outcome after bowel resection in infertile women with endometriosis. *Reprod Biomed Online.* 2010;20(5):602–9.

[93] Sun A jun, Luo M, Wang W, Chen R, Lang J he. Characteristics and efficacy of modified adenomyomectomy in the treatment of uterine adenomyoma. *Chin Med J (Engl).* 2011;124(9):1322–6.

[94] Osada H, Silber S, Kakinuma T, Nagaishi M, Kato K, Kato O. Surgical procedure to conserve the uterus for future pregnancy in patients suffering from massive adenomyosis. *Reprod Biomed Online.* 2011;22(1):94–9.

[95] Fujishita A, Masuzaki H, Khan KN, Kitajima M, Ishimaru T. Modified reduction surgery for adenomyosis. A preliminary report of the transverse H incision technique. *Gynecol Obstet Invest.* 2004;57(3):132–8.

[96] Nishida M, Takano K, Arai Y, Ozone H, Ichikawa R. Conservative surgical management for diffuse uterine adenomyosis. *Fertil Steril.* 2010;94(2):715–9.

[97] Wu R, Zeng L, Hu Q, Qu X, He F, Bao J, Wei W, Zhang W, Dai W, Li H, Du H, Li C. Outcome of uterine functional structures protection by fertility preservative PUSH surgery in diffuse adenomyosis. *Hum Fertil.* 2023;26(4):720–32.

[98] Athanasiou A, Fruscalzo A, Dedes I, Mueller MD, Londero AP, Marti C, Guani B, Feki A. Advances in Adenomyosis Treatment: High-Intensity Focused Ultrasound, Percutaneous Microwave Therapy, and Radiofrequency Ablation. *J Clin Med* 2024, Vol 13, Page 5828. 2024;13(19):5828.

[99] Liu L, Wang T, Lei B. Image-guided thermal ablation in the management of symptomatic adenomyosis: a systematic review and meta-analysis. *Int J Hyperthermia.* 2021;38(1):948–62.

[100] Yu J, Jiang L, Su X, Yang M, Yang C, Chen J. Comparison efficacy of ultrasound-guided HIFU for adenomyosis-associated dysmenorrhea with different signal intensity on T2-weighted MR imaging. *J Obstet Gynaecol Res.* 2023;49(4):1189–97.

[101] Marques ALS, Andres MP, Kho RM, Abrão MS. Is High-intensity Focused Ultrasound Effective for the Treatment of Adenomyosis? A Systematic Review and Meta-analysis. *J Minim Invasive Gynecol.* 2020;27(2):332–43.

[102] Popovic M, Puchner S, Berzaczy D, Lammer J, Bucek RA. Uterine artery embolization for the treatment of adenomyosis: A review. *J Vasc Interv Radiol.* 2011;22(7):901–9.

[103] Kröncke T. An update on uterine artery embolization for uterine leiomyomata and adenomyosis of the uterus. *Br J Radiol.* 2023;96(1143):20220121.

[104] Dedes I, Kolovos G, Fruscalzo A, Toub D, Vaineau C, Lanz S, Imboden S, Feki A, Mueller MD. Radiofrequency Ablation for Adenomyosis. *J Clin Med.* 2023;12(9):3069.

[105] Stepniewska AK, Baggio S, Clarizia R, Bruni F, Roviglione G, Ceccarello M, Manzone M, Guerriero M, Ceccaroni M. Heat can treat: long-term follow-up results after uterine-sparing treatment of adenomyosis with radiofrequency thermal ablation in 60 hysterectomy candidate patients. *Surg Endosc.* 2022;36(8):5803–11.

[106] Yang Y, Zhang J, Han Z yu, Ma X, Hao Y li, Xu C tao, Xu R fang, Zhang B song. Ultrasound-guided percutaneous microwave ablation for adenomyosis: efficacy of treatment and effect on ovarian function. *Sci Rep.* 2015;5:10034.

[107] Lin XL, Hai N, Zhang J, Han ZY, Yu J, Liu FY, Dong XJ, Liang P. Comparison between microwave ablation and radiofrequency ablation for treating symptomatic uterine adenomyosis. *Int J Hyperth.* 2020;37(1):151–6.

[108] Florio P, Nappi L, Mannini L, Pontrelli G, Fimiani R, Casadio P, Mazzon I, Gonzales G, Villani V, Franchini M, Gubbini G, Mereu L, Santangelo F, Sardo ADS. Prevalence of Infections After In-Office Hysteroscopy in Premenopausal and Postmenopausal Women. *J Minim Invasive Gynecol.* 2019;26(4):733–9.

[109] Florio P, Puzzutiello R, Filippeschi M, D'Onofrio P, Mereu L, Morelli R, Marianello D, Litta P, Mencaglia L, Petraglia F. Low-dose spinal anesthesia with hyperbaric bupivacaine with intrathecal fentanyl for operative hysteroscopy: a case series study. *J Minim Invasive Gynecol.* 2012;19(1):107–12.

[110] Molinas CR, Campo R. Office hysteroscopy and adenomyosis. *Best Pract Res Clin Obstet Gynaecol.* 2006;20(4):557–67.

[111] Vitale SG, Riemma G, Carugno J, Perez-Medina T, Alonso Pacheco L, Haimovich S, Parry JP, Di Spiezio Sardo A, De Franciscis P. Postsurgical barrier strategies to avoid the recurrence of intrauterine adhesion formation after hysteroscopic adhesiolysis: a network meta-analysis of randomized controlled trials. *Am J Obstet Gynecol.* 2022;226(4):487-498.e8.

[112] Vitale SG, Parry JP, Carugno J, Cholkeri-Singh A, Della Corte L, Cianci S, Schiattarella A, Riemma G, De Franciscis P. Surgical and Reproductive Outcomes

after Hysteroscopic Removal of Retained Products of Conception: A Systematic Review and Meta-analysis. *J Minim Invasive Gynecol.* 2021;28(2):204–17.

[113] McCausland V, McCausland A. The response of adenomyosis to endometrial ablation/resection. *Hum Reprod Update.* 1998;4(4):350–9.

[114] Vitale SG, Saponara S, Succu AG, Sicilia G, Martsidis K, D'Alterio MN, Angioni S. Efficacy and Safety of Non-Ablative Dual Wavelength Diode Laser Therapy for Genitourinary Syndrome of Menopause: A Single-Center Prospective Study. *Adv Ther.* 2024;41(12):4617–27.

[115] Vitale SG, Saponara S, Sicilia G, Klarić M, Sorrentino F, D'Alterio MN, Nappi L, Angioni S. Hysteroscopic diode laser myolysis: from a case series to literature review of incisionless myolysis techniques for managing heavy menstrual bleeding in premenopausal women. *Arch Gynecol Obstet.* 2024;309(3):949–59.

[116] Vitale SG, Moore O, Riemma G, Carugno J, Yarto ML, Haimovich S. Hysteroscopic laser ablation of symptomatic uterine fibroids: insights from a prospective study. *Climacteric.* 2023;26(5):497–502.

[117] Dueholm M. Minimally invasive treatment of adenomyosis. *Best Pract Res Clin Obstet Gynaecol.* 2018;51:119–37.

[118] Vitale SG, De Angelis MC, Della Corte L, Saponara S, Carugno J, Laganà AS, Török P, Tinelli R, Pérez-Medina T, Ertas S, Urman B, Angioni S. Uterine cervical stenosis: from classification to advances in management. Overcoming the obstacles to access the uterine cavity. *Arch Gynecol Obstet.* 2024;309(3):755–64.

[119] Vitale SG, Riemma G, Haimovich S, Carugno J, Alonso Pacheco L, Perez-Medina T, Parry JP, Török P, Tesarik J, Della Corte L, Cobellis L, Di Spiezio Sardo A, De Franciscis P. Risk of endometrial cancer in asymptomatic postmenopausal women in relation to ultrasonographic endometrial thickness: systematic review and diagnostic test accuracy meta-analysis. *Am J Obstet Gynecol.* 2023;228(1):22-35.e2.

[120] Chu Z, Jia L, Dai J, Wu Q, Tian F, Bai S. Effects of different treatment methods on clinical efficacy and fertility outcomes of patients with adenomyosis. *J Ovarian Res.* 2024;17(1):16.

Chapter 5

Chronic Endometritis

Laura Calles Sastre[1], MD
María Luna Arana[1], MD
Liliana Mereu[2], MD, PhD
Salvatore Giovanni Vitale[2], MD, PhD
and Tirso Pérez Medina[1,*], MD
[1]Puerta de Hierro University Hospital, Autónoma University of Madrid, Madrid, Spain
[2]Obstetrics and Gynecology Unit, "*Gaspare Rodolico*" University Hospital,
Department of General Surgery and Medical Surgical Specialties,
University of Catania, Catania, Italy

Abstract

Chronic endometritis (CE) is a localized, often asymptomatic inflammation of the endometrial mucosa, characterized by plasma cell infiltration, stromal edema, and dissociated maturation between epithelial and stromal cells. Its prevalence is highly variable, from 2.8% in the general population to 60-66% in women with recurrent pregnancy loss or repeated implantation failure (RIF). Infectious agents, such as *Streptococcus* species, *E. coli*, and *Ureaplasma*, are common causes, though non-infectious factors like retained products of conception and autoimmune responses also contribute.

CE significantly impacts fertility by altering uterine contractility, disrupting endometrial receptivity, and impairing embryo implantation, thereby contributing to unexplained infertility, RIF, and recurrent miscarriages. Histological examination with CD138 immunohistochemistry remains the diagnostic gold standard,

[*] Corresponding Author's Email: tirso.perez@uam.es

In: Endometrium and Related Endouterine Pathologies
Editors: Liliana Mereu and Salvatore Giovanni Vitale
ISBN: 979-8-89530-818-9

complemented by hysteroscopy and microbial cultures. Emerging molecular techniques, such as RT-PCR, provide promising diagnostic accuracy by identifying microbial DNA, though their clinical utility is still under investigation.
Treatment predominantly involves broad-spectrum antibiotics tailored to culture results, with regimens like doxycycline demonstrating high cure rates. Intrauterine therapies or endometrial curettage may be employed in resistant or persistent cases. Addressing CE improves reproductive outcomes, emphasizing the importance of accurate diagnosis and targeted therapy in affected women.
This review highlights the multifactorial etiology, diagnostic challenges, and therapeutic strategies for CE, underscoring its critical role in reproductive health.

Keywords: chronic endometritis, hysteroscopy, infertility

Introduction

Chronic endometritis (CE) is an often-overlooked condition within gynecological practice, primarily due to its subtle and nonspecific clinical presentation [1]. While traditionally considered a benign or secondary concern, accumulating evidence highlights its substantial role in reproductive health and its broader implications on uterine physiology [2].

Far from being a sterile cavity, the uterus is now understood to harbor a dynamic microbiome, where the interaction between microbial agents and the endometrial microenvironment can either maintain homeostasis or precipitate chronic inflammation [3]. Factors such as prior gynecological procedures, intrauterine devices, retained products of conception, or systemic conditions like immunosuppression further compound the risk of CE, underscoring its multifactorial origins [3].

Despite advancements in diagnostic modalities, including hysteroscopy, immunohistochemistry, and molecular biology techniques, chronic endometritis often remains underdiagnosed due to a lack of standardized criteria and awareness among clinicians [4]. Nevertheless, effective treatment strategies, particularly antibiotic regimens, have demonstrated the potential to restore uterine health and improve reproductive outcomes [5].

This chapter delves into the complexities of CE, exploring its pathophysiology, diagnostic challenges, and therapeutic innovations. It seeks to illuminate an area of gynecology that has long remained in the shadows, providing a foundation for improved clinical practice and research advancements.

5.1. Definition, Etiology and Risk Factors

5.1.1. Definition

Chronic endometritis (CE) is defined as localized inflammation of the endometrial mucosa characterized by the presence of edema, increased stromal cell density, dissociated maturation between epithelial cells and stroma fibroblasts, as well as the presence of plasma cell infiltrate in the stroma [1]. These changes at the level of the endometrial microenvironment could affect endometrial receptivity [6].

The CE estimated rate in the general population is hard to define due to the lack of a characteristic clinical manifestation.

In a prospective study published by Cicinelli et al. [7] in a total number of 2190 diagnostic hysteroscopy with different indications, they found a prevalence of 20% (438 patients) with CE, among whom 37% were also infertile. However, Kasius et al. [8] reported a prevalence of only 2.8% in 678 women. In comparison, in a selected group of women diagnosed with unexplained recurrent miscarriage or repeated implantation failure, it may be as high as 60% or 66%, respectively [5, 7, 8].

This wide range of reported CE prevalence results from the fact that its diagnosis depends on the detection method.

5.1.2. Etiology

Chronic endometritis results from infectious and non-infectious factors, leading to persistent endometrium inflammation. Below is a detailed overview of its etiology:

- Infectious causes

  The most frequent infectious agents are common bacteria frequently found in the urogenital area, such as Streptococcus (27%), E. coli (11%), Enterococcus faecalis (14%) and Ureaplasma urealyticum (11%) [7]. EC has classically been related to Chlamydia trachomatis and Neisseria gonorrhoeae but the presence of Chlamydia trachomatis is only 2.7%, and Neisseria gonorrhoeae is practically undetectable as causative in CE [9]. These findings are in line with the results of the PEACH study [10], showing that 60% of women with pelvic

inflammatory disease present non-gonococcal or Chlamydia infection.
In certain areas of the world, Mycobacterium tuberculosis is highly prevalent. It is considered the leading cause of infertility in 40-75% of cases since it causes implantation failure due to alteration of the immune response at the endometrial level, hormonal alterations, and release of antiphospholipid antibodies [11]. Today, it is well-accepted that the uterus is not a sterile cavity, and the presence of microorganisms does not equal inflammation [12]. The asymptomatic presence of bacteria in the endometrial cavity in either transcervical samples or cultures obtained in post-hysterectomy specimens has been reported by several investigators [13, 14]. More recently metagenomics, investigating hypervariable regions of the ribosomal 16S rRNA genes allow definition of genus order and species of bacteria, leading to confirm the presence of up to 12 different bacterial types in up to 95% of endometrial biopsies performed in patients undergoing hysterectomy for non-cancer indications [15]. As described by Espinoza et al. [16], accumulating evidences suggest that endometrium is continuously exposed to bacteria from the genital tract. Therefore, the presence of pathology is also determined by the interaction of the infectious agent with the endometrial microenvironment [17].

- Iatrogenic causes
    - Prolonged intrauterine devices can introduce pathogens into the uterine cavity, leading to chronic inflammation. Infections can be exacerbated by biofilms forming on the device's surface [18].
    - Procedures such as dilation and curettage, cesarean delivery, or uterine evacuation can introduce bacteria into the endometrial cavity, causing persistent low-grade infection [18].
- Non-Infectious causes
    - Foreign bodies or retained tissue: retained products of conception (placental fragments) or retained fetal tissue can result in persistent inflammation. Rarely, other foreign materials in the uterine cavity (e.g., sutures or remnants of prior instrumentation) may be implicated [18].
    - Endometrial pathology: Endometrial polyps, submucous myomas, or irregular growths may predispose the endometrium to chronic inflammation, possibly as a response to altered endometrial architecture or blood supply [19, 20].

- Autoimmune or Idiopathic factors: In some cases, CE may be related to an immune-mediated response, particularly in women with systemic autoimmune diseases [18].

5.1.3. Risk Factors

Taking into account these etiological factors, we can then define some risk factors that could predispose to chronic endometritis (Table 1):

Table 1. Chronic endometritis risk factors

Risk Factor	Description	Examples/Details
Sexual and Reproductive Behavior	Behaviors increasing exposure to infections.	Multiple sexual partners. Unprotected intercourse. History of STIs.
Use of Intrauterine Devices (IUDs)	IUDs can introduce pathogens and promote biofilm formation, leading to chronic infections.	Prolonged IUD use. Bacteria introduced during IUD insertion.
History of Obstetric or Gynecological Procedures	Medical procedures increasing the risk of bacterial introduction or retained tissue.	Dilation and curettage (D&C). Cesarean delivery. Hysteroscopy or endometrial biopsy.
Retained Products of Conception (RPOC)	Incomplete removal of tissue after delivery or abortion can lead to persistent inflammation and infection.	Postpartum placental fragments. Retained tissue after abortion (e.g., septic abortion).
Assisted Reproductive Technologies (ART)	Procedures that manipulate the uterus can introduce infections or exacerbate inflammation.	Embryo transfer. Repeated uterine interventions during ART cycles.
Immunosuppression	Reduced immune function increases vulnerability to infections, including chronic infections.	HIV/AIDS. Long-term use of corticosteroids or immunosuppressive medications.
Other Medical Conditions	Pre-existing conditions that predispose to chronic inflammation or infection of the endometrium.	Pelvic inflammatory disease (PID). Postmenopausal endometrial atrophy.
Socioeconomic and Geographic Factors	Limited healthcare access or geographic predisposition to specific infections increases CE risk.	Limited access to post-abortion or postpartum care. Genital tuberculosis in TB-endemic areas.

1) Sexual and reproductive behavior
   - Multiple Sexual Partners: Increases the risk of acquiring sexually transmitted infections (STIs) [21].
   - Unprotected Intercourse: Heightens exposure to pathogenic microorganisms that can ascend into the uterine cavity and cause chronic infections [22].
   - Previous History of STIs: Women with a history of pelvic infections are at greater risk due to potential lingering inflammation or untreated residual pathogens [21, 23].
2) Use of Intrauterine Devices (IUDs)
   - Prolonged Use: IUDs, especially if used for extended periods, can introduce bacteria into the endometrial cavity, leading to biofilm formation and persistent infections [24].
   - Insertion Procedure: the placement of an IUD itself carries a risk of introducing pathogens into the uterus, particularly if proper aseptic techniques are not followed [18].
3) History of Obstetric or Gynecological Procedures
   - Dilation and Curettage (D&C): frequently performed for miscarriage management, uterine evacuation, or abnormal uterine bleeding, D&C can introduce bacteria into the endometrial cavity or leave behind retained products of conception that contribute to inflammation [25]. Fortunately, the general trend in recent years is to abandon blind procedures and medical treatment in combination with hysteroscopy is increasingly used to manage abortions [26].
   - Cesarean delivery: women with cesarean sections may develop CE as a complication of postpartum infections, especially in cases of prolonged labor or membrane rupture [27].
   - Hysteroscopy or endometrial biopsy: like other gynecological procedures, hysteroscopy and endometrial biopsy can create a pathway for bacterial entry if performed under suboptimal conditions [28].
4) Retained Products of Conception (RPOC)
   - Postpartum period: retained placental fragments or other fetal tissues following delivery may lead to prolonged inflammation and chronic infection [29, 30].

- Post abortion: incomplete evacuation of the uterine cavity after an abortion is a significant risk factor for developing CE, especially in cases of septic abortion [30].

5) Assisted Reproductive Technologies (ART)
   - Embryo transfer and intrauterine manipulation: these procedures may introduce microorganisms into the uterine cavity, especially if pre-existing inflammation or subclinical infection is not addressed [18].
   - Recurrent implantation failure: Women undergoing repeated ART cycles are at risk of developing CE due to cumulative uterine trauma or infections [18].
6) Immunosuppression
   - HIV/AIDS: Immunosuppressed individuals are more vulnerable to chronic infections [31].
   - Corticosteroid or immunosuppressive therapy: Long-term use of these medications can suppress the immune response, allowing low-grade infections to persist and lead to CE [32].
7) Other medical conditions
   - Pelvic inflammatory disease: women with a history of PID may have a residual infection or low-grade inflammation extending to the endometrium [33].
   - Endometrial atrophy: in postmenopausal women, thinning of the endometrial lining can make it more susceptible to infection and chronic inflammation [34, 35].
   - Endometriosis is widely documented as an inflammatory disease with an abnormal immune response [36]. Takebayashi et al. [37] hypothesized that endometriosis may be related to chronic endometritis. They conducted a descriptive study finding a significantly higher incidence of chronic endometritis in the endometriosis group than in the non-endometriosis group. They found that only endometriosis significantly predicted chronic endometritis, suggesting a strong association between it and endometriosis.
8) Socioeconomic and geographic factors
   - Limited access to healthcare: in low-resource settings, lack of access to proper post-abortion care, postpartum follow-up, or treatment for STIs increases the risk of CE [38].

- Tuberculosis-Endemic Regions: In areas with high rates of tuberculosis, genital TB remains an important cause of CE [39].

5.2. Clinical Appearance

Although CE is usually asymptomatic, it can present with some nonspecific signs or symptoms such as:

- *Abnormal Uterine Bleeding (AUB):* this is the most common symptom of CE and it includes intermenstrual bleeding, heavy menstrual bleeding, or spotting [40].
- *Pelvic pain:* patients with CE can experience mild to moderate pelvic pain, which can be either chronic or intermittent. This pain is often diffuse or vague, making it difficult to pinpoint. In some cases, it may mimic other gynecological conditions like pelvic inflammatory disease or endometriosis [41].
- *Infertility:* CE is a significant cause of infertility, primarily due to impaired endometrial receptivity, which hinders the implantation of the embryo [42]. It is commonly identified in women undergoing evaluations for unexplained infertility or experiencing recurrent implantation failure during assisted reproductive technologies like in vitro fertilization [43]. The chronic inflammation alters the uterine microenvironment, making it less hospitable for embryo implantation and growth. CE is also associated with recurrent miscarriages, which occur due to chronic inflammation interfering with implantation or disrupting early pregnancy development [5, 44]. The persistent inflammatory response can impair vascularization, nutrient delivery, or hormone receptivity needed to sustain a pregnancy [5, 44].
- *Unusual vaginal discharge:* some women with CE may notice persistent or unusual vaginal discharge. This discharge is often described as yellow, brown, or blood-tinged and may be accompanied by mild pelvic discomfort or irritation [45].
- *Dyspareunia:* pain during sexual intercourse is an infrequent symptom but can occur in cases where the chronic inflammation spreads to deeper pelvic structures or causes localized tenderness [46].

Other less frequent symptoms, such as recurrent cystitis and mild gastro-intestinal discomfort, have been described in the literature [9].

5.3. Impact of Chronic Endometritis in Infertility

In recent years, the focus on chronic endometritis and its association with infertility has grown significantly, as demonstrated by the substantial increase in related publications. A search conducted on PubMed in 2024 identified 68 studies published between 2014 and 2019 and 191 studies published between 2019 and 2024.

This growing interest in chronic endometritis is primarily due to recent publications highlighting the increased prevalence of this condition in infertile patients, including those with unexplained infertility [5, 47], recurrent pregnancy loss [48–50], and repeated implantation failure (RIF) [44, 51].

Unexplained infertility is defined as the inability to conceive after 12 months of regular, unprotected sexual intercourse (or 6 months for women over 35) despite normal results in standard fertility evaluations. It is well known that CE modifies the pattern of uterine contractility in both the periovulatory and mid-luteal phases of the menstrual cycle [52]. Physiologically, in the proliferative phase, there is anterograde contractility from the fundus to the cervix, which facilitates removal of menstrual debris, followed by periovulatory and the luteal phase when there is a predominance of retrograde contraction in the opposite direction from the cervix to the fundus, which favors migration of the spermatozoa to the fallopian tubes. Conversely, during CE, there is a 3.3 times lower occurrence of retrograde contractility of the fallopian tubes [53]. This “altered peristalsis” induced by the presence of CE could impair, at least in part, fertility and contribute to some of the symptoms such as pelvic pain and dysmenorrhea [54].

The results of the retrospective study by Cicinelli et al. [55], in 2014, provided further evidence of the relationship between CE and unexplained infertility, finding a prevalence of CE in these patients of 66%. The study demonstrates that CE is a common finding in these patients and that common bacteria and mycoplasmas are the most frequent infectious agents involved. Furthermore, this study suggests that hysteroscopy is a proper diagnostic technique in patients with unexplained infertility, as it reliably detects and diagnoses the presence of CE. Additionally, reproductive outcomes in IVF improved significantly in patients whose antibiotic treatment successfully normalized both hysteroscopic findings and the histological endometrial pattern. It has also been suggested that untreated CE reduces success rates for both spontaneous conception and IVF cycles, in addition to contributing to adverse obstetric outcomes. Conversely, in their prospective study, Liu et al. [47], in their prospective study, propose the use of plasma cell counts, as will be explained in the corresponding section, since they believe that the prevalence rates of CE reported in previous studies may have been overestimated.

Recurrent pregnancy loss (RPL) defined as the loss of two or more consecutive pregnancies before 20 weeks of gestation, has also been strongly associated with CE. Several studies, such as those by Kitaya et al. [48], report significantly higher rates of CE in women with RPL of unknown causes. In one case-control study [50], secondary recurrent spontaneous abortion was associated with a CE prevalence of 83.9% histologically and 58.1% hysteroscopically, compared to much lower rates in fertile women.

With this data, we conclude that CE should be taken into consideration in those with unexplained RSA.

Similarly, CE has been implicated *in repeated implantation failure (RIF),* typically defined as the failure to achieve a clinical pregnancy after the transfer of at least three or more good-quality embryos in multiple assisted reproductive technology cycles, such as in vitro fertilization (IVF) or intracytoplasmic sperm injection [56].

The implantation consists of a physiological process involving mediators of inflammation such as leukocytes, cytokines, chemokines and other endometrial factors. All these cells and their mediators play an essential role in regulating the immune response and growth of the trophoblast [56].

The local expression of inflammatory response genes associated with endometrial receptivity, such as IL11 and CCL4, is decreased in the endometrium affected by EC compared to the endometrium without EC. These unusual gene expression patterns may explain the concomitant relationship between recurrent implantation failure and the presence of EC [56].

A systematic review and meta-analysis by Vitagliano et al. [57] demonstrates that CE therapy may improve IVF outcomes in patients suffering from RIF. Notably, the resolution of CE should be confirmed (at histology) before proceeding with IVF. The body of evidence on this topic is still insufficient to recommend routine CE screening as an intervention to improve clinical pregnancy rate and ongoing pregnancy rate/live birth rate in such patients.

It is also known that implantation rates are lower in patients with hydrosalpinx, which is believed to be related to the leakage of hydrosalpinx fluid, which contains leukocytes and inflammatory cytokines that impair the endometrial environment [58].

5.4. Pre-Hysteroscopic Diagnosis

As described in previous sections, chronic endometritis is an asymptomatic and silent condition. Clinical manifestations such as dyspareunia, leucorrhoea, pelvic pain and abnormal uterine bleeding, when they appear, are not specific to this pathology [18].

Despite being an inflammatory disease, inflammatory markers in peripheral blood (such as C-reactive protein, leptin, interleukin-6 and leukocytosis) cannot predict the presence of endometritis [42]. It is, therefore, a pathology with an absence of analytical markers.

Transvaginal ultrasound is also considered non-specific [59], as no typical findings have been identified [60].

Some studies have described hyperechoic areas in thinned endometrium in patients with chronic endometritis, representing foci of calcification or fibrosis [61, 62].

Alonso et al. [59] presented a clinical case of chronic endometritis confirmed by hysteroscopy and endometrial biopsy whose ultrasound findings on 3D ultrasound revealed the presence of several isoechogenic, round, well-demarcated structures within the endometrial cavity.

Similarly, Asherman's syndrome may sometimes accompany chronic endometritis, appearing on hysterosonography as linear echogenic bridges and irregular filling defects [62, 63].

The truth is that, to date, no other diagnostic tools are available to suspect or diagnose chronic endometritis. Thus, the current mainstays of diagnosis are still based on the classical techniques of histology, hysteroscopy and microbial culture.

5.5. Hysteroscopic Diagnosis

As previously mentioned, histological examination with identification of endometrial stromal plasma cells is considered the gold standard for CE diagnosis (Figure 1).

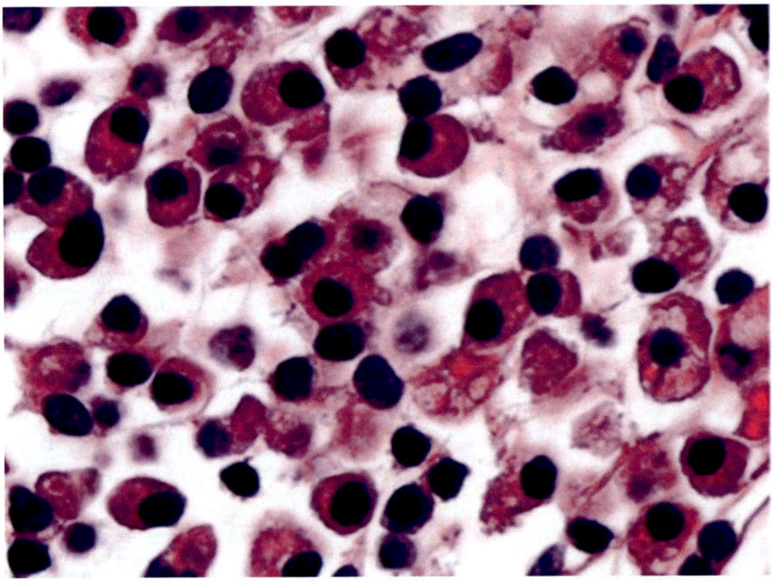

Figure 1. Hematoxylin–eosin staining of plasma cells in the endometrial stroma (× 400 pi) (©2023 Modified from *Pérez-Cejuela BA et al. Hysteroscopic versus histopathological agreement in the diagnosis of chronic endometritis: results from a retrospective observational study*. Licensed under the Creative Commons Attribution 4.0).

However, diagnostic difficulties persist due to this method's technical limitations and the lack of standardized histological diagnostic criteria [4].

Our proposal, aligned with the global trend of abandoning blind procedures, involves collecting samples for histological diagnosis under direct vision. This approach allows the clinician not only to assess potential signs of chronic endometritis but also to take samples for culture (with the advantage of being able to retrieve them through the working channel without contamination from the cervix or vagina) [4]. Additionally, it enables the collection of samples for histological analysis from the area most suspicious for endometritis.

In patients where hysteroscopy reveals other findings, such as retained products of conception, the presence of endometrial polyps, or uterine malformations that could interfere with their reproductive goals, the "see and treat" philosophy can be applied [64].

To ensure optimal outcomes, hysteroscopies should be performed during the follicular phase of the menstrual cycle (preferably between 3 and 7 days after menstruation) with a vaginoscopic approach and using saline solution as the distending medium [65, 66] The instruments needed are a rigid Hysteroscope with flexible biopsy forceps, introduced through a 5 Fr operative channel of the hysteroscope, and a fiber optic light cable. In detail, the forceps must be placed, with their jaws open, against the endometrium and pushed into the tissue for 0.5 to 1 cm [67]. Once a large portion of the mucosa is tangentially detached, the jaws are closed, and the entire hysteroscope is removed from the uterine cavity without pulling the instrument's tip back into the channel [68]. This method allowed us to collect a larger amount of tissue.

Hysteroscopy also allows for the identification of key inflammatory markers of CE on the endometrial surface, including focal or diffuse hyperemia, stromal edema, micropolyps, and the characteristic "strawberry-like" appearance [4].

Among these findings, *endometrial micropolyps* are considered one of the most distinctive features of CE (Figure 2). These small, vascularised protrusions are approximately 1–2 mm in diameter from the endometrial surface. These micropolyps cannot be visualised through ultrasound, hysterosonography, or hysterosalpingography. Their detection is straightforward, even for beginners, and is considered applicable in clinical practice. In 96 cases of micropolyps diagnosed via hysteroscopy, Cicinelli et al. reported a 94% correlation with histological findings for the diagnosis of CE [69].

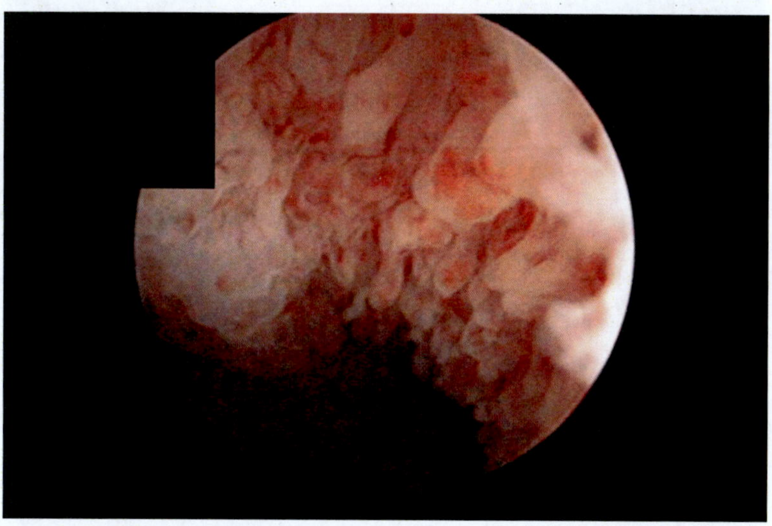

Figure 2. Micropolyps: Small protrusions visible in the endometrial surface, characteristic of an inflammatory response associated with Chronic Endometritis.

Micropolyps are constituted by small, vascularized ingrowths covered by endometrium. The stroma of micropolyps is characterized by an accumulation of inflammatory cells (lymphocytes, plasma cells or eosinophilic granulocytes) intermingled with normal stromal cells around small vessels and glandular structures [69].

They are very frequently associated with stromal edema, homogeneous or, more frequently, non-homogeneous endometrial thickening and focal or diffuse periglandular hyperemia [69].

Stromal edema another common feature, causes the endometrium to appear thickened and pale during the follicular phase, a pattern typically observed during the secretory phase (a normal finding in the secretory phase) [70] (Figure 3).

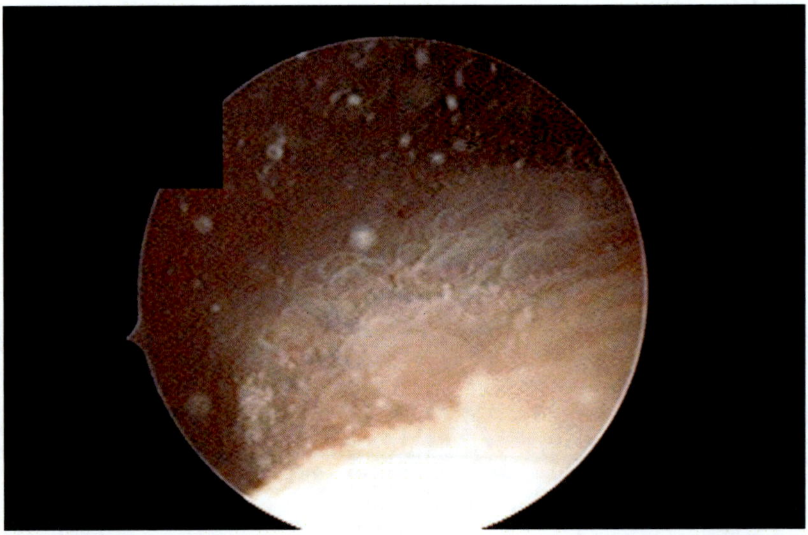

Figure 3. Edematous Changes in the Endometrium: Diffuse swelling and transparency of the endometrial mucosa, typically seen in cases of inflammation or Chronic Endometritis.

Meanwhile, *hyperemia* manifests as extensive or localized areas of redness, often accompanied by central pinpoint white spots or hemorrhagic patches [70] (Figure 4).

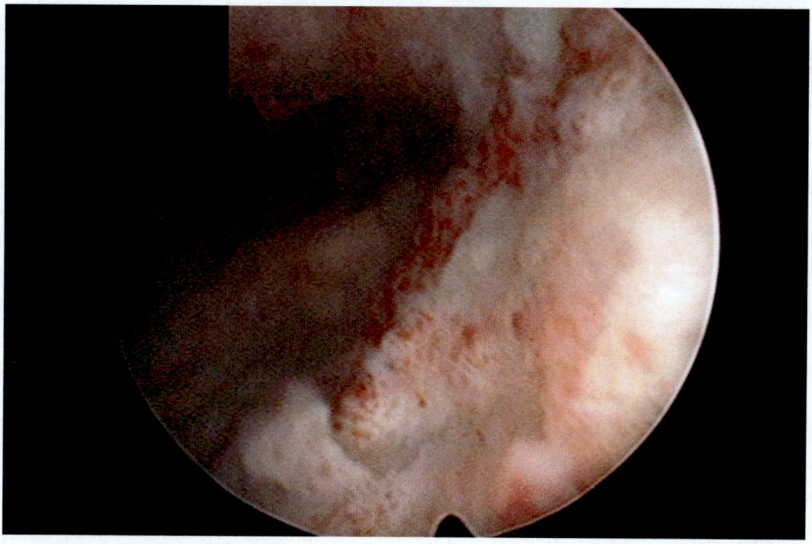

Figure 4. Typical Hemorrhagic spots of Chronic Endometritis (CE) in a focal pale area in the endometrium (©2023 Modified from *Pérez-Cejuela BA et al. Hysteroscopic versus histopathological agreement in the diagnosis of chronic endometritis: results from a retrospective observational study*. Licensed under the Creative Commons Attribution 4.0).

Since hysteroscopy is an operator-dependent technique, its diagnostic sensitivity and specificity are closely tied to the experience of the practitioner. To address this variability, the International Working Group for the Standardisation of the Diagnosis of Chronic Endometritis conducted a systematic review [70] and developed a set of standardized diagnostic hysteroscopic criteria, which include:

1) *Strawberry-like appearance:* extensive areas of hyperaemic endometrium with central whitish spots.
2) *Focal hyperemia:* small areas of hyperaemic endometrium.
3) *Hemorrhagic spots:* focal red areas with irregular borders, possibly continuous with capillaries.
4) *Micropolyp formation:* small endometrial protrusions <1 mm with a distinct vascular connective axis, distributed either in focal areas or across the entire endometrial surface.
5) *Thick and pale endometrial appearance during the follicular phase,* attributed to stromal edema (Figure 5).

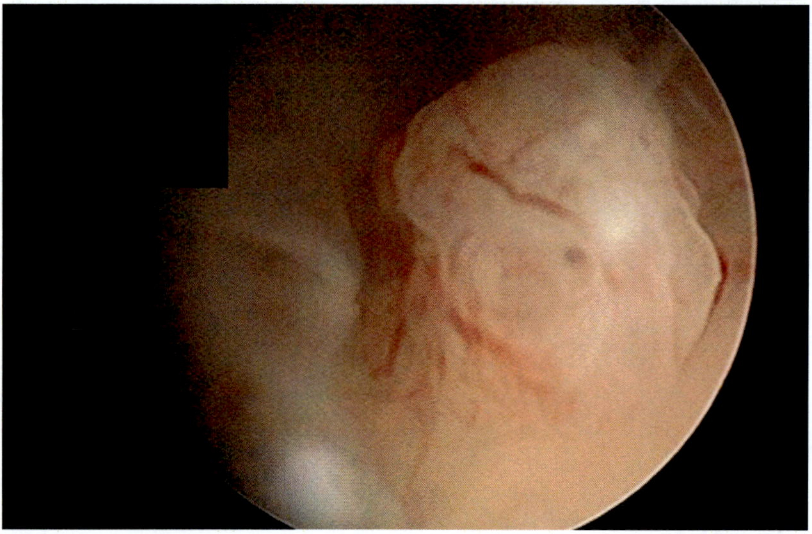

Figure 5. Localized pale area with tissue irregularity and inflammatory features suggestive of Focal Chronic Endometritis.

The authors conducted a randomized observational study to evaluate the reproducibility of these criteria among a group of professional participants [70]. The study revealed a positive impact of these criteria on the participants' ability to recognize CE.

5.6. Histological Diagnosis

The endometrium is a unique tissue containing a large variety of immunocompetent cells (except B lymphocytes and plasma cells which are rarely found), whose composition and density fluctuate periodically [71].

Chronic endometritis is a persistent inflammation of the endometrial mucosa, in which changes in the distribution and function of endometrial cells, elevation of proinflammatory cytokines and apoptosis phenomena will occur [72, 73].

Such an immune response provides an abnormal microenvironment, leading to the recruitment of circulating B-lymphocytes into the endometrial compartment. Of these, a fraction will differentiate into plasma cells, producing antibodies that potentially negatively impact the embryo implantation process [42].

Histological diagnosis, by identifying plasma cells in the endometrial stroma, is currently the gold standard for the diagnosis of chronic endometritis [72].

The main problem with histological diagnosis is that there are no standardized criteria and several limitations and controversies, which will be discussed below.

5.6.1. Limitations

One of the main limitations is the *subjectivity of sample analysis.* Staining with hematoxylin-eosin to identify the presence of plasma cells presents difficulties even for experienced pathologists. This is because plasma cells closely resemble stromal fibroblasts or mononuclear leukocytes resident in the endometrium [72]. Because of this, immunohistochemistry using the CD138 marker was introduced as a more accurate technique for diagnosis. CD138, also known as Syndecan-1, is a transmembrane protein antigen mainly expressed in mature plasma cells and skin cells [74]. An advantage of CD138 immunohistochemical staining is the ability to identify typical, round plasma cells with classic clock-shaped chromatin features and atypical spindle-shaped ones [75, 76]. This prevents them from going unnoticed.

Similarly, immunohistochemistry reduces the possibility of counting other cells by mistake, thus reducing the number of false positives [75]. A higher detection rate of chronic endometritis has been demonstrated using CD138 [77], decreasing inter-observer and intra-observer variability [78]. However, there is no standardised immunohistochemical technique, and results may vary depending on the type and duration of antigen retrieval, antibody dilution and selection, incubation time, tissue thickness of the section studied, or the number of sections examined [72]. Also, if the plasma cell count is based solely on CD138 staining, an overestimation of chronic endometritis can sometimes occur due to the background reaction [78, 79].

Another diagnostic difficulty is that although plasma cells in the endometrial stromal zone are considered a diagnostic hallmark, *it is possible to find such cells in healthy women* [72] or to indicate mild inflammation without clinical relevance [80]. Therefore, McQueen et al. [49] proposed that the diagnosis of chronic endometritis required both the presence of plasma cells and the presence of changes in the endometrial stroma (edema, areas of hypercellularity, deposition of disaggregated pigment, etc.) [81].

It is essential to *define the number of plasma cells necessary* to establish the diagnosis of chronic endometritis. Some authors consider the finding of one diagnostic plasma cell, others the finding of two or more, and others at least five.

All these proposed criteria are arbitrary and are not based on reference ranges derived from normal fertile populations.

First, it is necessary to define which quantification system has been used. Many researchers use different quantification methods.

Some use the number of plasma cells per whole section, and others the count of plasma cells per defined number of high magnification fields (HPF) [47].

Researchers who advocate examination of the whole sample argue that plasma cells are generally not present in the endometrium, and therefore, the finding of one or more cells is already considered diagnostic [82].

The drawback of this approach is that it does not consider tissue size, as one would expect that the larger the sample size, the greater the likelihood of finding plasma cells.

Therefore, the concept of plasma cell density was introduced to correct the size of the sample examined by examining ten or more HPFs chosen at random. However, the potential disadvantage of this approach is that plasma cells are often present in low numbers, so the inclusion of only ten selected HPFs may not be sufficient to produce a consistently reproducible result [82].

HPF's approach to counting CD138-positive cells is the most widely described. However, a new quantification method would probably be needed that counts all CD138+ cells in the whole section, then measures the area of the tissue section examined and expresses the result as plasma cell count per unit area [47].

Various cut-off points for the number of plasma cells diagnostic for chronic endometritis have been found in the literature (Table 2).

- Hirata et al. [83] conducted a prospective observational study that analyzed four plasma cell thresholds, concluding that chronic endometritis should be defined as the presence of ≥ 1 plasma cell per 10 HPF.
- Y. Liu et al. [47] conducted a prospective observational study of 220 patients of childbearing age to establish a reference range of plasma cell counts. The threshold level for three different quantification methods was 1.95 CD138 plasma cells per ten randomly selected HPF, 2.95 CD138 plasma cells per section, and 5.15 CD138 plasma cells per 0.1 mm2.

- On the other hand, Achilles et al. [80], who found that plasma cells were commonly present in the endometrium of asymptomatic, fertile, healthy women, suggest that the finding of one or more plasma cells could overdiagnose chronic endometritis.
- Vitagliano et al. [84] conducted a systematic review and concluded that, although the evidence is of low quality, the adverse effects of chronic endometritis on IVF outcomes may be primarily associated with severe cases (defined as ≥5 plasma cells per high-power field [HPF]). In contrast, the presence of 1-4 plasma cells per HPF does not appear to impair embryo implantation significantly.
- Similarly, Li et al. [85] conducted a retrospective study of 716 infertile patients who received IVF treatment. This study indicated that locally elevated CD138+ cells in the mid-luteal phase (≥5 plasma cells) were significantly associated with adverse pregnancy outcomes in infertile women.

Table 2. Plasma cells threshold

Study	Type	Threshold
Hirata et al. [83]	Prospective observational study	≥1 plasma cell/10 HPF
Liu et al. [47]	Prospective observational study	1.95 (10 HPF), 2.95 (per section), 5.15 (0.1 mm^2)
Achilles et al. [80]	Observational study	≥1 plasma cell
Vitagliano et al. [84]	Systematic review	≥5 plasma cells/HPF for severe cases
Li et al. [85]	Retrospective study	≥5 plasma cells

Another interesting aspect analyzed in Song's study was the correlation between the number of plasma cell counts and hysteroscopic findings. The study showed that the higher the plasma cell count per 10 HPF, the more likely the occurrence of hysteroscopic features of chronic endometritis [86].

In turn, Pérez-Cejuela et al. [87] conducted a retrospective observational study of 115 patients to evaluate the concordance rate between hysteroscopy and pathological examination in case of chronic endometritis. This study showed a concordance between histological and hysteroscopic findings of 75% in the presence of diffuse or focal hyperaemia, 53% in the presence of micropolyps only and 100% in the presence of hyperaemia and micropolyps.

Another diagnostic limitation is *the timing of sampling.* The menstrual cycle phase in which the biopsy is performed is of great importance. It has been shown that in 15% of samples during the secretory phase, plasma cells are only present in the basal stromal layer, making them unnoticed if not included in the biopsy [71]. Similarly, in the endometrial secretory phase, oedematous surface changes and increased stromal cell density occur, interfering with the identification of plasma cells [76, 88, 89]. A higher prevalence of chronic endometritis has therefore been demonstrated in the proliferative phase than in the secretory phase [84]. It will therefore be essential to know the time of the menstrual phase when the sample is obtained.

Endometrial sampling is usually performed using an endometrial biopsy device by hysteroscopy. However, when an endometrial biopsy is performed using a blind method, the diagnostic reliability may depend on the amount of endometrial tissue obtained, especially if the distribution of plasma cells is heterogeneous over the entire endometrial surface [84]. The diagnosis may be underestimated due to the random nature of tissue collection and the possible presence of chronic focal endometritis.

Therefore, defining the minimum amount of endometrial aspirate sample required is also important. All of this explains the enormous variability in the prevalence of chronic endometritis [90].

Histopathological examination is, for now, the gold standard for chronic endometritis, but it is vital to reach an international consensus on histopathological diagnostic criteria [90].

5.6.2. Molecular Biology

The concomitant use of histology, hysteroscopy and microbial culture could significantly impact diagnostic accuracy. However, their combined use considerably increases complexity and cost, and it has been shown that consistent and concordant results are only obtained using the three classical diagnostic methods in 20% of cases of chronic endometritis [9].

Both histology and hysteroscopy have an essential component of subjectivity [72]. Histopathological evaluation tends to underdiagnose endometritis and hysteroscopy to overdiagnose it.

Moreover, unlike microbial culture, these tools cannot identify the aetiological agent responsible.

The main advantage of microbial culture is the objective identification of endometrial pathogens and the possibility to administer a specific antibiogram-guided treatment. However, endometrial bacterial culture cannot be routinely performed due to its long turnaround time, and not all responsible bacteria are culturable under standard laboratory conditions [85, 91, 92].

On the other hand, it has been demonstrated that the endometrial cavity is not sterile under physiological conditions [75, 93–95]. Therefore, the modern pathophysiological concept of chronic endometritis focuses more on microbial and immune interaction than on the presence of bacteria in the uterine cavity [96].

Therefore, the replacement of the term endometritis (mainly caused by bacteria) by the term inflammatory altered endometrial status (IISE), which would directly indicate inflammation of the endometrium, regardless of the cause, is currently under review [71, 97].

Microbial infection is still believed to be the leading cause of persistent inflammation. The main finding supporting this theory is the efficacy of antibiotic treatment in the histopathologically confirmed resolution of this pathology [98].

In recent years, new molecular diagnostic methods have been a real breakthrough in detecting and characterizing microorganisms in various scientific fields. The use of quantitative polymerase chain reaction (RT-PCR) could provide a rapid and more accurate profile of the micro-organisms responsible for chronic endometritis (by facilitating the identification of culturable and non-culturable bacterial DNA) [61].

Molecular techniques allow the detection of low biomass uterine microbiota [75].

The study by Moreno in collaboration with Cicinelli [6], evaluated the diagnostic accuracy of molecular biology-based methods compared to traditional methods (histology, hysteroscopy and microbial culture) to diagnose chronic endometritis.

This molecular diagnostic tool reported a sensitivity of 75%, a specificity of 100%, and an accuracy of 77%. In other words, molecular microbiology provides similar results to using the 3 classical methods together, overcoming the bias of using any of the classical methods alone.

This demonstrated an opportunity to overcome the bias of classical diagnostic methods and provide new diagnostic tools.

RT-PCR can detect the intrauterine microbiome when histology is unfavorable, as it can identify and quantify very small amounts of bacterial DNA, regardless of its culturable or non-culturable nature, and is also valid for frozen or processed samples [82].

In turn, it can inform the choice of target therapy with turnaround times of hours rather than days.

However, by quantifying bacterial DNA rather than live bacteria, these procedures do not guarantee that the DNA found is from viable bacteria [99].

In addition, the minimum amount of bacterial DNA that causes pathology has not been determined. Therefore, the presence of such DNA in some women may be harmless, nor would it discriminate between acute or chronic endometritis [99].

Therefore, future studies will be needed to investigate these promising resources further and define both the technique and its clinical applications.

5.7. Treatment

As mentioned at the beginning, microorganisms detected in chronic endometritis include common bacteria (Streptococcus species, Escherichia coli, Enterococcus faecalis, and Staphylococcus species), mycoplasma/ ureaplasma species (Mycoplasma genitalium, Mycoplasma hominis, and Ureaplasma urealyticum), Proteus species, Klebsiella pneumoniae, Pseudomonas aeruginosa, Gardnerella vaginalis, Corynebacterium, and yeasts (Saccharomyces cerevisiae and Candida species) [2].

The positive impact of antibiotic therapy in achieving higher pregnancy and live birth rates in patients with chronic endometritis has been widely demonstrated [5, 9, 48, 55, 100].

In the treatment of chronic endometritis, broad-spectrum antibiotic regimens are used for 10-14 days, effective against the most prevalent pathogens mentioned above. Antibiotics are used depending on the results of the culture and Gram stain of the endometrial biopsy.

However, there is no defined antibiotic regimen for chronic endometritis. In the literature, we find different antibiotics and doses used.

Depending on the infectious agent isolated or if the culture is negative, antibiotic therapies can be classified into the following groups (Table 3):

- *Positive Culture:*
  For patients with chronic endometritis with positive culture for Gram-negative bacteria: an antibiotic regimen based on ciprofloxacin 500 mg twice daily for 10 days is recommended [5].
  Patients with chronic endometritis with positive culture for Gram-positive bacteria: an antibiotic regimen with amoxicillin-clavulanic acid 2 g once daily or 1 g every 12 hours for 8 days is recommended [5].
- *Mycoplasma or Ureaplasma:* Patients with chronic endometritis with isolation of Mycoplasma or Ureaplasma: treatment with josamycin 2 g per day for 12 days is recommended.
  In cases of resistance, use minocycline 200 mg daily for 12 days [5].

If these treatments are not available in our country, mycoplasma will be treated with the doxycycline regimen and ureoplasma with the azithromycin regimen.

- *Mycobacterium tuberculosis:* Patients with endometritis caused by Mycobacterium tuberculosis: antituberculous therapy is recommended. In a 60 kg adult, isoniazid 300mg/day, rifampicin 600mg/day, pyrazinamide 1600mg/day and ethambutol 1200mg/day for 2 months, followed by isoniazid 300mg/day plus rifampicin 600mg/day plus ethambutol 1200mg/day for 4 months [59, 101, 102].
- *Negative cultures:* Patients with chronic endometritis with negative cultures or of unknown aetiology: this is probably the most controversial or least standardised scenario in terms of antibiotic regimen.

  The rationale for treating cases with negative cultures is that many of the causative agents of chronic endometritis are not culturable under standard laboratory conditions.

  Some of the antibiotic guidelines found in the literature are:
- Johnston-MacAnanny et al. [103] suggest treatment with doxycycline 100 mg every 12 hours orally for 10-14 days in those patients with chronic endometritis of unknown aetiology. Revealing a cure rate of 70%.

  If the patient is allergic to doxycycline, they propose a five-day treatment with azithromycin 500 mg orally on the first day and 250 mg orally from the second to the fifth day.

  They also recommend in case of persistent endometritis, an antibiotic combination of ciprofloxacin 500mg every 12 hours (or ofloxacin 400 mg daily) plus metronidazole 500mg every 12 hours for 2 weeks [61, 103].

  It has been shown that oral doxycycline alone eradicated 92.3% of patients with chronic endometritis and reduced the detection rate of some pathogens such as corynebacterium, enterococcus, E. coli, Streptococcus agalactiae, U. urealyticum and Ureaplasma parvum [2].
- Kuroda et al. [104] proposed the same antibiotic regimen. They suggested endometrial curettage to remove the inflammatory endometrium in women who did not respond to the two previous treatments.

  Gentle endometrial curettage has been shown to significantly reduce the number of CD138-positive cells, improving pregnancy outcomes.

The use of morcelator or endometrial scratching as an alternative to curettage in patients with persistent endometritis is increasingly being discussed.

- Van Hoogenhuijze et al. [105] conducted a systematic literature search, including data from 4112 participants from 13 studies, on whether endometrial scratching in women undergoing IVF/ICSI influenced the likelihood of achieving higher live birth rates. They showed that endometrial scratching did indeed improve live birth rates in women undergoing IVF/ICSI.
  Also, although more imprecise, it was suggested that the timing of scratching in the luteal phase, natural cycle, may be superior to other timed and/or contraceptive cycle scratches.
- On the other hand, Cicinelli et al. [5] recommend a treatment based on Ceftriaxone 250 mg IM in a single dose plus doxycycline 100 mg orally twice a day for 14 days with Metronidazole 500 mg orally twice a day for 14 days.
  Repeat the same antibiotic regimen up to a maximum of 3 times in case of persistent endometritis.

Table 3. Chronic endometritis treatment

Category	Subcategory	Antibiotic/Treatment
Positive Cultures	Gram-negative bacteria	Ciprofloxacin 500 mg twice daily for 10 days.
	Gram-positive bacteria	Amoxicillin-clavulanic acid 2 g once daily or 1 g every 12 hours for 8 days.
	Mycoplasma/Ureaplasma	Josamycin 2 g/day for 12 days; alternatives: doxycycline or azithromycin.
Mycobacterium TB	-	Isoniazid, rifampicin, pyrazinamide, ethambutol (6-month regimen).
Negative Cultures	Unknown etiology	Doxycycline 100 mg every 12 hours for 10-14 days; azithromycin as alternative.
Persistent Cases	Endometritis resistant	Doxycycline 100 mg every 12 hours for 10-14 days; ciprofloxacin + metronidazole for 2 weeks.
	Inflammatory removal	Endometrial curettage, Morcellator, or scratching.
Novel Therapies	Intrauterine infusion	Antibiotics + dexamethasone; tailored based on culture sensitivity.
	Autologous PRP	Platelet-rich plasma (anti-inflammatory and antimicrobial properties).

Other antibiotic options proposed include the use of intracavitary antibiotics or the use of corticosteroids such as dexamethasone, and the administration of vaginal probiotics.

Zhang et al. [106] conducted a prospective study of 109 patients with chronic endometritis using combined intrauterine administration of antibiotic and dexamethasone as a treatment option, with histopathological cure rate rates of 77.98%, demonstrating that it could achieve the expected therapeutic effects and satisfactory pregnancy outcomes.

These patients received intrauterine infusion therapy with 20 mL of a self-made mixture containing an appropriate antibiotic based on the detected infectious agent and antibiotic sensitivity testing, dexamethasone (DXM 5 mg), hyaluronidase (1500 U) and saline (added up to 20 mL).

For gram-negative bacteria, 80 mg gentamicin at 20 mL was used. In cases of gram-positive bacteria, clindamycin 60 mg was used. In case of isolation of Mycoplasma and urealyticum they were treated with minocycline 6 mg. Finally, women with negative cultures were treated with a mixture of several antibiotics, including gentamicin 80 mg, clindamycin 60 mg and metronidazole 80 mg.

At this stage, it cannot be excluded that oral antibiotics are more effective than intrauterine infusion therapy, and further research is needed.

Recently, another new therapeutic technique has emerged based on treatment with autologous platelet-rich plasma, especially in patients who do not respond to conventional antibiotic regimens [107], due to its anti-inflammatory and antimicrobial properties [108].

We are therefore faced with new and novel therapeutic lines, which will require further studies to confirm and position their therapeutic action.

Conclusion

Chronic endometritis (CE) remains an underdiagnosed yet impactful condition in gynecological and reproductive health. Its silent and often asymptomatic presentation belies the significant role it plays in infertility, recurrent pregnancy loss, and implantation failure. Through advancements in diagnostic techniques, including hysteroscopy, immunohistochemistry, and molecular biology tools, the understanding of CE has grown, paving the way for more accurate detection and targeted treatments.

The multifactorial etiology of CE underscores the importance of a comprehensive clinical approach that considers infectious, non-infectious, and iatrogenic factors. Tailored antibiotic regimens have proven effective in resolving the condition, particularly when guided by microbial cultures and advanced diagnostic techniques. Emerging therapies, such as intrauterine treatments and platelet-rich plasma, offer promising alternatives for resistant cases, although further research is needed to validate their efficacy.

As the field evolves, standardizing diagnostic criteria and therapeutic protocols will be critical to improving outcomes for women affected by CE.

References

[1] Michels TC. Chronic endometritis. *Am Fam Physician.* 1995;52(1):217–222.

[2] Kitaya K, Takeuchi T, Mizuta S, Matsubayashi H, Ishikawa T. Endometritis: new time, new concepts. *Fertil Steril.* 2018;110(3):344–50.

[3] Chen Q, Zhang X, Hu Q, Zhang W, Xie Y, Wei W. The alteration of intrauterine microbiota in chronic endometritis patients based on 16S rRNA sequencing analysis. *Ann Clin Microbiol Antimicrob.* 2023;22(1):1–10.

[4] Saponara S, Angioni S, Parry JP, Pacheco LA, Carugno J, Moawad N, Haimovich S, Lasmar RB, Dealberti D, Aksakal E, Urman B, Nappi L, Vitale SG. The Pivotal role of hysteroscopy in diagnosing subtle uterine lesions in infertile patients: Seeing the unseen can make the difference. *European Journal of Obstetrics and Gynecology and Reproductive Biology.* 2025;305:132–41.

[5] Cicinelli E, Matteo M, Tinelli R, Lepera A, Alfonso R, Indraccolo U, Marrocchella S, Greco P, Resta L. Prevalence of chronic endometritis in repeated unexplained implantation failure and the IVF success rate after antibiotic therapy. *Hum Reprod.* 2015;30(2):323–30.

[6] Wiesenfeld HC, Hillier SL, Meyin LA, Amortegui AJ, Sweet RL. Subclinical pelvic inflammatory disease and infertility. *Obstet Gynecol.* 2012;120(1):37–43.

[7] Cicinelli E, Ziegler D, Nicoletti R, Tinelli R, Saliani N, Resta L. Poor reliability of vaginal and endocervical cultures for evaluating microbiology of endometrial cavity in women with chronic endometritis. *Gynecol Obstet Invest.* 2009;68(2):108–115.

[8] Kasius JC, Broekmans FJ, Sie-Go DM, Bourgain C, Eijkemans MJ, Fauser BC. The reliability of the histological diagnosis of endometritis in asymptomatic IVF cases: a multicenter observer study. *Hum Reprod.* 2012;27(1):153–158.

[9] Moreno I, Cicinelli E, Garcia-Grau I, Gonzalez-Monfort M, Bau D, Vilella F, De Ziegler D, Resta L, Valbuena D, Simon C. The diagnosis of chronic endometritis in infertile asymptomatic women: a comparative study of histology, microbial cultures, hysteroscopy, and molecular microbiology. *Am J Obstet Gynecol.* 2018;218(6):602.e1-602.e16.

[10] Ness RB, Soper DE, Holley RL, Peipert J, Randall H, Sweet RL, Sondheimer SJ, Hendrix SL, Amortegui A, Trucco G, Songer T, Lave JR, Hillier SL, Bass DC, Kelsey SF. Effectiveness of inpatient and outpatient treatment strategies for women

with pelvic inflammatory disease: Results from the Pelvic Inflammatory Disease Evaluation and Clinical Health (PEACH) Randomized Trial. *Am J Obstet Gynecol.* 2002;186(5):929–37.

[11] Jindal UN, Verma S, Bala Y. Favorable infertility outcomes following anti-tubercular treatment prescribed on the sole basis of a positive polymerase chain reaction test for endometrial tuberculosis. *Hum Reprod.* 2012;27(5):1368–1374.

[12] Verstraelen H, Vilchez-Vargas R, Desimpel F, Jauregui R, Vankeirsbilck N, Weyers S. Characterisation of the human uterine microbiome in non-pregnant women through deep sequencing of the V1-2 region of the 16S rRNA gene. *Peer J.* 2015;4:1602.

[13] Cowling P, McCoy DR, Marshall RJ, Padfield CJ, Reeves DS. Bacterial colonization of the non-pregnant uterus: a study of pre-menopausal abdominal hysterectomy specimens. *Eur J Clin Microbiol Infect Dis.* 1992;11(2):204–205.

[14] Møller BR, Kristiansen F V, Thorsen P, Frost L, Mogensen SC. Sterility of the uterine cavity. *Acta Obstet Gynecol Scand.* 1995;74(3):216–219.

[15] Mitchell CM, Haick A, Nkwopara E, Garcia R, Rendi M, Agnew K. Colonization of the upper genital tract by vaginal bacterial species in nonpregnant women. *Am J Obstet Gynecol.* 2015;212(5):611 1–9.

[16] Espinoza J, Erez O, Romero R. Preconceptional antibiotic treatment to prevent preterm birth in women with a previous preterm delivery. *Am J Obstet Gynecol.* 2006;194(3):630–637.

[17] Eckert LO, Moore DE, Patton DL, Agnew KJ, Eschenbach DA. Relationship of vaginal bacteria and inflammation with conception and early pregnancy loss following in-vitro fertilization. *Infect Dis Obstet Gynecol.* 2003;11(1):11–17.

[18] Kimura F, Takebayashi A, Ishida M, Nakamura A, Kitazawa J, Morimune A, Hirata K, Takahashi A, Tsuji S, Takashima A, Amano T, Tsuji S, Ono T, Kaku S, Kasahara K, Moritani S, Kushima R, Murakami T. Review: Chronic endometritis and its effect on reproduction. *J Obstet Gynaecol Res.* 2019;45(5):951–60.

[19] Vitale SG, Moore O, Riemma G, Carugno J, Yarto ML, Haimovich S. Hysteroscopic laser ablation of symptomatic uterine fibroids: insights from a prospective study. *Climacteric.* 2023;26(5):497–502.

[20] Vitale SG, Saponara S, Sicilia G, Klarić M, Sorrentino F, D'Alterio MN, Nappi L, Angioni S. Hysteroscopic diode laser myolysis: from a case series to literature review of incisionless myolysis techniques for managing heavy menstrual bleeding in premenopausal women. *Arch Gynecol Obstet.* 2024;309(3):949–59.

[21] Wiesenfeld HC, Hillier SL, Krohn MA, Amortegui AJ, Heine RP, Landers D V., Sweet RL. Lower genital tract infection and endometritis: Insight into subclinical pelvic inflammatory disease. *Obstetrics and Gynecology.* 2002;100(3):456–63.

[22] Shi Y, Zhu Y, Fan S, Vitagliano A, Liu X, Liao Y, Liang Y, Vitale SG. Clinical Characteristics and Antifungal Susceptibility of Candida nivariensis from Vulvovaginal Candidiasis. *Gynecol Obstet Invest.* 2020;85(1):88–93.

[23] Cai T, Mazzoli S, Migno S, Malossini G, Lanzafame P, Mereu L, Tateo S, Wagenlehner FM, Pickard RS, Bartoletti R. Development and validation of a nomogram predicting recurrence risk in women with symptomatic urinary tract infection. *Int J Urol.* 2014;21(9):929–34.

[24] Vitale SG, Di Spiezio Sardo A, Riemma G, De Franciscis P, Alonso Pacheco L, Carugno J. In-office hysteroscopic removal of retained or fragmented intrauterine device without anesthesia: a cross-sectional analysis of an international survey. *Updates Surg.* 2022;74(3):1079–85.

[25] Vitale SG, Riemma G, Carugno J, Perez-Medina T, Alonso Pacheco L, Haimovich S, Parry JP, Di Spiezio Sardo A, De Franciscis P. Postsurgical barrier strategies to avoid the recurrence of intrauterine adhesion formation after hysteroscopic adhesiolysis: a network meta-analysis of randomized controlled trials. *Am J Obstet Gynecol.* 2022;226(4):487-498.e8.

[26] Villegas-Echeverri JD, Pope R, Robert M, Meinhold-Heerlein I, Haimovich S, Carugno J, Pacheco LA, Sardo ADS. FIGO-GCH joint consensus statement on the current status and recommendations for the use of blind intrauterine procedures in the evaluation and management of women with suspected intrauterine pathologies. *International Journal of Gynecology and Obstetrics.* 2025;168(2):493–6.

[27] Kawakita T, Landy HJ. Surgical site infections after cesarean delivery: epidemiology, prevention and treatment. *Matern Health Neonatol Perinatol.* 2017;3(1):12.

[28] Vitale SG, Angioni S, Saponara S, Sicilia G, Etrusco A, D'Alterio MN, Cobellis L, De Franciscis P, Riemma G. TikTok as a platform for hysteroscopy information: An analytical video-based cross-sectional study to assess quality, reliability, and accuracy. *International Journal of Gynecology and Obstetrics.* 2025;168(1):353–61.

[29] Vitale SG, Parry JP, Carugno J, Cholkeri-Singh A, Della Corte L, Cianci S, Schiattarella A, Riemma G, De Franciscis P. Surgical and Reproductive Outcomes after Hysteroscopic Removal of Retained Products of Conception: A Systematic Review and Meta-analysis. *J Minim Invasive Gynecol.* 2021;28(2):204–17.

[30] Rouse CE, Eckert LO, Muñoz FM, Stringer JSA, Kochhar S, Bartlett L, Sanicas M, Dudley DJ, Harper DM, Bittaye M, Meller L, Jehan F, Maltezou HC, Šubelj M, Bardaji A, Kachikis A, Beigi R, Gravett MG. Postpartum endometritis and infection following incomplete or complete abortion: Case definition & guidelines for data collection, analysis, and presentation of maternal immunization safety data. *Vaccine.* 2019;37(52):7585–95.

[31] Corrado G, Vizza E, Perrone AM, Mereu L, Cela V, Legge F, Hilaris G, Pasciuto T, D'Indinosante M, La Fera E, Certelli C, Bruno V, Kogeorgos S, Fanfani F, De Iaco P, Scambia G, Gallotta V. Comparison Between Laparoscopic and Robotic Surgery in Elderly Patients With Endometrial Cancer: A Retrospective Multicentric Study. *Front Oncol.* 2021;11:724886.

[32] Ali DES, Shah M, Ali A, Malik MO, Rehman F, Badshah H, Ehtesham E, Vitale SG. Treatment with Metformin and Combination of Metformin plus Pioglitazone on Serum Levels of IL-6 and IL-8 in Polycystic Ovary Syndrome: A Randomized Clinical Trial. *Hormone and Metabolic Research.* 2019;51(11):714–22.

[33] Corrado G, Mereu L, Bogliolo S, Cela V, Gardella B, Sperduti I, Certelli C, Pellegrini A, Posar G, Zampa A, Tateo S, Gadducci A, Spinillo A, Vizza E. Comparison between single-site and multiport robot-assisted hysterectomy in

obese patients with endometrial cancer: An Italian multi-institutional study. *Int J Med Robot.* 2020;16(2):e2066.

[34] Vitale SG, Riemma G, Haimovich S, Carugno J, Alonso Pacheco L, Perez-Medina T, Parry JP, Török P, Tesarik J, Della Corte L, Cobellis L, Di Spiezio Sardo A, De Franciscis P. Risk of endometrial cancer in asymptomatic postmenopausal women in relation to ultrasonographic endometrial thickness: systematic review and diagnostic test accuracy meta-analysis. *Am J Obstet Gynecol.* 2023;228(1):22-35.e2.

[35] Vitale SG, Saponara S, Succu AG, Sicilia G, Martsidis K, D'Alterio MN, Angioni S. Efficacy and Safety of Non-Ablative Dual Wavelength Diode Laser Therapy for Genitourinary Syndrome of Menopause: A Single-Center Prospective Study. *Adv Ther.* 2024;41(12):4617–27.

[36] Angioni S, Saponara S, Vitale SG. Metabolomics analysis in endometriosis patients: is it a step toward the future? *Gynecological Endocrinology.* 2023;39(1):2227276.

[37] Takebayashi A, Kimura F, Kishi Y, Ishida M, Takahashi A, A Y. The association between endometriosis and chronic endometritis. *PLoS One.* 2014;9(2):e88354.

[38] Corrado G, Vizza E, Cela V, Mereu L, Bogliolo S, Legge F, Ciccarone F, Mancini E, Gallotta V, Baiocco E, Monterossi G, Perri MT, Zampa A, Pasciuto T, Scambia G. Laparoscopic versus robotic hysterectomy in obese and extremely obese patients with endometrial cancer: A multi-institutional analysis. *European Journal of Surgical Oncology.* 2018;44(12):1935–41.

[39] Sikenis M, Prajapati B, Singh AK, Yadav K, Rahman A, Pandey MK, Nema RK, Sikenis M, Prajapati B, Singh AK, Yadav K, Rahman A, Pandey MK, Nema RK. Genital tuberculosis: A silent contributor to infertility and adverse pregnancy outcomes. *Journal of Reproductive Healthcare and Medicine.* 2024;5:17.

[40] Vitale SG, Angioni S, D'Alterio MN, Ronsini C, Saponara S, De Franciscis P, Riemma G. Risk of endometrial malignancy in women treated for breast cancer: the BLUSH prediction model–evidence from a comprehensive multicentric retrospective cohort study. *Climacteric.* 2024;25(5):482–8.

[41] Angioni S, Saponara S, Succu AG, Sigilli M, Scicchitano F, D'Alterio MN. Metabolomic Characteristics in Endometriosis Patients. In: Genazzani AR, Nisolle M, Petraglia F, Taylor RN, editors. *Endometriosis pathogenesis, clinical impact and management ISGE series.* Cham: Springer; 2021.

[42] Espinós JJ, Fabregues F, Fontes J, García-Velasco JA, Llácer J, Requena A, Checa M, Bellver J. Impact of chronic endometritis in infertility: a SWOT analysis. *Reprod Biomed Online.* 2021;42(5):939–51.

[43] Chiofalo B, Palmara V, Vilos GA, Pacheco LA, Lasmar RB, Shawki O, Giacobbe V, Alibrandi A, Di Guardo F, Vitale SG. Reproductive outcomes of infertile women undergoing "see and treat" office hysteroscopy: a retrospective observational study. *Minimally Invasive Therapy and Allied Technologies.* 2021;30(3):147–53.

[44] Bouet PE, El Hachem H, Monceau E, Gariépy G, Kadoch IJ, Sylvestre C. Chronic endometritis in women with recurrent pregnancy loss and recurrent implantation

failure: prevalence and role of office hysteroscopy and immunohistochemistry in diagnosis. *Fertil Steril.* 2016;105(1):106–10.

[45] Lozano FM, Bernabeu A, Lledo B, Morales R, Diaz M, Aranda FI, Llacer J, Bernabeu R. Characterization of the vaginal and endometrial microbiome in patients with chronic endometritis. *Eur J Obstet Gynecol Reprod Biol.* 2021;263:25–32.

[46] Vitale SG, Caruso S, Rapisarda AMC, Valenti G, Rossetti D, Cianci S, Cianci A. Biocompatible porcine dermis graft to treat severe cystocele: impact on quality of life and sexuality. *Arch Gynecol Obstet.* 2016;293(1):125–31.

[47] Liu Y, Chen X, Huang J, Wang CC, Yu MY, Laird S, Li TC. Comparison of the prevalence of chronic endometritis as determined by means of different diagnostic methods in women with and without reproductive failure. *Fertil Steril.* 2018;109(5):832–9.

[48] Kitaya K. Prevalence of chronic endometritis in recurrent miscarriages. *Fertil Steril.* 2011;95(3):1156–8.

[49] McQueen DB, Maniar KP, Hutchinson A, Confino R, Bernardi L, Pavone ME. Redefining chronic endometritis: the importance of endometrial stromal changes. *Fertil Steril.* 2021;116(3):855–61.

[50] Zolghadri J, Momtahan M, Aminian K, Ghaffarpasand F, Tavana Z. The value of hysteroscopy in diagnosis of chronic endometritis in patients with unexplained recurrent spontaneous abortion. *Eur J Obstet Gynecol Reprod Biol.* 2011;155(2):217–20.

[51] Cicinelli E, Resta L, Nicoletti R, Tartagni M, Marinaccio M, Bulletti C, Colafiglio G. Detection of chronic endometritis at fluid hysteroscopy. *J Minim Invasive Gynecol.* 2005;12(6):514–8.

[52] Pinto V, Matteo M, Tinelli R, Mitola PC, De Ziegler D, Cicinelli E. Altered uterine contractility in women with chronic endometritis. *Fertil Steril.* 2015;103(4):1049–52.

[53] Coughlan C, Ledger W, Wang Q, Liu F, Demirol A, Gurgan T. Recurrent implantation failure: definition and management. *Reprod Biomed Online.* 2014;28(1):14–38.

[54] Török P, Molnár S, Herman T, Jashanjeet S, Lampé R, Riemma G, Vitale SG. Fallopian tubal obstruction is associated with increased pain experienced during office hysteroscopy: a retrospective study. *Updates Surg.* 2020;72(1):213–8.

[55] Cicinelli E, Matteo M, Tinelli R, Pinto V, Marinaccio M, Indraccolo U, De Ziegler D, Resta L. Chronic endometritis due to common bacteria is prevalent in women with recurrent miscarriage as confirmed by improved pregnancy outcome after antibiotic treatment. *Reproductive Sciences.* 2014;21(5):640–7.

[56] Buzzaccarini G, Vitagliano A, Andrisani A, Santarsiero CM, Cicinelli R, Nardelli C, Ambrosini G, Cicinelli E. Chronic endometritis and altered embryo implantation: a unified pathophysiological theory from a literature systematic review. *J Assist Reprod Genet.* 2020;37(12):2897–911.

[57] Vitagliano A, Saccardi C, Noventa M, Di Spiezio Sardo A, Saccone G, Cicinelli E, Pizzi S, Andrisani A, Litta PS. Effects of chronic endometritis therapy on in vitro

fertilization outcome in women with repeated implantation failure: a systematic review and meta-analysis. *Fertil Steril.* 2018;110(1):103-112.e1.
[58] Strandell A, Lindhard A. Why does hydrosalpinx reduce fertility? The importance of hydrosalpinx fluid. *Hum Reprod.* 2002;17(5):1141–5.
[59] Alonso Pacheco L, Carugno J. Chronic Endometritis: Three-dimensional Ultrasound and Hysteroscopy Correlation. *J Minim Invasive Gynecol.* 2020;27(5):993–4.
[60] Prisco MG, Zannoni GF, De Stefano I, Vellone VG, Tortorella L, Fagotti A, Mereu L, Scambia G, Gallo D. Prognostic role of metastasis tumor antigen 1 in patients with ovarian cancer: a clinical study. *Hum Pathol.* 2012;43(2):282–8.
[61] Singh N, Sethi A. Endometritis - Diagnosis,Treatment and its impact on fertility - A Scoping Review. *JBRA Assist Reprod.* 2022;26(3):538–46.
[62] Shah HU, Sannananja B, Baheti AD, Udare AS, Badhe P V. Hysterosalpingography and ultrasonography findings of female genital tuberculosis. *Diagn Interv Radiol.* 2015;21(1):1386–9.
[63] Urman B, Yakin K, Ertas S, Alper E, Aksakal E, Riemma G, Angioni S, Vitale SG. Fertility and anatomical outcomes following hysteroscopic adhesiolysis: An 11-year retrospective cohort study to validate a new classification system for intrauterine adhesions (Urman-Vitale Classification System). *International Journal of Gynecology and Obstetrics*. 2024;165(2):644–54.
[64] Florio P, Puzzutiello R, Filippeschi M, D'Onofrio P, Mereu L, Morelli R, Marianello D, Litta P, Mencaglia L, Petraglia F. Low-dose spinal anesthesia with hyperbaric bupivacaine with intrathecal fentanyl for operative hysteroscopy: a case series study. *J Minim Invasive Gynecol.* 2012;19(1):107–12.
[65] Vitale SG, Angioni S, Saponara S, Sicilia G, Mignacca A, Caiazzo A, De Franciscis P, Riemma G. Hysteroscopic metroplasty and its reproductive impact among the social networks: A cross-sectional analysis on video quality, reliability and creators' opinions on YouTube, TikTok and Instagram. *Int J Med Inform.* 2025;195:105776.
[66] Vitale SG, Laganà AS, Török P, Lasmar RB, Carugno J, Palumbo M, Tesarik J. Virtual sonographic hysteroscopy in assisted reproduction: A retrospective cost-effectiveness analysis. *Int J Gynaecol Obstet.* 2022;156(1):112–8.
[67] Vitale SG. The Biopsy Snake Grasper Sec. VITALE: A New Tool for Office Hysteroscopy. *J Minim Invasive Gynecol.* 2020;27(6):1414–6.
[68] Vitale SG, Laganà AS, Caruso S, Garzon S, Vecchio GM, La Rosa VL, Casarin J, Ghezzi F. Comparison of three biopsy forceps for hysteroscopic endometrial biopsy in postmenopausal patients (HYGREB-1): A multicenter, single-blind randomized clinical trial. *Int J Gynaecol Obstet.* 2021;155(3):425–32.
[69] Cicinelli E, Resta L, Nicoletti R, Zappimbulso V, Tartagni M, Saliani N. Endometrial micropolyps at fluid hysteroscopy suggest the existence of chronic endometritis. *Hum Reprod.* 2005;20(5):1386–9.
[70] Cicinelli E, Vitagliano A, Kumar A, Lasmar RB, Bettocchi S, Haimovich S, Kitaya K, de Ziegler D, Simon C, Moreno I, Andrisani A, Ambrosini G, Bouet PE, Hackem H el, Kushnir VA, Alviggi C, Francescato R, Fascilla F, Vitale SG, Tulandi T, Shrem G, Ferrari A, di Spiezio Sardo A. Unified diagnostic criteria for

chronic endometritis at fluid hysteroscopy: proposal and reliability evaluation through an international randomized-controlled observer study. *Fertil Steril.* 2019;112(1):162-173.e2.

[71] Puente E, Alonso L, Laganà AS, Ghezzi F, Casarin J, Carugno J. Chronic Endometritis: Old Problem, Novel Insights and Future Challenges. *Int J Fertil Steril.* 2020;13(4):250–6.

[72] Marín-Montes A, Azcárraga-Sapena A, Martínez-Massa A, Abril-Pérez J, González-Timoneda A, Cortés-Sierra L. Endometritis crónica y reproducción: revisión de la literatura. *Revista Iberoamericana de Fertilidad y Reproducción Humana.* 2021;38(1).

[73] Pignata S, Ferrandina G, Scarfone G, Scollo P, Odicino F, Cormio G, Katsaros D, Frigerio L, Mereu L, Ghezzi F, Manzione L, Lauria R, Breda E, Alletti DG, Ballardini M, Vernaglia A, Sorio R, Tumolo S, Musso P, Magni G, Pisano C, Morabito A. Poor outcome of elderly patients with platinum-sensitive recurrent ovarian cancer: results from the SOCRATES retrospective study. *Crit Rev Oncol Hematol.* 2009;71(3):233–41.

[74] Palaiologou M, Delladetsima I, Tiniakos D. CD138 (syndecan-1) expression in health and disease. *Histol Histopathol.* 2014;29(2):177–89.

[75] Klimaszyk K, Svarre Nielsen H, Wender-Ozegowska E, Kedzia M. Chronic endometritis - is it time to clarify diagnostic criteria? *Ginekol Pol.* 2023;94(2):152–157.

[76] Kannar V, Lingaiah HK, Sunita V. Evaluation of endometrium for chronic endometritis by using syndecan-1 in abnormal uterine bleeding. *J Lab Physicians.* 2012;4(2):69–73.

[77] McQueen DB, Perfetto CO, Hazard FK, Lathi RB. Pregnancy outcomes in women with chronic endometritis and recurrent pregnancy loss. *Fertil Steril.* 2015;104(4):927–31.

[78] Kitaya K, Yasuo T. Inter-observer and intra-observer variability in immunohistochemical detection of endometrial stromal plasmacytes in chronic endometritis. *Exp Ther Med.* 2013;5(2):485–8.

[79] Cicinelli E, Haimovich S, De Ziegler D, Raz N, Ben-Tzur D, Andrisani A, Ambrosini G, Picardi N, Cataldo V, Balzani M, Cicinelli R, Noventa M, Marin L, Greco P, Resta L, Saccardi C, Buzzaccarini G, Vitagliano A. MUM-1 immunohistochemistry has high accuracy and reliability in the diagnosis of chronic endometritis: a multi-centre comparative study with CD-138 immunostaining. *J Assist Reprod Genet.* 2022;39(1):219.

[80] Achilles SL, Amortegui AJ, Wiesenfeld HC. Endometrial plasma cells: do they indicate subclinical pelvic inflammatory disease? *Sex Transm Dis.* 2005;32(3):185–8.

[81] Greenwood SM, Moran JJ. Chronic endometritis: morphologic and clinical observations. *Obstet Gynecol.* 1981;58(2):176–84.

[82] Santoro A, Travaglino A, Inzani F, Angelico G, Raffone A, Maruotti GM, Straccia P, Arciuolo D, Castri F, D'Alessandris N, Scaglione G, Valente M, Cianfrini F, Masciullo V, Zannoni GF. The Role of Plasma Cells as a Marker of Chronic

Endometritis: A Systematic Review and Meta-Analysis. *Biomedicines.* 2023;11(6):1714.

[83] Hirata K, Kimura F, Nakamura A, Kitazawa J, Morimune A, T H. Histological diagnostic criterion for chronic endometritis based on the clinical outcome. *BMC Womens Health.* 2021;21(1):94.

[84] Vitagliano A, Laganà AS, Ziegler D, Cicinelli R, Santarsiero CM, Buzzaccarini G. Chronic Endometritis in Infertile Women: Impact of Untreated Disease, Plasma Cell Count and Antibiotic Therapy on IVF Outcome-A Systematic Review and Meta-Analysis. *Diagnostics.* 2022;12(9):2250.

[85] Li Y, Xu S, Yu S, Huang C, Lin S, W C. Diagnosis of chronic endometritis: How many CD138+ cells/HPF in endometrial stroma affect pregnancy outcome of infertile women? *Am J Reprod Immunol.* 2021;85(5):e13369.

[86] Song D, Li TC, Zhang Y, Feng X, Xia E, X H. Correlation between hysteroscopy findings and chronic endometritis. *Fertil Steril.* 2019;111(4):772–9.

[87] Pérez-Cejuela BA, Vitale SG, Pérez-Medina T, Rios-Vallejo M, Della Corte L, AR V. Hysteroscopic versus histopathological agreement in the diagnosis of chronic endometritis: results from a retrospective observational study. *Arch Gynecol Obstet.* 2023;308(6):1817–22.

[88] Kitaya K, Yasuo T. Immunohistochemistrical and clinicopathological characterization of chronic endometritis. *Am J Reprod Immunol.* 2011;66(4):410–5.

[89] Bayer-Garner IB, Nickell JA, Korourian S. Routine syndecan-1 immunohistochemistry aids in the diagnosis of chronic endometritis. *Arch Pathol Lab Med.* 2004;128(9):1000–3.

[90] Klimaszyk K, Nielsen HS, Wender-Ozegowska E, Kedzia M. Chronic endometritis - is it time to clarify diagnostic criteria? *Ginekol Pol.* 2023;94(2):152–7.

[91] Khan KN, Fujishita A, Kitajima M, Hiraki K, Nakashima M, Masuzaki H. Intra-uterine microbial colonization and occurrence of endometritis in women with endometriosis. *Hum Reprod.* 2014;29(11):2446–56.

[92] Cicinelli E, De Ziegler D, Nicoletti R, Colafiglio G, Saliani N, Resta L, Rizzi D, De Vito D. Chronic endometritis: correlation among hysteroscopic, histologic, and bacteriologic findings in a prospective trial with 2190 consecutive office hysteroscopies. *Fertil Steril.* 2008;89(3):677–84.

[93] Chen C, Song X, Wei W, Zhong H, Dai J, Z L. The microbiota continuum along the female reproductive tract and its relation to uterine-related diseases. *Nat Commun.* 2017;8(1):875.

[94] Ding T, Schloss PD. Dynamics and associations of microbial community types across the human body. *Nature.* 2014;509(7500):357–60.

[95] Moreno I, Codoñer FM, Vilella F, Valbuena D, Martinez-Blanch JF, Jimenez-Almazán J, Alonso R, Alamá P, Remohí J, Pellicer A, Ramon D, Simon C. Evidence that the endometrial microbiota has an effect on implantation success or failure. *Am J Obstet Gynecol.* 2016;215(6):684–703.

[96] D'Ippolito S, Nicuolo F, Pontecorvi A, Gratta M, Scambia G, Simone N. Endometrial microbes and microbiome: Recent insights on the inflammatory and

immune "players" of the human endometrium. *Am J Reprod Immunol.* 2018;80(6):e13065.

[97] Matteo M, Cicinelli E, Greco P, Massenzio F, Baldini D, T F. Abnormal pattern of lymphocyte subpopulations in the endometrium of infertile women with chronic endometritis. *Am J Reprod Immunol.* 2009;61(5):322–9.

[98] Song D, He Y, Wang Y, Liu Z, Xia E, X H. Impact of antibiotic therapy on the rate of negative test results for chronic endometritis: a prospective randomized control trial. *Fertil Steril.* 2021;115(6):1549–56.

[99] Garcia-Grau I, Simon C, Moreno I, Gardner DK. Uterine microbiome-Low biomass and high expectations. *Biol Reprod.* 2019;101(6):1102–14.

[100] Pirtea P, Cicinelli E, Nola R, Ziegler D, Ayoubi JM. Endometrial causes of recurrent pregnancy losses: endometriosis, adenomyosis, and chronic endometritis. *Fertil Steril.* 2021;115(3):546–60.

[101] Arora R, Rajaram P, Oumachigui A, Arora VK. Prospective analysis of short course chemotherapy in female genital tuberculosis. *Int J Gynaecol Obstet.* 1992;38(4):311–4.

[102] Sharma J, Singh N, Dharmendra S, Singh U, Vanamail P, Kumar S, Hari S, Iyer V, Sharma S. Six months versus nine months anti-tuberculous therapy for female genital tuberculosis: a randomized controlled trial. *Eur J Obstet Gynecol Reprod Biol.* 2016;203:264–73.

[103] Johnston-MacAnanny EB, Hartnett J, Engmann LL, Nulsen JC, Sanders MM, Benadiva CA. Chronic endometritis is a frequent finding in women with recurrent implantation failure after in vitro fertilization. *Fertil Steril.* 2010;93(2):437–41.

[104] Kuroda K, Ishiyama S, Shiobara K, Nakao K, Moriyama A, Kataoka H, Horikawa T, Ojiro Y, Takamizawa S, Nakagawa K, Sugiyama R. Therapeutic efficacy of gentle endometrial curettage on antibiotic-resistant chronic endometritis in infertile women. *Reprod Med Biol.* 2023;22(1):e12525.

[105] van Hoogenhuijze NE, Casarramona GL, Lensen S, Farquhar C, Kamath MS, Kunjummen AT, Raine-Fenning N, Berntsen S, Pinborg A, Mackens S, Inal ZO, Ng EHY, Mak JSM, Narvekar SA, Martins WP, Olesen MS, Torrance HL, Mol BW, Eijkemans MJC, Wang R, Broekmans FJM. Endometrial scratching in women undergoing IVF/ICSI: an individual participant data meta-analysis. *Hum Reprod Update.* 2023;29(6):721–40.

[106] Zhang Y, Xu H, Liu Y, Zheng S, Zhao W, D W. Confirmation of chronic endometritis in repeated implantation failure and success outcome in IVF-ET after intrauterine delivery of the combined administration of antibiotic and dexamethasone. *Am J Reprod Immunol.* 2019;82(5):e13177.

[107] Sfakianoudis K, Simopoulou M, Nitsos N, Lazaros L, Rapani A, Pantou A, Koutsilieris M, Nikas Y, Pantos K. Successful Implantation and Live Birth Following Autologous Platelet-rich Plasma Treatment for a Patient with Recurrent Implantation Failure and Chronic Endometritis. *In Vivo* (Brooklyn). 2019;33(2):515–21.

[108] Woodall J, Tucci M, Mishra A, Benghuzzi H. Cellular effects of platelet rich plasma: A study on HL-60 macrophage-like cells. *Biomed Sci Instrum.* 2007;43:266–71.

Chapter 6

Uterine Synechiae: Cause or Effect?

Salvatore Giovanni Vitale[1,*], MD, PhD
Stefano Di Michele[2], MD
Stefania Saponara[2], MD
Ricardo Bassil Lasmar[3], MD, PhD
Bernardo Portugal Lasmar[4], MD
Luis Alonso Pacheco[5], MD
Péter Török[6], MD, PhD
and Liliana Mereu[1], MD, PhD

[1]Obstetrics and Gynecology Unit, "*Gaspare Rodolico*" University Hospital, Department of General Surgery and Medical Surgical Specialties, University of Catania, Catania, Italy
[2]Division of Gynecology and Obstetrics, Department of Surgical Sciences, University of Cagliari, Cagliari, Italy
[3]Department of Surgery and Specialities, Federal Fluminense University, Rio de Janeiro, Brazil
[4]Maternal-Infant Department, Faculty of Medicine, Fluminense Federal University, UFF, Rio de Janeiro, Brazil
[5]Unidad Histeroscopia, Hospital Quirón, Málaga, Spain
[6]Faculty of Medicine, Institute of Obstetrics and Gynecology, University of Debrecen, Debrecen, Hungary

* Corresponding Author's Email: salvatoreg.vitale@unict.it

In: Endometrium and Related Endouterine Pathologies
Editors: Liliana Mereu and Salvatore Giovanni Vitale
ISBN: 979-8-89530-818-9

Abstract

Uterine synechiae, or intrauterine adhesions (IUA), represent a significant condition in gynecology characterized by the formation of fibrous tissue bands within the uterine cavity. These adhesions often result from endometrial trauma, including uterine surgeries, infections, or pregnancy-related complications. Clinical manifestations range from menstrual irregularities and pelvic pain to infertility and pregnancy complications, such as recurrent miscarriage and abnormal placental development. Diagnosis commonly involves hysteroscopy, transvaginal ultrasound, or hysterosalpingography, with classification systems aiding in severity assessment and treatment planning. The pathophysiology of IUAs is multifaceted, involving impaired endometrial receptivity, implantation failure, and abnormal placentation, which contribute to infertility and adverse reproductive outcomes. Hysteroscopic adhesiolysis remains the gold standard for treatment, enabling precise visualization and dissection of adhesions. However, recurrence rates remain high, necessitating postoperative strategies like anti-adhesion barriers, estrogen therapy, and second-look hysteroscopy to improve outcomes. Emerging techniques, including stem cell therapy and tissue engineering, show promise in preventing recurrence and restoring endometrial functionality. Innovations, such as the Urman-Vitale and Lasmar classifications, offer advanced frameworks for categorizing adhesions and tailoring interventions, enhancing diagnostic and therapeutic precision.

Preventive strategies are crucial in managing IUAs, with mechanical barriers, anti-adhesion agents, and hormonal treatments demonstrating efficacy in reducing recurrence. Further research into regenerative therapies and standardization of surgical protocols is essential to optimize patient care and improve fertility outcomes. This chapter underscores the importance of early diagnosis, personalized treatment, and preventive measures in addressing the complex challenges posed by intrauterine adhesions.

Keywords: intrauterine adhesions, uterine synechiae, hysteroscopy, infertility, adhesiolysis, endometrial regeneration, classification systems, reproductive outcomes

Introduction

Uterine synechiae, also referred to as intrauterine adhesions or Asherman's syndrome, are fibrous bands that partially or completely obliterate the uterine cavity, leading to clinical manifestations such as menstrual irregularities, infertility, and recurrent pregnancy loss [1]. They were first described by Fritsch in 1894 and later characterized in detail by Asherman in 1948 [1, 2]. The most frequent etiopathogenetic factor is trauma to the endometrial basalis, commonly following curettage for retained products of conception, postpartum, or post-abortion [3]. Severe infections (e.g., genital tuberculosis) and iatrogenic causes like hysteroscopic surgeries can also trigger the fibrotic healing response [3, 4]. Given the significant impact on reproductive outcomes, timely recognition and effective management of uterine synechiae are crucial [5].

6.1. Definition and Etiopathogenetic Aspects

Uterine synechiae, commonly called intrauterine adhesions (IUA), involve the formation of fibrous tissue bands within the uterine cavity. Heinrich Fritsch first characterized this condition in 1894, and it was later refined by Joseph Asherman in 1948 [1, 2]. The term "*Asherman's Syndrome*" is specifically applied when these adhesions lead to clinical symptoms such as menstrual irregularities, infertility, or recurrent pregnancy loss [3, 4]. IUA results from trauma to the basal layer of the endometrium, typically following uterine instrumentation or infections. The adhesions may vary in severity from thin, filmy bands to dense fibrous tissue, which can obliterate the uterine cavity partially or entirely [5].

The development of intrauterine synechiae is predominantly linked to mechanical or infectious injury to the endometrial basalis. Common causes include:

- Pregnancy-related trauma, such as post-abortion or postpartum curettage, with incidences reported between 19% and 40% in cases involving retained products of conception [6].
- Iatrogenic causes, including hysteroscopic surgeries, such as myomectomy, septal resection, endometrial ablation [3], or retained or fragmented intrauterine devices [7].
- Infections, notably genital tuberculosis and severe endometritis predispose the endometrium to fibrotic healing [8].

The pathophysiology involves an initial injury that causes endometrial damage, followed by an inflammatory response and subsequent fibroblast proliferation. This culminates in the formation of adhesions that may distort the uterine architecture, causing varying degrees of uterine cavity obliteration and impairing its function [4]. Figures 1 and 2 show different types of intrauterine adhesions.

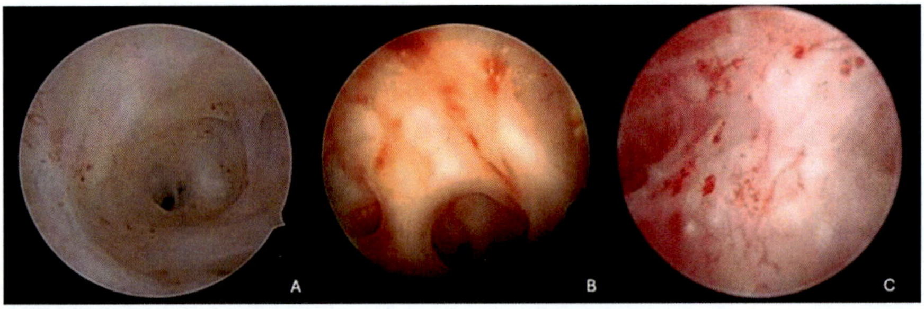

Figure 1. Hysteroscopic view of Intrauterine Adhesions. (A) Mild Adhesions; (B) Moderate Adhesions; (C) Severe Adhesions.

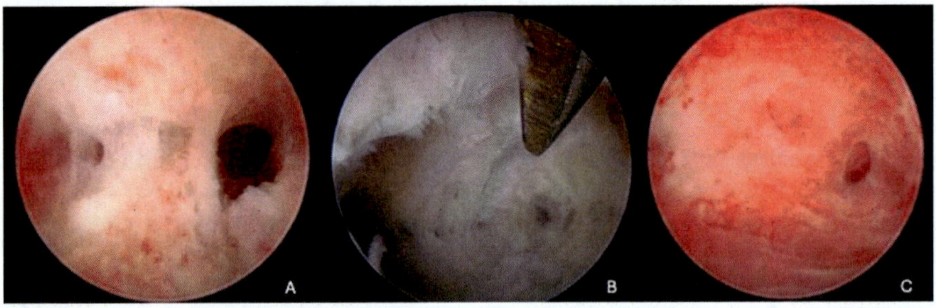

Figure 2. Hysteroscopic view of Intrauterine Adhesions. (A) Filmy Adhesions; (B) Cold scissors hysteroscopic adhesiolysis; (C) Thick Adhesions.

6.2. Comparative Classifications

Numerous classification systems for IUA have been developed to assess their severity and predict clinical outcomes with a practical need so that it can serve as a guide to the prognosis after a treatment, which is linked to the disease severity [9]. These systems are primarily based on hysteroscopic and radiologic findings, though a universally accepted standard is still lacking [10].

6.2.1. March and Israel Classification (1978)

One of the earliest systems, proposed by March and Israel, categorizes IUA into mild, moderate, or severe. Mild adhesions involve less than one-quarter of the uterine cavity, moderate adhesions affect one to three-quarters, and severe adhesions involve more than three-quarters, often with dense fibrous bands. This classification system is still used because it is simple to use and easy to remember. However, it has shortcomings: There is no correlation with clinical symptoms, and post-treatment success was not defined [11].

6.2.2. Hamou Classification (1983)

It has introduced a classification system that went beyond simple hysteroscopic evaluation. It included the extent and histological nature of the adhesions, an assessment of the surrounding glandular endometrium, and the degree of uterine cavity distortion. They described three types of adhesions: endometrial adhesions, which are white and have vascularization similar to the surrounding endometrium; fibrous adhesions, which are transparent, poorly vascularized, and bridge-like; and myometrial adhesions, which are highly vascular and extensive. These characteristics categorized adhesions as mild, moderate, or severe [12].

6.2.3. Valle and Sciarra Classification (1988)

They proposed a classification system emphasizing the correlation between treatment success and disease severity, as measured by improved menstrual patterns and reproductive outcomes. This system considered the extent of endometrial cavity involvement and the type of adhesions present [13].

6.2.4. American Fertility Society Classification (1988)

The American Fertility Society (AFS, 1988) developed one of the most widely accepted classification systems (see Table 1). This system incorporated clinical symptoms, particularly menstrual patterns, as indicators of disease severity. It introduced a scoring method that assigned points to various characteristics, including the extent of cavity obliteration, adhesion type, and menstrual status. Based on the total score, patients were categorized into mild, moderate, or severe stages [14].

Table 1. American Society for reproductive medicine classification of intrauterine adhesions

Patient's name ______		Date ______		Chart______		Chart______	
Age ______	G ______	P ______	Sp Ab ______	VTP ______	Ectopic ______	Infertile yes ______	No ______
Other significant history (i.e., surgery, infection, etc.) ______							
HSG ______		Sonography ______		Photography ______		Laparoscopy ____	Laparotomy ____
Extent of cavity involved	<1/3	1/3–2/3	>2/3				
	1	2	4				
Type of adhesions	Filmy	Filmy and dense	Dense				
	1	2	4				
Menstrual pattern	Normal	Hypomenorrhea	Amenorrhea				
	0	2	4				
Prognostic classification		HSG Score	Hysteroscopy Score	Additional findings			
Stage I (mild)	1–4	____	____	______			
Stage II (moderate)	5–8	____	____	______			
Stage III (severe)	9–12	____	____	______			

6.2.5. European Society of Hysteroscopy (ESH) Classification (1989)

The ESH classification system evaluates adhesions based on type, consistency, and location, assigning grades from I (thin, easily breakable adhesions) to IV (extensive fibrous bands causing complete cavity obliteration) [15].

6.2.6. Donnez and Nisolle classification (1994)

They highlighted the importance of integrating hysterosalpingography (HSG) with hysteroscopic findings. They developed a classification system that divided adhesions into three main groups and six subgroups based on the type of adhesion and the degree of uterine involvement [16].

6.2.7. Nasr Classification (2000)

Nasr and colleagues developed a system incorporating clinical symptoms such as menstrual patterns and reproductive history. They provide a prognosis based on a scoring system: mild (0–4), moderate (5–10), and severe (11–22). This system emphasized the type of adhesions and the visualization of the tubal ostia, with a specific focus on isthmic fibrosis, which was recognized as a separate entity capable of affecting endometrial function and causing amenorrhea [17].

6.2.8. The Urman-Vitale Classification (2024)

The Urman-Vitale Classification is a recent system proposed to evaluate intrauterine adhesions (IUA). As shown in Table 2, this classification aims to improve the prediction of both reproductive and anatomical outcomes following hysteroscopic adhesiolysis. It considers multiple factors, including the extent and density of adhesions, uterine cavity distortion, and healthy endometrial tissue. A retrospective study spanning 11 years validated this classification, highlighting its efficacy in predicting post-adhesiolysis outcomes. Its comprehensive approach allows for more accurate tailoring of therapeutic strategies, thereby optimizing patient care and enhancing fertility outcomes [18].

Table 2. Urman-Vitale classification system for classification of intrauterine adhesions based on symptoms, early follicular phase hysterosalpingography, and a preovulatory or luteal phase 2D/3D ultrasound examination; proposed treatments and prognoses are suggested

	Symptoms	HSG	TV US	Treatment	Prognosis[a]
Class 1	Patients in this group may be amenorrheic (adhesions at the level of the internal os blocking the menstrual blood flow), hypomenorrheic, or eumenorrheic (centrally located adhesions).	Adhesions at the level of the internal cervical os and/or centrally located adhesions sparing the uterine cavity sidewalls and the fundus.	Adhesions at the level of the internal cervical os may give the false impression of a total cavity occlusion. Endometrial stripe in the upper cavity is normal. Centrally located adhesions present with interruption of the endometrial stripe on 2D and 3D ultrasound.	Hysteroscopic adhesiolysis (ultrasound Excellent guidance is advised to prevent opening of a false passage when the adhesions block the cervical canal). Adjuvants are not necessary.	Excellent
Class 2	Patients in this group are usually hypomenorrheic.	Adhesions involving the uterine cavity sidewalls or a dysmorphic uterus appearance (T-shaped or I-shaped) after endometrial trauma.	Endometrial stripe is usually thin. May appear regular or irregular depending on the location of the adhesions.	Hysteroscopic adhesiolysis. Postoperative estrogen treatment and intrauterine adjuvants (balloon, Foley catheter, gel) should be considered. Second-look hysteroscopy[b] may be necessary.	Good
Class 3	Patients in this group are usually hypomenorrheic.	Adhesions involving the upper cavity and the fundal area. One of the corneal areas is occluded with lack of tubal patency.	Endometrial stripe is irregular and usually thin.	Hysteroscopic adhesiolysis under ultrasound guidance. Postoperative estrogen treatment and intrauterine adjuvants (balloon, Foley catheter, gel) should be considered. Second-look hysteroscopy[b] is usually necessary.	Fair

	Symptoms	HSG	TV US	Treatment	Prognosis[a]
Class 4	Patients in this group are usually hypomenorrheic or amenorrheic.	Adhesions involving the upper uterine cavity and the fundus resulting in bilateral cornual occlusion. The cavity is small and constricted. Patients with a pseudoseptum and blocked tubes most commonly ascribed to genital tuberculosis should be regarded in this group.	Endometrial stripe is irregular and usually thin.	Hysteroscopic adhesiolysis under ultrasound guidance. Pre- and postoperative estrogen treatment and intrauterine adjuvants (balloon, Foley catheter, gel) should be considered. Repeat hysteroscopies are always necessary. Consideration should be given to endometrium rejuvenating treatments such as PRP, stem cells etc.	Poor
Class 5	These patients are usually amenorrheic.	Total cavity occlusion. Only the cervical canal below the internal os is visible.	Endometrial stripe is very thin and irregular. May contain hypoechogenic and hyperechogenic islands.	Hysteroscopic adhesiolysis under ultrasound guidance. Pre- and postoperative estrogen treatment and intrauterine adjuvants (balloon, Foley catheter, gel) should be considered. Repeat hysteroscopies are always necessary. Consideration should be given to endometrium rejuvenating treatments such as PRP, stem cells etc.	Poor

Abbreviations: 2D/3D, two-dimensional/three-dimensional; HSG, hysterosalpingography; PR, Pregnancy rate; PRP, platelet-rich plasma; TV-US, transvaginal ultrasound.

[a]Prognosis: Excellent—Postoperative PRs equivalent to what is to be expected in women of similar age and the presence or absence of other infertility factors. Good—Postoperative PRs slightly less than what is to be expected in women of similar age and the presence or absence of other infertility factors. Fair—PRs depend on the extent of remaining adhesions after repeat hysteroscopies; lower than what is to be expected in women of similar age and the presence or absence of other infertility factors; abnormal placentation is common. Poor—Pregnancies are uncommon; miscarriage rates are high; abnormal placentation is common.

[b]A postoperative HSG is recommended to document the extent of cavity restoration.

6.2.9. Lasmar Classification System (2024)

This novel classification system for intrauterine IUA provides an innovative and structured approach to categorizing adhesion sites within the uterine cavity. This system divides the uterus into nine distinct regions, using a "tic-tac-toe" grid for visualization. The upper third includes regions 1 (right cornual), 2 (fundus), and 3 (left cornual); the middle third comprises regions 4 (right lateral), 5 (central), and 6 (left lateral); and the lower third consists of regions 7 (right margin), 8 (internal os), and 9 (left margin). Adhesions are further classified based on tissue type as endometrial (E), fibrotic (F), or myometrial (M), reflecting the depth and nature of tissue involvement. This classification enhances communication among healthcare providers, facilitates personalized surgical planning, and simplifies the documentation of adhesions, enabling tailored interventions such as intrauterine devices (IUDs) or anti-adhesion barriers. Furthermore, its visual and numerical framework aids in patient understanding and allows precise monitoring of outcomes, optimizing management strategies for IUAs. Figure 3 shows this user-friendly system holds promise for improving surgical outcomes and advancing research in adhesion-related fertility management [19].

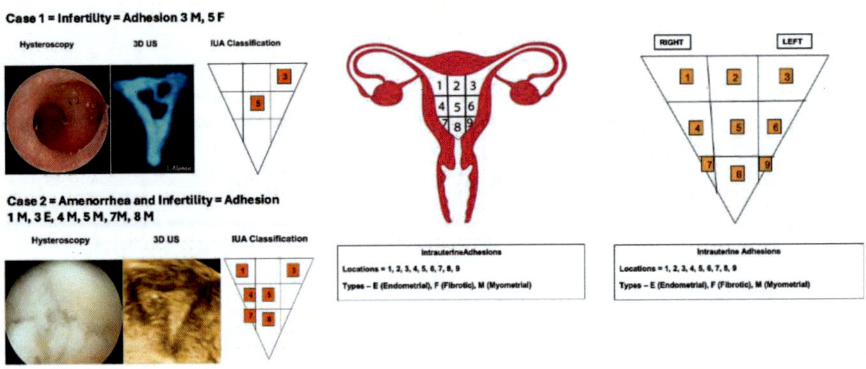

Figure 3. Lasmar Classification System and Practical example of the applicability.

6.3. Clinical Manifestations

IUA may present with a spectrum of clinical manifestations that can significantly impact a woman's reproductive health.

- Menstrual Irregularities: Patients often experience changes in their menstrual cycles, including hypomenorrhea (reduced menstrual flow) or amenorrhea (absence of menstruation). These alterations are frequently associated with the extent and severity of the adhesions [20].
- Pelvic Pain: Some women report pelvic discomfort or dysmenorrhea (painful menstruation), which may be linked to the presence of adhesions within the uterine cavity [21]. Furthermore, infections, particularly those involving resistant pathogens, can exacerbate endometrial inflammation and impair uterine health. Recent studies have highlighted the clinical challenges posed by less common pathogens, such as *Candida nivariensis*, which demonstrate significant antifungal resistance and complicate the management of vulvovaginal infections [22]. Such infections, when untreated, may indirectly influence uterine health by altering the endometrial microenvironment.
- Infertility: IUA is a notable cause of infertility, as adhesions can obstruct the uterine cavity, hindering embryo implantation or increasing the risk of miscarriage [21].
- Pregnancy Complications: Even when conception occurs, women with IUA may face challenges such as recurrent pregnancy loss, preterm delivery, or abnormal placental development, including placenta previa or accreta [23].

It's important to note that some individuals with intrauterine adhesions may remain asymptomatic, with the condition only being discovered during evaluations for infertility or other reproductive issues [24].

Intrauterine adhesions can obscure the endometrial cavity, complicating the diagnosis of coexisting pathologies such as atypical hyperplasia or endometrial carcinoma. Hysteroscopically guided biopsies improve diagnostic accuracy, even in challenging cases where the endometrial architecture is altered [25].

In patients with a history of breast cancer, particularly those treated with tamoxifen, endometrial surveillance is crucial due to the increased risk of developing endometrial pathologies. A recent study demonstrated the utility of a predictive model incorporating hysteroscopic and ultrasonographic findings to improve the early detection of premalignant or malignant endometrial changes, which may also aid in identifying adhesions that obscure diagnostic accuracy [26]. Indeed, ultrasound of the uterus and ovaries is essential in detecting morphological variations in the whole gynecological life, providing insights into reproductive outcomes [27].

6.4. Uterine Synechiae and Infertility

IUA, in its severe form, represents a significant cause of infertility and recurrent pregnancy loss. Therefore, reducing any risk factor associated with forming this disease is fundamental [28].

The pathophysiology of infertility in IUA involves multiple interconnected mechanisms:

1) Sperm Transport Impairment: IUAs can distort the cervical canal and uterine cavity, impairing sperm transport. Reducing endometrial and cervical mucus quality further hinders sperm migration, reducing the likelihood of successful fertilization [21]. Additionally, chronic inflammation is increasingly recognized as contributing to endometrial dysfunction in IUA. Elevated pro-inflammatory cytokines such as IL-6 and IL-8 are frequently observed in conditions like polycystic ovary syndrome (PCOS), which shares overlapping inflammatory pathways with IUA. A randomized trial demonstrated that treatments targeting these cytokines, such as metformin or pioglitazone, can significantly reduce systemic inflammation and improve metabolic profiles in PCOS patients [29]. These findings underscore the critical role of inflammation in impairing endometrial receptivity and fertility.
2) Endometrial Receptivity Deficiency: The endometrium in patients with IUAs is often characterized by fibrosis and an atrophic, avascular structure. These changes impair its ability to respond to hormonal stimulation and hinder the cyclical regeneration required for successful implantation. A thin endometrium, commonly observed in these patients, correlates with lower implantation rates and higher miscarriage rates [30].
3) Implantation Failure: Adequate endometrial receptivity and uterine contractility are crucial for embryo implantation. IUAs alter uterine contractile patterns and disrupt the molecular dialog between the embryo and endometrium, which is critical for implantation success [31, 32].

4) Placentation Disorders: Abnormal placental implantation, such as placenta accreta, is more common in women with IUAs. This is attributed to deficient decidualization and abnormal trophoblastic invasion, which can lead to severe obstetric complications, including postpartum hemorrhage [33].

Virtual sonographic hysteroscopy (VSH) has proven effective in identifying intrauterine pathologies, including adhesions, which can compromise uterine receptivity. By detecting and addressing these anomalies before assisted reproductive treatments, VSH may improve pregnancy outcomes, highlighting its potential role in the management and prevention of recurrent intrauterine adhesions in high-risk populations [34].

Even after surgical adhesiolysis, reproductive outcomes in women with IUAs remain suboptimal compared to the general population. Studies indicate that while adhesiolysis improves menstrual and fertility outcomes, a substantial proportion of patients continue to experience infertility or recurrent pregnancy loss due to persistent or recurrent adhesions [3].

Understanding the multifaceted impact of IUAs on fertility underscores the importance of preventive measures during uterine surgeries, early diagnosis, and effective management strategies. Hysteroscopic adhesiolysis remains the gold standard for treatment, but the high recurrence rate of adhesions postoperatively necessitates the development of advanced preventive and regenerative therapies [35].

IUAs pose a significant challenge in reproductive medicine, with complex mechanisms impairing fertility. Advancements in diagnostic and therapeutic approaches are essential to improve reproductive outcomes and mitigate the long-term impacts of this condition.

6.5. Treatment and Restoration of Uterine Functionality

Treatment strategies largely depend on the gynecologist's experience and are tailored to each patient's needs. Historically, the management of intrauterine adhesions involved blind adhesiolysis, a technique that lacked adequate visualization of the adhesions and could lead to frequent potential risks. Surgery has been the criterion standard in managing Asherman syndrome; however, no RCTs compare surgical intervention and expectant management, nor are there RCTs comparing different methods of surgical interventions for Asherman syndrome. The limited data supporting a role for expectant management published many decades ago demonstrated the resumption of menstruation in as many as 78% within 7 years from diagnosis of IUAs and pregnancy in 45.5% of women [32].

Dilation and curettage or cervical probing have been used with or without ultrasound guidance before the widespread use of hysteroscopy. Hysteroscopic treatment enables the lysis of IUAs to be performed under direct vision and magnification. On the other hand, mild adhesions may be separated during hysteroscopy due to the effect of the distension medium; the tip of the hysteroscope can also be used to separate the adhesions gently [36]. The more lateral the adhesions are and the greater their density, the more complex the dissection is and the greater the risk of complications such as uterine perforation [36, 37]. While some gynecologists prefer using hysteroscopic scissors for adhesiolysis due to their lower risk of endometrial injury, others advocate for the use of monopolar or bipolar energy sources despite their higher risk of damaging the remaining endometrium [38, 39]. Different techniques used to lyse adhesions under direct vision have been described, including Monopolar [13, 40], bipolar [41, 42], and the NdYAG laser electrosurgical instruments [43], with the advantages of precise cutting and good hemostasis. In minimally invasive surgery settings, using various types of energy has shown significant benefits in reducing tissue damage and improving reproductive outcomes [44]. Disadvantages include potential visceral damage if uterine perforation occurs [9], further endometrial damage predisposing to recurrence of IUAs [45], cost, and the degree of cervical dilation required to accommodate operative instruments. None of these techniques have been compared; consequently, there is no evidence that one method is superior. Additional Guiding Techniques for Hysteroscopy Fluoroscopically guided blunt dissection of severe adhesions has been described using a hysteroscopically directed Tuohy needle under image intensifier control with the patient under general anesthesia [46]. This technique is no longer used, is costly, exposes the patient to ionizing radiation, and is technically challenging.

Laparoscopic guidance is reported to aid hysteroscopically directed division of severe IUAs and enable concurrent inspection of the pelvic organs, but its practical use faces higher operative time and costs [23]. Intervention may not be necessary in asymptomatic patients who are not seeking to conceive [32]. The primary goal of treatment is to restore the normal anatomy of the uterine cavity while implementing measures to prevent the recurrence of adhesions. In cases involving severe and dense adhesions, the risk of creating a false passage is heightened, and such procedures are best performed under ultrasonographic guidance [47]. Restoration of uterine functionality often mirrors outcomes observed in other pelvic surgeries. For instance, transvaginal bilateral sacrospinous fixation for recurrent vaginal vault prolapse has proven effective not only in anatomical restoration but also in significantly improving patients' quality of life and sexual well-being. These outcomes underline the importance of personalized approaches in gynecological surgery to address both physical and psychosocial aspects of recovery [48].

A key element of hysteroscopic treatment is minimal invasiveness; reducing the diameter of new instruments allows lower cervical dilatation, limiting operative time and complications [49]. Moreover, the use of new technologies applied in the gynecology field concerning different kinds of available energy sources [50], like diode lasers, boosts the preciseness and safety of hysteroscopic treatment in a way that has never been seen before [51].

Anesthesia plays a pivotal role in operative hysteroscopy, ensuring patient comfort and facilitating the completion of complex intrauterine procedures. Various factors influence the choice of anesthetic technique, including the type of intervention, patient comorbidities, and the setting where the procedure is performed (office-based vs. inpatient) [52].

For minor procedures such as diagnostic hysteroscopy or polypectomy, local anesthesia or minimal sedation may suffice. However, more extensive interventions, including myomectomy or adhesiolysis, often require regional or general anesthesia to provide adequate pain control and immobilization [49].

Recently, there has been a growing interest in optimizing anesthetic protocols to reduce perioperative risks and enhance patient recovery. Techniques such as low-dose spinal anesthesia have emerged as promising options, particularly for patients at high surgical risk [53].

On some occasions, IUA can be incidentally diagnosed in postmenopausal women presenting with abnormal uterine bleeding or endometrial thickening enrolled for endometrial biopsy. The presence of adhesions, especially in nulliparous patients, may lead to painful procedures. Therefore, it is fundamental to use proper and efficient instruments to facilitate adhesiolysis and endometrial biopsy as quickly as possible [54, 55].

In fertile women, hysteroscopic procedures are best performed when the endometrium is thin because the operating time is lessened and fluid absorption decreases, making surgery easier. Therefore, in this population, endometrial preparation before undergoing hysteroscopy is highly recommended, with a vast choice of drugs that can be used [56, 57].

Regarding infertility, office hysteroscopy is a feasible and highly effective diagnostic and therapeutic procedure for cervical-isthmic and intrauterine adhesions, as well as for small polyps, allowing the resolution of female infertility related to these pathologies without trauma and with only minimal discomfort [58].

Among its many uses, hysteroscopy seems to be an efficient method of removing retained products of conception in a single surgical step. It has low complication rates and subsequent fecundity restoration, with appropriate clinical pregnancy and live birth rates [59].

Hysteroscopists need to ease and act as painlessly as possible during any office hysteroscopy exam; for instance, knowing any potential tubal patency of the treated woman and its higher associated pain during the exam may guide the gynecologist to use milder intrauterine pressure of fluid distention medium to reduce discomfort [60].

6.6. Prevention of Recurrences: The Real Solution

Preventing the recurrence of IUA after treatment is critical to managing this condition. Despite successful hysteroscopic adhesiolysis, recurrence rates remain high, emphasizing the need for effective preventive strategies [61]. Several approaches have been developed to address this challenge, combining surgical precision with innovative postoperative care.

6.6.1. Mechanical Barriers and Anti-Adhesion Agents

Mechanical barriers, such as intrauterine balloons and devices (IUDs), have prevented adhesion reformation [62]. In addition, advanced surgical materials have shown promise in reducing adhesion recurrence. For instance, biocompatible grafts, such as porcine dermis, used primarily in repairing severe cystoceles, have improved anatomical outcomes and patients' quality of life, suggesting potential applicability in intrauterine procedures [63].

These devices help maintain uterine cavity patency during the healing phase. Anti-adhesion agents, particularly those based on cross-linked hyaluronic acid, provide additional protection by creating a temporary barrier over the endometrium. A recent network meta-analysis of randomized controlled trials evaluated various postsurgical barrier strategies to prevent the recurrence of intrauterine adhesions (IUA) after hysteroscopic adhesiolysis.

The study identified that using cross-linked hyaluronic acid gel, with or without a copper intrauterine device, was among the most effective methods in reducing adhesion recurrence and improving fertility outcomes [64].

Estrogen therapy significantly promotes endometrial regeneration and reduces the likelihood of postoperative adhesion recurrence. This hormonal approach enhances endometrial thickness and vascularity, fostering a conducive environment for tissue repair [65].

Second-look hysteroscopy is recommended within weeks after the initial adhesiolysis to evaluate the uterine cavity and remove any residual adhesions. This practice has been associated with improved reproductive outcomes by enabling early intervention and preventing the consolidation of new adhesions [66].

Emerging methods such as stem cell therapy and tissue engineering hold promise for more robust prevention of IUA. These techniques aim to regenerate endometrial tissue, providing a long-term solution to adhesion formation. Stem cell therapy has shown promising results in animal and human models. Exogenous and endogenous stem cells, gene modulation, and intrauterine stents are some of the units of stem cell therapy [67].

Endometrial surveillance plays a critical role in preventing malignancies in high-risk populations. A recent systematic review demonstrated that using lower endometrial thickness thresholds for biopsy increases the sensitivity of detecting atypical hyperplasia and carcinoma, which is crucial in recurrent intrauterine adhesions [47].

Patient perception and understanding of hysteroscopic procedures, including those aimed at diagnosing or treating intrauterine adhesions, can significantly influence procedural outcomes. A recent analysis of TikTok videos revealed that misinformation is prevalent, particularly in content created by non-healthcare professionals. This can potentially exacerbate patient anxiety and distrust toward gynecologists [68, 69].

Advances in every minimally invasive surgery field can be an inspirational model for developing innovative and standardized treatment strategies in complex gynecological conditions [70]. Combining these strategies in a comprehensive approach minimizes recurrence rates and improves the overall prognosis for patients with IUA. Further research is essential to refine these methods and establish standardized protocols for optimal care.

Conclusion

Despite advancements in hysteroscopic adhesiolysis, currently the gold standard for treating intrauterine adhesions, recurrence remains a significant concern [3, 9, 21]. Multiple preventive measures, including the use of anti-adhesion barriers, estrogen therapy, and second-look hysteroscopy, have demonstrated efficacy in reducing re-adhesion and improving fertility outcomes [9, 32, 57]. Moreover, regenerative approaches like stem cell therapy may enhance endometrial restoration and long-term reproductive success. Overall, an integrated strategy focusing on early detection, minimally invasive treatment, and robust postoperative interventions is essential for optimizing uterine function and reproductive results in women affected by intrauterine adhesions [21, 32, 57].

References

[1] Asherman JG. Amenorrhoea traumatica (atretica). *J Obstet Gynaecol Br Emp.* 1948;55(1):23–30.

[2] Asherman JG. Traumatic intra-uterine adhesions. *J Obstet Gynaecol Br Emp.* 1950;57(6):892–6.

[3] Yu D, Wong YM, Cheong Y, Xia E, Li TC. Asherman syndrome--one century later. *Fertil Steril.* 2008;89(4):759–79.

[4] Taskin O, Sadik S, Onoglu A, Gokdeniz R, Erturan E, Burak F, Wheeler JM. Role of endometrial suppression on the frequency of intrauterine adhesions after resectoscopic surgery. *J Am Assoc Gynecol Laparosc.* 2000;7(3):351–4.

[5] Matevossian K, Cholkeri A. Uterine Synechiae and Postoperative Care. In: Tandulwadkar S, Pal B, editors. *Hysteroscopy Simplified by Masters.* Singapore: Springer; 2021. p. 133–9.

[6] Westendorp IC, Ankum WM, Mol BW, Vonk J. Prevalence of Asherman's syndrome after secondary removal of placental remnants or a repeat curettage for incomplete abortion. *Hum Reprod Oxf Engl.* 1998;13(12):3347–50.

[7] Vitale SG, Di Spiezio Sardo A, Riemma G, De Franciscis P, Alonso Pacheco L, Carugno J. In-office hysteroscopic removal of retained or fragmented intrauterine device without anesthesia: a cross-sectional analysis of an international survey. *Updat Surg.* 2022;74(3):1079–85.

[8] Conforti A, Alviggi C, Mollo A, De Placido G, Magos A. The management of Asherman syndrome: a review of literature. *Reprod Biol Endocrinol RBE.* 2013;11:118.

[9] Magos A. Hysteroscopic treatment of Asherman's syndrome. *Reprod Biomed Online.* 2002;4 Suppl 3:46–51.

[10] March CM. Management of Asherman's syndrome. *Reprod Biomed Online.* 2011;23(1):63–76.

[11] March CM, Israel R, March AD. Hysteroscopic management of intrauterine adhesions. *Am J Obstet Gynecol.* 1978;130(6):653–7.

[12] Hamou J, Salat-Baroux J, Siegler AM. Diagnosis and treatment of intrauterine adhesions by microhysteroscopy. *Fertil Steril.* 1983;39(3):321–6.

[13] Valle RF, Sciarra JJ. Intrauterine adhesions: hysteroscopic diagnosis, classification, treatment, and reproductive outcome. *Am J Obstet Gynecol.* 1988;158(6 Pt 1):1459–70.

[14] The American Fertility Society classifications of adnexal adhesions, distal tubal occlusion, tubal occlusion secondary to tubal ligation, tubal pregnancies, müllerian anomalies and intrauterine adhesions. *Fertil Steril.* 1988;49(6):944–55.

[15] Manchanda R, Rathore A. Intrauterine Adhesions: Classification Systems. In: Manchanda R, editor. *Intra Uterine Adhesions: Diagnostic and Therapeutic Insight.* Singapore: Springer; 2021. p. 21–32.

[16] Donnez J, Nisolle M. Hysteroscopic lysis of intrauterine adhesions (Asherman's syndrome). editor. *Atlas of Laser Operative Laparoscopy and Hysteroscopy.* Press-Parthenon; New York, NY, USA: 1994. pp. 305–322.

[17] Nasr AL, Al-Inany HG, Thabet SM, Aboulghar M. A clinicohysteroscopic scoring system of intrauterine adhesions. *Gynecol Obstet Invest.* 2000;50(3):178–81.

[18] Urman B, Yakin K, Ertas S, Alper E, Aksakal E, Riemma G, Angioni S, Vitale SG. Fertility and anatomical outcomes following hysteroscopic adhesiolysis: An 11-year retrospective cohort study to validate a new classification system for intrauterine adhesions (Urman-Vitale Classification System). *Int J Gynaecol Obstet Off Organ Int Fed Gynaecol Obstet.* 2024;165(2):644–54.

[19] Lasmar RB, Lasmar BP, Haimovich S, Pacheco LA, Moawad NS. Proposal for a new classification of intrauterine adhesions by sites. *Int J Gynaecol Obstet.* 2025;169(1):9-14.

[20] Leung RKK, Lin Y, Liu Y. Recent Advances in Understandings Towards Pathogenesis and Treatment for Intrauterine Adhesion and Disruptive Insights from Single-Cell Analysis. *Reprod Sci.* 2021;28(7):1812–26.

[21] Hooker AB, Leeuw RA de, Emanuel MH, Mijatovic V, Brolmann HAM, Huirne JA. The link between intrauterine adhesions and impaired reproductive performance: a systematic review of the literature. *BMC Pregnancy Childbirth.* 2022;22:837.

[22] Shi Y, Zhu Y, Fan S, Vitagliano A, Liu X, Liao Y, Liang Y, Vitale SG. Clinical Characteristics and Antifungal Susceptibility of Candida nivariensis from Vulvovaginal Candidiasis. *Gynecol Obstet Invest.* 2020;85(1):88–93.

[23] AAGL Elevating Gynecologic Surgery. AAGL practice report: practice guidelines on intrauterine adhesions developed in collaboration with the European Society of Gynaecological Endoscopy (ESGE). *Gynecol Surg.* 2017;14(1):6.

[24] Lee WL, Liu CH, Cheng M, Chang WH, Liu WM, Wang PH. Focus on the Primary Prevention of Intrauterine Adhesions: Current Concept and Vision. *Int J Mol Sci.* 2021;22(10):5175.

[25] Garuti G, Angioni S, Mereu L, Calzolari S, Mannini L, Scrimin F, Casadio P, De Alberti D, Nappi L, Busato E, Leone FPG, Perrini G, Cela V, Luerti M. Hysteroscopic view with targeted biopsy in the assessment of endometrial carcinoma. What is the rate of underestimatated diagnosis? The results of a multicenter Italian trial. *Gynecol Surg.* 2020;17(1):10.

[26] Vitale SG, Angioni S, D'Alterio MN, Ronsini C, Saponara S, De Franciscis P, Riemma G. Risk of endometrial malignancy in women treated for breast cancer: the BLUSH prediction model - evidence from a comprehensive multicentric retrospective cohort study. *Climacteric.* 2024;27(5):482–8.

[27] Fulghesu AM, Di Michele S, Zangaris I, Cordella M, Pittui E, Scalise G, Vitale SG, Angioni S. Clinical and Ultrasound Features of Normocyclic Non-Hyperandrogenic Adolescents in Early Gynecological Life. *Gynecol Obstet Invest.* 2024;1–9.

[28] Hooker AB, Lemmers M, Thurkow AL, Heymans MW, Opmeer BC, Brölmann HAM, Mol BW, Huirne JAF. Systematic review and meta-analysis of intrauterine adhesions after miscarriage: prevalence, risk factors and long-term reproductive outcome. *Hum Reprod* Update. 2014;20(2):262–78.

[29] Ali DES, Shah M, Ali A, Malik MO, Rehman F, Badshah H, Ehtesham E, Vitale S G. Treatment with Metformin and Combination of Metformin Plus Pioglitazone on Serum Levels of IL-6 and IL-8 in Polycystic Ovary Syndrome: A Randomized Clinical Trial. *Horm Metab.* 2019;51(11):714–22.

[30] Malhotra N, Bahadur A, Kalaivani M, Mittal S. Changes in endometrial receptivity in women with Asherman's syndrome undergoing hysteroscopic adhesiolysis. *Arch Gynecol Obstet.* 2012;286(2):525–30.

[31] Fukuda M, Fukuda K. Uterine endometrial cavity movement and cervical mucus. *Hum Reprod Oxf Engl.* 1994;9(6):1013–6.

[32] Schenker JG, Margalioth EJ. Intrauterine adhesions: an updated appraisal. *Fertil Steril.* 1982;37(5):593–610.

[33] Capella-Allouc S, Morsad F, Rongières-Bertrand C, Taylor S, Fernandez H. Hysteroscopic treatment of severe Asherman's syndrome and subsequent fertility. *Hum Reprod Oxf Engl*. 1999;14(5):1230–3.

[34] Vitale SG, Laganà AS, Török P, Lasmar RB, Carugno J, Palumbo M, Tesarik J. Virtual sonographic hysteroscopy in assisted reproduction: A retrospective cost-effectiveness analysis. *Int J Gynaecol Obstet.* 2022;156(1):112–8.

[35] Hooker AB, de Leeuw RA, Twisk JWR, Brölmann HAM, Huirne JAF. Reproductive performance of women with and without intrauterine adhesions following recurrent dilatation and curettage for miscarriage: long-term follow-up of a randomized controlled trial. *Hum Reprod Oxf Engl.* 2021;36(1):70–81.

[36] Sugimoto O. Diagnostic and therapeutic hysteroscopy for traumatic intrauterine adhesions. *Am J Obstet Gynecol.* 1978;131(5):539–47.

[37] Deans R, Abbott J. Review of intrauterine adhesions. *J Minim Invasive Gynecol.* 2010;17(5):555–69.

[38] Cararach M, Penella J, Ubeda A, Labastida R. Hysteroscopic incision of the septate uterus: scissors versus resectoscope. *Hum Reprod Oxf Engl.* 1994;9(1):87–9.

[39] Kodaman PH, Arici A. Intra-uterine adhesions and fertility outcome: how to optimize success? *Curr Opin Obstet Gynecol.* 2007;19(3):207–14.

[40] Pabuçcu R, Atay V, Orhon E, Urman B, Ergün A. Hysteroscopic treatment of intrauterine adhesions is safe and effective in restoring normal menstruation and fertility. *Fertil Steril.* 1997;68(6):1141–3.

[41] Touboul C, Fernandez H, Deffieux X, Berry R, Frydman R, Gervaise A. Uterine synechiae after bipolar hysteroscopic resection of submucosal myomas in patients with infertility. *Fertil Steril.* 2009;92(5):1690–3.

[42] Fernandez H, Gervaise A, de Tayrac R. Operative hysteroscopy for infertility using normal saline solution and a coaxial bipolar electrode: a pilot study. *Hum Reprod Oxf Engl.* 2000;15(8):1773–5.

[43] Newton JR, MacKenzie WE, Emens MJ, Jordan JA. Division of uterine adhesions (Asherman's syndrome) with the Nd-YAG laser. *Br J Obstet Gynaecol.* 1989;96(1):102–4.

[44] Di Michele S, Bramante S, Angioni S, Bernassola M, De Vita T, Iaccarino DA, Giannoni L, Rosati M. Superficial Peritoneal Endometriosis Vaporization Using a CO2 Laser: A Long-Term Single-Center Experience. *J Clin Med.* 2024;13(6):1722.

[45] Roge P, D'Ercole C, Cravello L, Boubli L, Blanc B. Hysteroscopic management of uterine synechiae: a series of 102 observations. *Eur J Obstet Gynecol Reprod Biol.* 1996;65(2):189–93.

[46] Broome JD, Vancaillie TG. Fluoroscopically guided hysteroscopic division of adhesions in severe Asherman syndrome. *Obstet Gynecol.* 1999;93(6):1041–3.

[47] Vitale SG, Riemma G, Haimovich S, Carugno J, Alonso Pacheco L, Perez-Medina T, Parry JP, Török P, Tesarik J, Della Corte L, Corbellis L, Di Spiezio Sardo A, De Franciscis P. Risk of endometrial cancer in asymptomatic postmenopausal women in relation to ultrasonographic endometrial thickness: systematic review and diagnostic test accuracy meta-analysis. *Am J Obstet Gynecol.* 2023;228(1):22-35.e2.

[48] Vitale SG, Laganà AS, Noventa M, Giampaolino P, Zizolfi B, Butticè S, La Rosa VL, Gullo G, Rossetti D. Transvaginal Bilateral Sacrospinous Fixation after Second Recurrence of Vaginal Vault Prolapse: Efficacy and Impact on Quality of Life and Sexuality. *BioMed Res Int.* 2018;2018:5727165.

[49] Mencaglia L, Carri G, Prasciolu C, Giunta G, Albis Florez ED, Cofelice V, Mereu L. Feasibility and complications in bipolar resectoscopy: preliminary experience. *Minim Invasive Ther Allied Technol.* 2013;22(1):50–5.

[50] Vitale SG, Saponara S, Succu AG, Sicilia G, Martsidis K, D'Alterio MN, Angioni S. Efficacy and Safety of Non-Ablative Dual Wavelength Diode Laser Therapy for Genitourinary Syndrome of Menopause: A Single-Center Prospective Study. *Adv Ther.* 2024;41(12):4617–27.

[51] Vitale SG, Moore O, Riemma G, Carugno J, Yarto ML, Haimovich S. Hysteroscopic laser ablation of symptomatic uterine fibroids: insights from a prospective study. Climacteric. 2023;26(5):497–502.

[52] Cicinelli E. Hysteroscopy without anesthesia: review of recent literature. *J Minim Invasive Gynecol.* 2010;17(6):703–8.

[53] Florio P, Puzzutiello R, Filippeschi M, D'Onofrio P, Mereu L, Morelli R, Marianello D, Litta P, Mencaglia L, Petraglia F. Low-dose spinal anesthesia with hyperbaric bupivacaine with intrathecal fentanyl for operative hysteroscopy: a case series study. *J Minim Invasive Gynecol.* 2012;19(1):107–12.

[54] Vitale SG, Laganà AS, Caruso S, Garzon S, Vecchio GM, La Rosa VL, Casarin J, Ghezzi F. Comparison of three biopsy forceps for hysteroscopic endometrial biopsy in postmenopausal patients (HYGREB-1): A multicenter, single-blind randomized clinical trial. *Int J Gynaecol Obstet.* 2021;155(3):425–32.

[55] Vitale SG. The Biopsy Snake Grasper Sec. VITALE: A New Tool for Office Hysteroscopy. *J Minim Invasive Gynecol.* 2020;27(6):1414–6.

[56] Mereu L, Giunta G, Carri G, Prasciolu C, Albis Florez ED, Mencaglia L. Nomegestrol acetate versus combined oral contraceptive as rapid endometrial preparation for operative hysteroscopy: a prospective randomised pilot study. *Gynecol Surg.* 2012;9(4):401–4.

[57] Florio P, Filippeschi M, Imperatore A, Mereu L, Franchini M, Calzolari S, Mencaglia L, Litta P. The practicability and surgeons' subjective experiences with vaginal danazol before an operative hysteroscopy. *Steroids.* 2012;77(5):528–33.

[58] Chiofalo B, Palmara V, Vilos GA, Pacheco LA, Lasmar RB, Shawki O, Giacobbe V, Alibrandi A, Di Guardo F, Vitale SG. Reproductive outcomes of infertile women undergoing "see and treat" office hysteroscopy: a retrospective observational study. *Minim Invasive Ther Allied Technol.* 2021;30(3):147–53.

[59] Vitale SG, Parry JP, Carugno J, Cholkeri-Singh A, Della Corte L, Cianci S, Schiattarella A, Riemma G, De Franciscis P. Surgical and Reproductive Outcomes after Hysteroscopic Removal of Retained Products of Conception: A Systematic Review and Meta-analysis. *J Minim Invasive Gynecol.* 2021;28(2):204–17.

[60] Török P, Molnár S, Herman T, Jashanjeet S, Lampé R, Riemma G, Vitale SG. Fallopian tubal obstruction is associated with increased pain experienced during office hysteroscopy: a retrospective study. *Updat Surg.* 2020;72(1):213–8.

[61] Yang JH, Chen CD, Chen SU, Yang YS, Chen MJ. The influence of the location and extent of intrauterine adhesions on recurrence after hysteroscopic adhesiolysis. *BJOG Int J Obstet Gynaecol.* 2016;123(4):618–23.

[62] Yang X, Liu Y, Li TC, Xia E, Xiao Y, Zhou F, Song D, Zhou Q. Durations of intrauterine balloon therapy and adhesion reformation after hysteroscopic adhesiolysis: a randomized controlled trial. *Reprod Biomed Online.* 2020;40(4):539–46.

[63] Vitale SG, Caruso S, Rapisarda AMC, Valenti G, Rossetti D, Cianci S, Cianci A. Biocompatible porcine dermis graft to treat severe cystocele: impact on quality of life and sexuality. *Arch Gynecol Obstet.* 2016;293(1):125–31.

[64] Vitale SG, Riemma G, Carugno J, Perez-Medina T, Alonso Pacheco L, Haimovich S, Parry JP, Di Spiezio Sardo A, De Franciscis P. Postsurgical barrier strategies to avoid the recurrence of intrauterine adhesion formation after hysteroscopic adhesiolysis: a network meta-analysis of randomized controlled trials. *Am J Obstet Gynecol.* 2022;226(4):487-498.e8.

[65] Feng L, Sun Y, Zhang S, Qian Y, Fang S, Yang B, Xu L, Li Y, Niu Y, Zhang L, Chen J. A novel intrauterine estrogen-releasing system for preventing the postoperative recurrence of intrauterine adhesion: a multicenter randomized controlled study. *BMC Med.* 2024;22(1):395.

[66] Sebbag L, Even M, Fay S, Naoura I, Revaux A, Carbonnel M, Pirtea P, de Ziegler D, Ayoubi JM. Early Second-Look Hysteroscopy: Prevention and Treatment of Intrauterine Post-surgical Adhesions. *Front Surg.* 2019;6:50.

[67] Parashar S, Pajai S, Tarang T. Recent Advancement in the Management of Intrauterine Adhesions Using Stem Cell Therapy: A Review Article. *Cureus.* 2023;15(8):e43553.

[68] Vitale SG, Angioni S, Saponara S, Sicilia G, Etrusco A, D'Alterio MN, Cobellis L, De Franciscis P, Riemma G. TikTok as a platform for hysteroscopy information: An analytical video-based cross-sectional study to assess quality, reliability, and accuracy. *Int J Gynecol Obstet.* 2025;168(1):353-361.

[69] Vitale SG, Angioni S, Saponara S, Sicilia G, Mignacca A, Caiazzo A, De Franciscis P, Riemma G. Hysteroscopic metroplasty and its reproductive impact among the social networks: A cross-sectional analysis on video quality, reliability and creators' opinions on YouTube, TikTok and Instagram. *Int J Med Inf.* 2024;195:105776.

[70] Di Michele S, Bramante S, Rosati M. A Systematic Review of Ureteral Reimplantation Techniques in Endometriosis: Laparoscopic Versus Robotic-Assisted Approach. *J Clin Med.* 2024;13(19):5677.

Chapter 7

Endometrial Hyperplasia

Ozge Kahramanoglu[1,*], MD, PhD
Stefania Saponara[2], MD
and Ilker Kahramanoglu[3], MD, PhD
[1]Department of Obstetrics and Gynecology, Sancaktepe Sehit Prof. Dr. Ilhan Varank Research and Training Hospital, Istanbul, Turkey
[2]Division of Gynecology and Obstetrics, Department of Surgical Sciences, University of Cagliari, Cagliari, Italy
[3]Department of Gynecologic Oncology, Biruni University Medical School, Istanbul, Turkey

Abstract

Endometrial hyperplasia (EH) is a significant pathological condition characterized by abnormal proliferation of the endometrial glands, driven primarily by prolonged exposure to unopposed estrogen. As a precursor lesion for endometrial cancer, EH occupies a critical position in gynecological practice, necessitating timely diagnosis, risk stratification, and appropriate management. With an increasing prevalence influenced by rising rates of obesity and metabolic disorders, the importance of understanding EH's pathogenesis, clinical presentation, diagnostic pathways, and therapeutic strategies cannot be overstated. Advances in diagnostic modalities, including hysteroscopy and molecular markers, as well as evolving guidelines for conservative and definitive management, have transformed the care landscape for women with EH. This chapter aims to provide a comprehensive overview of the epidemiology, risk factors, diagnostic limitations, and current international management strategies, while emphasizing the role of combined conservative

* Corresponding Author's Email: ilkerkahramanoglu@gmail.com

In: Endometrium and Related Endouterine Pathologies
Editors: Liliana Mereu and Salvatore Giovanni Vitale
ISBN: 979-8-89530-818-9

therapies, particularly hysteroscopy, in addressing patients' clinical and reproductive needs.

Keywords: endometrial hyperplasia, hysteroscopy, endometrial cancer, atypical hyperplasia

Introduction

Endometrial hyperplasia (EH) represents a critical pathological condition in gynecological practice, defined by the aberrant proliferation of endometrial glands relative to the stromal component, primarily driven by sustained exposure to unopposed estrogen. Recognized as a precursor lesion to endometrial carcinoma, EH warrants rigorous diagnostic evaluation, stratified risk assessment, and evidence-based therapeutic intervention [1].

The increasing global prevalence of EH, influenced by rising rates of obesity and associated metabolic disorders, underscores the importance of a nuanced understanding of its pathogenesis, clinical presentation, diagnostic methodologies, and management paradigms. Advances in diagnostic techniques, including hysteroscopy and molecular profiling, coupled with evolving therapeutic strategies, have substantially refined the care pathway for affected women [2].

This chapter endeavors to provide a detailed examination of the epidemiology, etiological factors, and diagnostic challenges associated with EH. Furthermore, it explores the latest international management guidelines and highlights the role of hysteroscopic approaches as part of a multidisciplinary strategy to address both oncological safety and the reproductive aspirations of patients.

7.1. Epidemiology and Risk Factors

Endometrial hyperplasia is characterized by the abnormal proliferation of the endometrial glands, leading to an increased gland-to-stroma ratio of over 50% [3]. This condition is strongly linked to prolonged exposure to unopposed estrogen, which stimulates endometrial growth without the counteractive effects of progesterone. Key risk factors include obesity, polycystic ovary syndrome (PCOS), nulliparity, early menarche, and late menopause [4].

Additionally, tamoxifen use, Lynch syndrome, and a history of anovulation are notable contributors [5].

The incidence of endometrial hyperplasia varies widely, with studies estimating between 130 and 800 cases per 100,000 women annually for all forms, and 5 to 23 per 100,000 for atypical hyperplasia [3, 5]. The latter, a precancerous condition, is most commonly diagnosed in postmenopausal women aged 60-64, whereas non-atypical hyperplasia frequently occurs in women aged 50-54. These demographic variations emphasize the importance of targeted screening strategies [6].

The escalating prevalence of obesity worldwide has further exacerbated the incidence of endometrial hyperplasia, particularly among younger women [7]. Obesity contributes to chronic low-grade inflammation and increased peripheral conversion of androgens to estrogen, perpetuating endometrial hyperplasia's pathogenesis. Given these findings, public health initiatives focusing on weight management could significantly reduce the burden of this condition [8].

The risk factors for endometrial hyperplasia closely align with those for endometrial cancer, with unopposed estrogen exposure forming the cornerstone of these risks (Table 1).

Table 1. Risk factors for endometrial hyperplasia

Advanced age
Prolonged unopposed estrogen exposure
Use of tamoxifen
Obesity
Early menarche
Late menopause
Estrogen-secreting tumors
Lynch Syndrome
Cowden Syndrome

7.2. Clinical Appearance

The clinical manifestation of endometrial hyperplasia often revolves around abnormal uterine bleeding (AUB), which is the most common presenting symptom [9]. This may include heavy menstrual bleeding, intermenstrual spotting, or postmenopausal bleeding. Less commonly, patients may report pelvic pain or discomfort, though some cases remain asymptomatic and are diagnosed incidentally during evaluations for infertility or other gynecological concerns [2].

Premenopausal women with persistent AUB, particularly those with risk factors for endometrial hyperplasia such as obesity and PCOS, warrant prompt evaluation [10–12]. Postmenopausal bleeding, though less common, carries a higher index of suspicion for endometrial pathology and necessitates immediate investigation. Clinical guidelines underscore the importance of thorough history-taking and risk stratification to guide diagnostic pathways [13]. In women without any symptoms, the diagnosis can occasionally be made through the detection of abnormal endometrial glandular cells in cervical cytology [14]. Atypical glandular cells (AGC) observed on cervical cytology are less frequently encountered compared to abnormal squamous cells and are typically derived from the glandular epithelium of the endocervix or, less commonly, the endometrium. Patients presenting with AGC require comprehensive evaluation to identify potential premalignant or malignant conditions involving the cervix, uterus, and, in rare cases, the ovaries or fallopian tubes. Studies have shown that the majority of AGC cases arise from either the endocervix or endometrium. Reviews of approximately 3,890 AGC tests revealed 1% of endometrial hyperplasia cases [15].

7.3. Current Diagnostic Perspectives and Limitations

Diagnosing endometrial hyperplasia requires a combination of clinical evaluation, imaging, and histopathological confirmation. Endometrial hyperplasia is diagnosed histologically through the evaluation of tissue obtained via endometrial biopsy, dilation and curettage (D&C), or hysterectomy specimens. Key diagnostic tools include:

- *Transvaginal Ultrasound (TVUS):* TVUS is a non-invasive and widely available modality, often used as the first-line diagnostic tool (Figure 1). It provides critical information about endometrial thickness, with a threshold of >4 mm in women with postmenopausal bleeding necessitating further evaluation. However, its sensitivity is limited in detecting focal lesions or distinguishing between benign and malignant conditions [16].

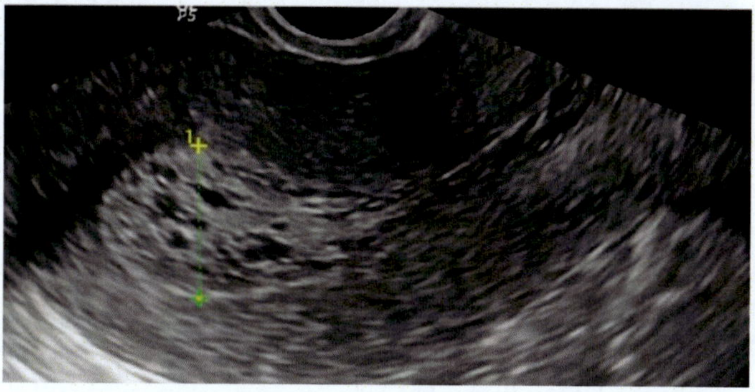

Figure 1. Sagittal view by TVUS showing a thickened homogenous echogenic endometrium, measuring about 12.5 mm in maximal anteroposterior diameter, with regular borders, preserving subendometrial halo and few variable sized cysts. Histopathology result of the endometrial biopsy was consistent with endometrial hyperplasia. *(© 2019 From Hetta WM et al. Role of transvaginal ultrasound in detection of endometrial changes in breast cancer patients under hormonal therapy. Licensed under the Creative Commons Attribution 4.0).*

- *Dilatation and curettage (D&C):* D&C is performed under anesthesia and is known for its high diagnostic accuracy, exceeding 98% for endometrial cancer. Its sensitivity for diagnosing atypical hyperplasia is approximately 90% [16]. The indications for D&C can be summarized as follows:

  - Inability to tolerate office biopsy due to pain or anxiety [17–19],
  - Cases suspected of endometrial cancer where the office biopsy yields insufficient results,
  - Persistent bleeding symptoms despite benign findings on office biopsy,
  - Presence of lesions occupying the endometrial cavity, such as polyps,
  - Situations where another surgical procedure is planned concurrently with the biopsy.

The likelihood of obtaining insufficient material or missing an existing malignancy with D&C is less than 5% [20]. The most common complication associated with D&C is uterine perforation, with rates ranging between 0.3% and 5%. For diagnostic procedures, the risk is 0.3% in premenopausal women and increases to 2.6% in postmenopausal women [21]. Other potential complications include bleeding, cervical injuries, infections, and the development of intrauterine adhesions [22].

- *Pipelle Biopsy:* Pipelle biopsy is a procedure that can be performed in an office setting. Its primary advantages include the absence of a need for anesthesia or, in some cases, the use of only local anesthesia, as well as the lack of cervical dilation requirements and its lower cost compared to alternative methods. Studies have shown that the sensitivity of Pipelle biopsy for detecting endometrial hyperplasia and cancer exceeds 90% [20].

  A meta-analysis comparing Pipelle biopsy with dilation and curettage (D&C) and hysteroscopic biopsy reported that all three methods demonstrated a sensitivity of over 98% for diagnosing cancer. However, the sensitivity of Pipelle biopsy for atypical hyperplasia was found to be 81% [23]. A prospective study involving 130 patients with abnormal uterine bleeding who underwent both Pipelle biopsy and subsequent D&C under anesthesia found that the diagnostic accuracy of Pipelle biopsy, compared to D&C, was 97% [24].
- *Hysteroscopy:* Hysteroscopy combines direct visualization with the ability to perform targeted biopsies [25, 26]. It is particularly useful in cases of focal abnormalities detected on imaging or in patients with inconclusive biopsy results [27, 28]. Despite its advantages, hysteroscopy's role in potentially disseminating malignant cells remains a subject of ongoing debate [29]. Although positive peritoneal cytology does not alter the staging of endometrial cancer, it is considered a poor prognostic factor. A meta-analysis comparing cases of endometrial cancer diagnosed with and without the use of hysteroscopy found no statistically significant difference in the incidence of positive peritoneal cytology (OR 1.64, 95% CI 1.0-28) [30]. Similarly, some studies have reported no significant differences in survival outcomes between patients diagnosed via hysteroscopy and those diagnosed using other methods [31]. The role of hysteroscopy in diagnosing endometrial hyperplasia remains a subject of ongoing discussion in the medical literature [8]. Key hysteroscopic features that may suggest the presence of endometrial hyperplasia include localized or widespread thickening of the endometrium, a papillary or polypoid appearance, irregular vascular patterns, glandular cysts, and abnormal glandular outlets with atypical structural characteristics [32, 33] (Figure 2-3).

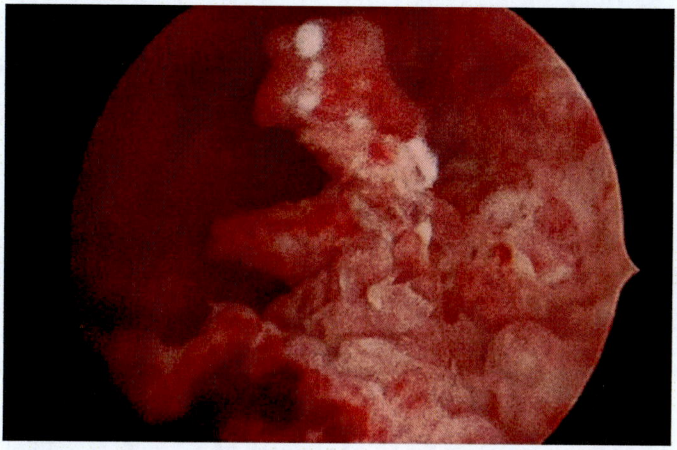

Figure 2. Hysteroscopic findings compatible with endometrial hyperplasia. Focal endometrial thickening with heterogeneous morphology, vascular course distortion, and multiple capillary aggregations. *(© 2022 Modified from Biswas D et al. Diagnostic hysteroscopy is a better method for diagnosis and management of abnormal uterine bleeding than traditional methods – An Indian perspective. Licensed under the Creative Commons Attribution 4.0).*

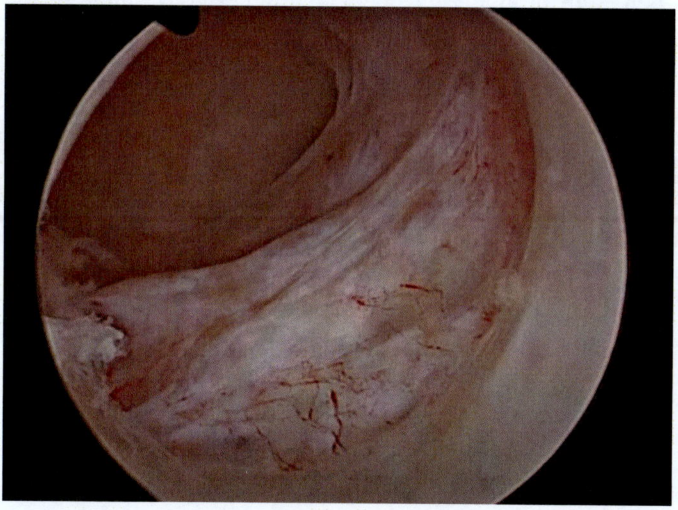

Figure 3. Hysteroscopic view of endometrial hyperplasia, showing a thickened and irregular endometrial lining with increased vascularization and abnormal capillary distribution. The surface appears opaque with signs of tissue proliferation, indicative of increased glandular and stromal density.

However, these diagnostic indicators are derived primarily from retrospective studies rather than robust evidence from randomized controlled trials (RCTs), leaving their reliability open to question. A meta-analysis assessing the effectiveness of hysteroscopy in detecting hyperplasia and cancer in women with abnormal uterine bleeding found that its sensitivity for diagnosing endometrial hyperplasia was limited to 78%. In contrast, hysteroscopy was shown to be more reliable in identifying endometrial cancer [34]. However, hysteroscopy offers the unique benefit of serving both diagnostic and therapeutic purposes for managing endometrial cancer and atypical hyperplasia [35]. This dual functionality makes it an invaluable tool in gynecological practice. Moreover, it provides the ability to thoroughly assess the uterine cavity and tubal lumen, which is particularly beneficial for evaluating and planning potential future pregnancies [36].

The definitive diagnosis of endometrial hyperplasia is fundamentally reliant on histopathological examination, as it requires a detailed analysis of endometrial tissue samples (Figure 4). Immunohistochemical evaluation may play an essential role in distinguishing between benign endometrial hyperplasia, atypical hyperplasia, and endometrial carcinoma [8].

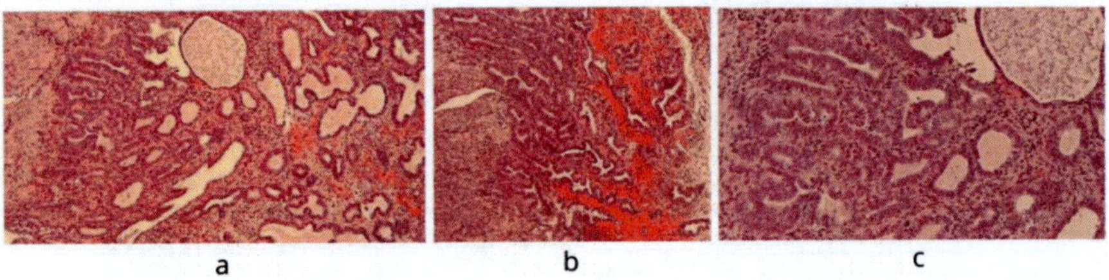

Figure 4. Histopathological images of atypical endometrial hyperplasia. (a) Irregular proliferation of glandular structures with loss of normal architecture; (b) Glandular crowding and stromal invasion with increased vascularization; (c) Glands showing nuclear atypia and altered gland-to-stroma ratio. *(© 2022 Modified from Pace L et al. Clinical, Sonographic, and Hysteroscopic Features of Endometrial Carcinoma Diagnosed after Hysterectomy in Patients with a Preoperative Diagnosis of Atypical Hyperplasia: A Single-Center Retrospective Study. Licensed under the Creative Commons Attribution 4.0)*.

A critical marker in this process is the protein phosphatase and tensin homolog (PTEN), a well-established tumor suppressor that is instrumental in the early stages of endometrial cancer development and progression [37]. The guidelines from the European Society of Gynaecological Oncology/the

European Society for Radiotherapy & Oncology and the European Society of Pathology emphasize the importance of PTEN immunohistochemistry in differentiating benign hyperplasia from malignant and premalignant lesions [38]. However, the lack of standardized criteria for its application continues to pose challenges in routine clinical practice.

7.4. Appropriate Management According to International Clinical Guidelines

Treatment strategies for endometrial hyperplasia are dictated by the presence or absence of atypia and the patient's reproductive goals. The overarching aim is to reverse hyperplasia, reduce malignancy risk, and address patient symptoms.

The primary international guidelines addressing appropriate management include those from the American College of Obstetricians and Gynecologists (ACOG), the European Society of Gynaecological Oncology/European Society of Human Reproduction and the European Society for Gynaecological Endoscopy (ESGO/ESHRE/ESGE), and the Royal College of Obstetricians and Gynaecologists (RCOG). Each guideline emphasizes the importance of histological diagnosis, individualizing treatment plans, and regular follow-up [38–40]. To prevent overtreatment or undertreatment, distinguishing between hyperplasia without atypia and with atypia is crucial.

- *Non-Atypical Hyperplasia:* Endometrial hyperplasia without atypia has a low risk of progressing to endometrial cancer, estimated to be under 5%, with the majority of cases showing spontaneous regression during follow-up [41]. This condition is managed conservatively with progestin therapy, either orally or via a levonorgestrel-releasing intrauterine system (LNG-IUS). Weight loss and management of underlying metabolic conditions, such as diabetes or PCOS, are essential adjuncts to therapy. Surveillance with repeat endometrial sampling is recommended every 3-6 months until regression is confirmed [40].
- *Atypical Hyperplasia:* Before initiating treatment for endometrial hyperplasia, it is essential to counsel women about the potential risks of underlying malignancy and the possibility of progression to endometrial cancer. Pretreatment evaluations should be conducted to exclude the presence of invasive endometrial cancer or co-existing

ovarian malignancies [42]. For women who have completed their reproductive plans, hysterectomy should be considered due to the high likelihood of disease recurrence [43]. Fertility-sparing treatments include hormonal therapy, hysteroscopic interventions, or a combination of both. Hormonal therapy typically involves the use of oral progestins, such as megestrol acetate or medroxyprogesterone acetate, or the levonorgestrel-releasing intrauterine system (LNG-IUS) [44]. As a premalignant condition, atypical hyperplasia necessitates more aggressive management. Fertility-preserving approaches, such as high-dose oral progestins or LNG-IUS, are appropriate for younger women desiring future pregnancies. Definitive treatment with hysterectomy is advised for postmenopausal women or those who have completed childbearing [45, 46]. Emerging evidence supports the use of combined therapies, including hysteroscopic resection followed by hormonal treatment, in select cases [33].

The international guidelines from ACOG, ESGO/ESHRE/ESGE, and RCOG converge on key principles: early identification of hyperplasia, individualized management plans, and the central role of progestin therapy for fertility preservation. Hysterectomy remains the definitive treatment for atypical hyperplasia, while LNG-IUS emerges as the preferred conservative option [47, 48]. Regular surveillance and lifestyle modifications, particularly weight loss, are integral to achieving favorable outcomes. This harmonized approach ensures optimal patient care tailored to risk profiles and fertility desires [49]. A comparison of recommendations of ACOG and RCOG guidelines is presented in Table 2.

Table 2. Comparison of International guidelines for EH treatment

Feature	ACOG [39]	RCOG [40]
EH without atypia		
Management	Not directly specified	Recommend weight loss, stopping HRT, and observation alone, as spontaneous regression can occur. Women should be informed that the risk of progression to cancer is <5% over 20 years. LNG-IUD is the preferred first-line treatment due to its higher regression rates and better bleeding profile.

Feature	ACOG [39]	RCOG [40]
EH without atypia		
		Continuous progestogens should be used (medroxyprogesterone 10–20 mg/day or norethisterone 10–15 mg/day) for women who decline the LNG-IUD. Cyclic progestins should not be used.
Duration of treatment	Not directly specified	Treatment with oral progestogens or the LNG-IUD should be for a minimum of 6 months in order to induce histological regression
		If adverse effects are tolerable and fertility is not desired, women should be encouraged to retain the LNG-IUD for up to 5 years as this reduces the risk of relapse
Surveillance & Follow-up	Not directly specified	Endometrial biopsy every 6 months until two consecutive negative results; for high-risk patients (BMI ≥35, oral progestin users), consider annual biopsy.
Indications for Surgical Treatment	Not directly specified	Hysterectomy is not a first-line option; recommended if progression to atypia, persistence after 12 months, relapse after treatment, or persistent bleeding occurs.
EH with atypia		
Definitive Treatment	Hysterectomy. The decision for oophorectomy should be individualized.	Total hysterectomy BSO for postmenopausal women, salpingectomy for premenopausal women
Fertility preservation Options	Fertility-sparing options can be considered, but thorough evaluation to exclude concurrent carcinoma is necessary.	Fertility-sparing treatment can be considered for women desiring pregnancy, but malignancy should be excluded through histology and imaging.
First-Line Medical Treatment for Fertility Preservation	LNG-IUD or oral progestins or combined. Lifestyle modifications.	LNG-IUD is the first-line treatment due to higher regression rates and better tolerability compared to oral progestins. Continuous oral progestins (medroxyprogesterone 10–20 mg/day or norethisterone 10–15 mg/day) are second-line options. For a minimum of 6 months
Surveillance	Endometrial biopsy every 3–6 months to monitor response.	Every 3 months until two consecutive negative biopsies are obtained. In asymptomatic women with a uterus and evidence of histological disease regression, based upon a minimum of two consecutive negative endometrial biopsies, long-term follow-up with endometrial biopsy every 6–12 months is recommended until a hysterectomy is performed Hysterecomy after no desire of fertility

BSO: Bilateral salpingo-oophorectomy. EH: Endometrial hyperplasia. HRT: Hormon replacement therapy. LNG-IUD: Levonorgestrel releasing intrauterine device.

7.5. Combined Conservative Therapies: The Role of Hysteroscopy

The treatment of endometrial hyperplasia (EH) and atypical endometrial hyperplasia (AEH) has evolved significantly over the past decades, with a growing emphasis on fertility preservation in young women of reproductive age. Among the conservative therapies available, hysteroscopy has emerged as a pivotal tool due to its dual capability for diagnosis and targeted treatment [50, 51]. The integration of operative hysteroscopy with hormonal therapy has demonstrated promising outcomes in achieving disease regression while preserving the endometrial structure for future pregnancies [8]. This sub-section explores the intricate role of hysteroscopy in conservative management, including its diagnostic accuracy, therapeutic applications, and combined approaches with medical therapies, while evaluating its safety, efficacy, and clinical implications.

7.5.1. Hysteroscopy as a Diagnostic and Therapeutic Tool

Hysteroscopy offers a direct visualization of the uterine cavity, enabling precise assessment and targeted biopsy of focal or diffuse lesions [52, 53]. Compared to blind methods like dilation and curettage (D&C) or Pipelle biopsy, hysteroscopy increases diagnostic accuracy by avoiding sampling errors and allowing targeted resection of suspicious areas. Studies have highlighted its superiority in identifying atypical or precancerous changes in the endometrium, particularly in women presenting with abnormal uterine bleeding (AUB), which is the hallmark symptom of EH and AEH [54].

In terms of therapeutic intervention, hysteroscopy facilitates the complete removal of hyperplastic or atypical lesions while preserving the underlying myometrium. The Mazzon technique, a standardized approach developed for hysteroscopic treatment, involves the three-step resection of endometrial lesions: resection of the visible lesion, surrounding endometrium, and the myometrial layer beneath the lesion. This approach ensures the thorough removal of abnormal tissue, thereby reducing the risk of persistence or recurrence [55]. The technique is particularly advantageous in achieving histological confirmation of the diagnosis while simultaneously providing treatment.

7.5.2. Combined Therapy: Hysteroscopy and Hormonal Treatments

The success of hysteroscopic interventions is significantly enhanced when combined with hormonal therapies. Progestin therapy, delivered orally, systemically, or locally via the levonorgestrel-releasing intrauterine device

(LNG-IUD), remains the cornerstone of conservative management for EH and AEH. Progestins act by counteracting unopposed estrogenic stimulation, inducing glandular atrophy and halting the progression of hyperplastic changes to malignancy [44].

Numerous studies have reported favorable outcomes when hysteroscopic resection is followed by progestin therapy. A meta-analysis demonstrated that hysteroscopic resection combined with hormonal treatment achieved a complete regression rate of up to 98% for AEH, significantly surpassing the regression rates seen with progestin therapy alone (77%) [56]. The combination approach also resulted in higher live birth rates, with approximately 52% of patients achieving successful pregnancies compared to 33% with progestin monotherapy. These findings underscore the synergistic effect of hysteroscopic resection and hormonal therapy in both oncologic and reproductive outcomes [57].

The LNG-IUD has emerged as a preferred modality for localized progestin delivery owing to its sustained release of medication directly to the endometrium. Compared to oral progestins, LNG-IUD offers superior compliance, minimal systemic side effects, and higher rates of lesion regression. When combined with hysteroscopic resection, LNG-IUD therapy not only improves remission rates but also reduces recurrence, particularly in obese patients or those with insulin resistance [58].

7.5.3. Safety and Complications of Hysteroscopic Procedures

Hysteroscopy is a minimally invasive procedure associated with a favorable safety profile. Complications such as uterine perforation, bleeding, infection, or intrauterine adhesions are rare, occurring in less than 1% of cases. A meta-analysis reviewing hysteroscopic management for EH and AEH reported no serious adverse events across multiple studies [32]. Additionally, concerns regarding the dissemination of malignant cells during hysteroscopic resection have not been substantiated in clinical practice, particularly when appropriate operative techniques and fluid management strategies are employed.

However, there remains a theoretical risk of positive peritoneal cytology following hysteroscopic procedures in patients with underlying endometrial cancer. Several studies have investigated this concern, concluding that hysteroscopy does not significantly increase the incidence of positive peritoneal cytology or impact survival outcomes in women with early-stage endometrial cancer [44]. As such, hysteroscopy remains a safe and effective option for fertility-preserving treatment when performed in carefully selected patients [59].

7.5.4. Oncologic and Reproductive Outcomes

The primary goal of conservative management in EH and AEH is to achieve complete remission while preserving fertility. Hysteroscopic resection, when combined with hormonal therapy, has demonstrated superior oncologic outcomes compared to hormonal therapy alone. Complete remission rates range from 80% to 100%, with the majority of patients achieving histologic regression within 6 to 12 months of treatment [32]. Factors associated with favorable outcomes include lesion size <2 cm, body mass index (BMI) <25 kg/m^2, and absence of myometrial invasion on imaging.

In terms of reproductive outcomes, combined hysteroscopic and hormonal therapy has been associated with promising pregnancy rates [60]. Studies have reported cumulative pregnancy rates ranging from 25% to 67%, with live birth rates exceeding 50% in some series [61, 62]. Assisted reproductive technologies (ART), including ovulation induction, intrauterine insemination, and in vitro fertilization, play a critical role in optimizing fertility outcomes for women undergoing conservative management. Importantly, obesity and insulin resistance remain significant predictors of reduced fertility, emphasizing the need for weight management and metabolic optimization as adjunctive strategies [63].

7.5.5. The Role of Metformin in Combined Therapy

Emerging evidence supports the addition of metformin to progestin therapy in patients with AEH, particularly those with polycystic ovary syndrome (PCOS) or metabolic disorders. Metformin, an insulin-sensitizing agent, enhances the efficacy of progestins by reducing peripheral estrogen production, improving endometrial receptivity, and exerting direct antiproliferative effects on the endometrium. A phase II study evaluating metformin and medroxyprogesterone acetate (MPA) reported significantly higher complete response rates compared to MPA alone, particularly in non-obese, insulin-sensitive patients [58]. The integration of metformin into combined conservative therapies represents a promising strategy for improving both oncologic and metabolic outcomes in women with AEH.

7.5.6. Follow-up and Surveillance

Close surveillance is essential during and after conservative treatment to monitor for disease persistence, progression, or recurrence. Current guidelines recommend histologic evaluation of the endometrium every 3 to 6 months during treatment [39, 40] Hysteroscopy plays a central role in follow-up, allowing for direct visualization of the uterine cavity and targeted biopsy of any residual or recurrent lesions [64]. Imaging modalities such as transvaginal ultrasound and magnetic resonance imaging (MRI) may complement hysteroscopic evaluation in assessing endometrial thickness and myometrial invasion.

Long-term follow-up is particularly important for women who achieve complete remission but remain at high risk for recurrence, including those with obesity, metabolic syndrome, or Lynch syndrome [65]. Once childbearing is complete, definitive treatment with hysterectomy is strongly recommended to mitigate the risk of progression to endometrial cancer [66, 67].

Hysteroscopy has revolutionized the conservative management of endometrial hyperplasia and atypical hyperplasia, offering a precise, minimally invasive approach for diagnosis and treatment. When combined with hormonal therapies such as LNG-IUD or oral progestins, hysteroscopic resection significantly improves remission rates, reduces recurrence, and enhances fertility outcomes [68]. Emerging strategies, including the integration of metformin for metabolic optimization, further expand the therapeutic potential of combined conservative therapies [69].

The safety, efficacy, and reproducibility of hysteroscopic interventions have been well-documented, with minimal risk of complications or adverse oncologic outcomes. Nevertheless, standardized protocols for hysteroscopic resection, hormonal therapy, and surveillance are needed to optimize patient care and ensure long-term success. Future research should focus on refining patient selection criteria, investigating novel therapeutic combinations, and evaluating the cost-effectiveness of hysteroscopic management in diverse clinical settings. With continued advancements, hysteroscopy will remain a cornerstone of fertility-preserving treatment for endometrial hyperplasia and atypical hyperplasia, balancing oncologic safety with reproductive aspirations [70].

Conclusion

Endometrial hyperplasia represents a significant clinical challenge with profound implications for cancer prevention and reproductive health. Advances in diagnostic modalities, including molecular markers and hysteroscopy, have enhanced our ability to tailor management strategies to individual patient needs. The integration of conservative therapies, particularly hysteroscopic resection combined with hormonal treatment, offers promising outcomes for patients desiring fertility preservation.

Future research should focus on standardizing hysteroscopic techniques, exploring novel therapeutic agents, and refining surveillance protocols to optimize patient outcomes. By adopting a multidisciplinary approach, clinicians can ensure that patients with endometrial hyperplasia receive comprehensive, evidence-based care that aligns with their clinical and personal goals.

References

[1] Lacey JV., Chia VM. Endometrial hyperplasia and the risk of progression to carcinoma. *Maturitas.* 2009;63(1):39–44.

[2] Sanderson PA, Critchley HOD, Williams ARW, Arends MJ, Saunders PTK. New concepts for an old problem: The diagnosis of endometrial hyperplasia. *Hum Reprod Update.* 2017;23(2):232–54.

[3] Sobczuk K, Sobczuk A. New classification system of endometrial hyperplasia WHO 2014 and its clinical implications. *Prz Menopauzalny.* 2017;16(3):107–111.

[4] Vitale SG, Saponara S, Succu AG, Sicilia G, Martsidis K, D'Alterio MN, Angioni S. Efficacy and Safety of Non-Ablative Dual Wavelength Diode Laser Therapy for Genitourinary Syndrome of Menopause: A Single-Center Prospective Study. *Adv Ther.* 2024;41(12):4617–27.

[5] Lacey J, Chia V, Rush B, Carreon D, Richesson D, Ioffe OB, Ronnett BM, Chatterjee N, Langholz B, Sherman ME, Glass AG. Incidence rates of endometrial hyperplasia, endometrial cancer and hysterectomy from 1980 to 2003 within a large prepaid health plan. *Int J Cancer.* 2012;131(8):1921–9.

[6] Gressel G, Parkash V, Pal L. Management options and fertility-preserving therapy for premenopausal endometrial hyperplasia and early-stage endometrial cancer. *Int J Gynaecol Obs.* 2015;131(3):234–9.

[7] Corrado G, Vizza E, Cela V, Mereu L, Bogliolo S, Legge F, Ciccarone F, Mancini E, Gallotta V, Baiocco E, Monterossi G, Perri MT, Zampa A, Pasciuto T, Scambia G. Laparoscopic versus robotic hysterectomy in obese and extremely obese patients with endometrial cancer: A multi-institutional analysis. *Eur J Surg Oncol.* 2018;44(12):1935–41.

[8] Vitale SG, Riemma G, Carugno J, Chiofalo B, Vilos GA, Cianci S, Budak MS, Lasmar BP, Raffone A, Kahramanoglu I. Hysteroscopy in the management of endometrial hyperplasia and cancer in reproductive aged women: new developments and current perspectives. *Transl Cancer Res.* 2020;9(12):7767–77.

[9] Kahramanoglu I. Hysteroscopic treatments for endometrial malignancies and premalignancies: state of the art. *Minim Invasive Ther Allied Technol.* 2021;30(5):272–7.

[10] Ali DES, Shah M, Ali A, Malik MO, Rehman F, Badshah H, Ehtesham E, Vitale SG. Treatment with Metformin and Combination of Metformin plus Pioglitazone on Serum Levels of IL-6 and IL-8 in Polycystic Ovary Syndrome: A Randomized Clinical Trial. *Horm Metab Res.* 2019;51(11):714–22.

[11] Cai T, Mazzoli S, Migno S, Malossini G, Lanzafame P, Mereu L, Tateo S, Wagenlehner FM, Pickard RS, Bartoletti R. Development and validation of a nomogram predicting recurrence risk in women with symptomatic urinary tract infection. *Int J Urol.* 2014;21(9):929–34.

[12] Prisco MG, Zannoni GF, De Stefano I, Vellone VG, Tortorella L, Fagotti A, Mereu L, Scambia G, Gallo D. Prognostic role of metastasis tumor antigen 1 in patients with ovarian cancer: a clinical study. *Hum Pathol.* 2012;43(2):282–8.

[13] Pignata S, Ferrandina G, Scarfone G, Scollo P, Odicino F, Cormio G, Katsaros D, Frigerio L, Mereu L, Ghezzi F, Manzione L, Lauria R, Breda E, Alletti DG, Ballardini M, Vernaglia A, Sorio R, Tumolo S, Musso P, Magni G, Pisano C, Morabito A. Poor outcome of elderly patients with platinum-sensitive recurrent ovarian cancer: results from the SOCRATES retrospective study. *Crit Rev Oncol Hematol.* 2009;71(3):233–41.

[14] Shi Y, Zhu Y, Fan S, Vitagliano A, Liu X, Liao Y, Liang Y, Vitale SG. Clinical Characteristics and Antifungal Susceptibility of Candida nivariensis from Vulvovaginal Candidiasis. *Gynecol Obstet Invest.* 2020;85(1):88–93.

[15] Schnatz PF, Guile M, O'Sullivan DM, Sorosky JI. Clinical significance of atypical glandular cells on cervical cytology. *Obs Gynecol.* 2006;107(3):701–8.

[16] Mahajan NN, Mahajan K, Soni R. Endometrial thickness screening in premenopausal women with abnormal uterine bleeding. *J Obstet Gynaecol Res.* 2007;33(6):886.

[17] Török P, Molnár S, Herman T, Jashanjeet S, Lampé R, Riemma G, Vitale SG. Fallopian tubal obstruction is associated with increased pain experienced during office hysteroscopy: a retrospective study. *Updates Surg.* 2020;72(1):213–8.

[18] Penzias A, Azziz R, Bendikson K, Cedars M, Falcone T, Hansen K, Hill M, Jindal S, Kalra S, Mersereau J, Racowsky C, Reindollar R, Shannon CN, Steiner A, Stovall D, Tanrikut C, Taylor H, Yauger B. Fertility evaluation of infertile women: a committee opinion. *Fertil Steril.* 2021;116(5):1255–65.

[19] Florio P, Puzzutiello R, Filippeschi M, D'Onofrio P, Mereu L, Morelli R, Marianello D, Litta P, Mencaglia L, Petraglia F. Low-dose spinal anesthesia with hyperbaric bupivacaine with intrathecal fentanyl for operative hysteroscopy: a case series study. *J Minim Invasive Gynecol.* 2012;19(1):107–12.

[20] Van Hanegem N, Prins MMC, Bongers MY, Opmeer BC, Sahota DS, Mol BWJ, Timmermans A. The accuracy of endometrial sampling in women with postmenopausal bleeding: A systematic review and meta-analysis. *Eur J Obstet Gynecol Reprod Biol.* 2016;197:147–55.

[21] Hefler L, Lemach A, Seebacher V, Polterauer S, Tempfer C, Reinthaller A. The intraoperative complication rate of nonobstetric dilation and curettage. *Obs Gynecol.* 2009;113(6):1268–71.

[22] Urman B, Yakin K, Ertas S, Alper E, Aksakal E, Riemma G, Angioni S, Vitale SG. Fertility and anatomical outcomes following hysteroscopic adhesiolysis: An 11-year retrospective cohort study to validate a new classification system for intrauterine adhesions (Urman-Vitale Classification System). *Int J Gynecol Obstet.* 2024;165(2):644–54.

[23] Dijkhuizen FP, Mol BW, Brölmann HA, Heintz AP. The accuracy of endometrial sampling in the diagnosis of patients with endometrial carcinoma and hyperplasia: a meta-analysis. *Cancer.* 2000;89(8):1765–72.

[24] Sanam M, Majid MM. Comparison the Diagnostic Value of Dilatation and Curettage Versus Endometrial Biopsy by Pipelle--a Clinical Trial. *Asian Pac J Cancer Prev.* 2015;16(12):4971–5.

[25] Vitale SG, Angioni S, Saponara S, Sicilia G, Mignacca A, Caiazzo A, De Franciscis P, Riemma G. Hysteroscopic metroplasty and its reproductive impact among the social networks: A cross-sectional analysis on video quality, reliability and creators' opinions on YouTube, TikTok and Instagram. *Int J Med Inform.* 2025;195:105776.

[26] Vitale SG, Di Spiezio Sardo A, Riemma G, De Franciscis P, Alonso Pacheco L, Carugno J. In-office hysteroscopic removal of retained or fragmented intrauterine device without anesthesia: a cross-sectional analysis of an international survey. *Updates Surg.* 2022;74(3):1079–85.

[27] Vitale SG. The Biopsy Snake Grasper Sec. VITALE: A New Tool for Office Hysteroscopy. *J Minim Invasive Gynecol.* 2020;27(6):1414–6.

[28] Saponara S, Angioni S, Parry JP, Pacheco LA, Carugno J, Moawad N, Haimovich S, Lasmar RB, Dealberti D, Aksakal E, Urman B, Nappi L, Vitale SG. The Pivotal role of hysteroscopy in diagnosing subtle uterine lesions in infertile patients: Seeing the unseen can make the difference. *Eur J Obstet Gynecol Reprod Biol.* 2025;305:132–41.

[29] Vitale SG, Angioni S, Saponara S, Sicilia G, Etrusco A, D'Alterio MN, Cobellis L, De Franciscis P, Riemma G. TikTok as a platform for hysteroscopy information: An analytical video-based cross-sectional study to assess quality, reliability, and accuracy. *Int J Gynecol Obstet.* 2025;168(1):353–61.

[30] Yazbeck C, Dhainaut C, Batallan A, Benifla JL, Thoury A, Madelenat P. Diagnostic hysteroscopy and risk of peritoneal dissemination of tumor cells. *Gynecol Obs Fertil.* 2005;33(4):247–52.

[31] Ben-Arie A, Tamir S, Dubnik S, Gemer O, Ben Shushan A, Dgani R, Peer G, Barnett-Griness O, Lavie O. Does hysteroscopy affect prognosis in apparent early-stage endometrial cancer? *Int J Gynecol Cancer.* 2008;18(4):247–52.

[32] Bilir E, Kahramanoğlu İ. The role of hysteroscopy in fertility preservation in endometrial cancer and atypical endometrial hyperplasia: a semi-systematic literature review. *Arch Gynecol Obs.* 2024;308(4):1113–26.

[33] Bilir E, Kacperczyk-Bartnik J, Bizzarri N, Kahramanoğlu İ. Current practice with operative hysteroscopy for fertility preservation in endometrial cancer and endometrial premalignancies. *Arch Gynecol Obs.* 2024;309(6):2267–78.

[34] Clark TJ, Voit D, Gupta JK, Hyde C, Song F, Khan KS. Accuracy of Hysteroscopy in the Diagnosis of Endometrial Cancer and Hyperplasia. *Jama.* 2002;288(13).

[35] Vitale SG, Angioni S, D'Alterio MN, Ronsini C, Saponara S, De Franciscis P, Riemma G. Risk of endometrial malignancy in women treated for breast cancer: the BLUSH prediction model–evidence from a comprehensive multicentric retrospective cohort study. *Climacteric.* 2024;25(5):482–8.

[36] Vitale SG, Riemma G, Haimovich S, Carugno J, Alonso Pacheco L, Perez-Medina T, Parry JP, Török P, Tesarik J, Della Corte L, Cobellis L, Di Spiezio Sardo A, De

Franciscis P. Risk of endometrial cancer in asymptomatic postmenopausal women in relation to ultrasonographic endometrial thickness: systematic review and diagnostic test accuracy meta-analysis. *Am J Obstet Gynecol.* 2023;228(1):22-35.e2.

[37] Mutter GL, Monte NM, Neuberg D, Ferenczy A, Eng C. Emergence, involution, and progression to carcinoma of mutant clones in normal endometrial tissues. *Cancer Res.* 2014;74(10):2796–802.

[38] Rodolakis A, Scambia G, Planchamp F, Acien M, Di Spiezio Sardo A, Farrugia M, Grynberg M, Pakiz M, Pavlakis K, Vermeulen N, Zannoni G, Zapardiel I, Macklon KLT. ESGO/ESHRE/ESGE Guidelines for the fertility-sparing treatment of patients with endometrial carcinoma. *Hum Reprod open.* 2023;2023(1).

[39] Management of Endometrial Intraepithelial Neoplasia or Atypical Endometrial Hyperplasia: ACOG Clinical Consensus No. 5. *Obstet Gynecol.* 2023;142(3):735–44.

[40] Royal College of Obstetricians & Gynaecologists, The British Society for Gynaecological Endoscopy. *Management of Endometrial Hyperplasia* [Internet]. Green-top Guideline No. 67. 2016 [cited 2025 Jan 12]. Available from: https://www.bsge.org.uk/wp-content/uploads/2016/03/gtg_67_endometrial_hyperplasia.pdf.

[41] Lacey J V., Sherman ME, Rush BB, Ronnett BM, Ioffe OB, Duggan MA, Glass AG, Richesson DA, Chatterjee N, Langholz B. Absolute risk of endometrial carcinoma during 20-year follow-up among women with endometrial hyperplasia. *J Clin Oncol.* 2010;28(5):788–92.

[42] Buda A, Gasparri ML, Puppo A, Mereu L, De Ponti E, Di Martino G, Novelli A, Tateo S, Muller M, Landoni F, Papadia A. Lymph node evaluation in high-risk early stage endometrial cancer: A multi-institutional retrospective analysis comparing the sentinel lymph node (SLN) algorithm and SLN with selective lymphadenectomy. *Gynecol Oncol.* 2018;150(2):261–6.

[43] Angioni S, Pontis A, Pisanu A, Mereu L, Roman H. Single-port access subtotal laparoscopic hysterectomy: A prospective case-control study. *J Minim Invasive Gynecol.* 2015;22(5):807–12.

[44] Cavaliere AF, Perelli F, Zaami S, D'indinosante M, Turrini I, Giusti M, Gullo G, Vizzielli G, Mattei A, Scambia G, Vidiri A, Signore F. Fertility Sparing Treatments in Endometrial Cancer Patients: The Potential Role of the New Molecular Classification. *Int J Mol Sci.* 2021;22(22):12248.

[45] Schipa C, Ripa M, Gallotta V, Russo A, Polidori L, Fanfani F, Capomacchia FM, Corrado G, Vizza E, Perrone AM, Mereu L, Cela V, Legge F, Hilaris G, Pasciuto T, D'Indinosante M, La Fera E, Certelli C, Bruno V, Kogeorgos S, De Iaco P, Lathouras K, Sollazzi L, Scambia G, Aceto P. Can the Modified Frailty Index (mFI) Predict Intraoperative and Postoperative Complications in Older Women with Endometrial Cancer Undergoing Laparoscopic or Robotic Surgery? A Multicenter Observational Study. *J Clin Med.* 2023;12(23):7205.

[46] Tateo S, Nozza A, Del Pezzo C, Mereu L. Robotic single-site pelvic lymphadenectomy. *Gynecol Oncol.* 2014;134(3):631.

[47] Mereu L, Berlanda V, Surico D, Gardella B, Pertile R, Spinillo A, Tateo S. Evaluation of quality of life, body image and surgical outcomes of robotic total

laparoscopic hysterectomy and sentinel lymph node mapping in low-risk endometrial cancer patients – A Robotic Gyne Club study. *Acta Obstet Gynecol Scand.* 2020;99(9):1238–45.

[48] Imboden S, Mereu L, Siegenthaler F, Pellegrini A, Papadia A, Tateo S, Mueller MD. Oncological safety and perioperative morbidity in low-risk endometrial cancer with sentinel lymph-node dissection. *Eur J Surg Oncol.* 2019;45(9):1638–43.

[49] Bogani G, Scambia G, Cimmino C, Fanfani F, Costantini B, Loverro M, Ferrandina G, Landoni F, Bazzurini L, Grassi T, Vitobello D, Siesto G, Perrone AM, Zanagnolo V, De Iaco P, Multinu F, Ghezzi F, Casarin J, Berretta R, Capozzi VA, Zupi E, Centini G, Pellegrino A, Corso S, Stevenazzi G, Montoli S, Boschi AC, Comerci G, Greco P, Martinello R, Sopracordevole F, Giorda G, Simoncini T, Caretto M, Sartori E, Ferrari F, Cianci A, Sarpietro G, Matarazzo MG, Zullo F, Bifulco G, Morelli M, Ferrero A, Biglia N, Barra F, Ferrero S, Maggiore ULR, Cianci S, Chiantera V, Ercoli A, Sozzi G, Martoccia A, Schettini S, Orlando T, Cannone FG, Ettore G, Puppo A, Borghese M, Martinelli C, Muzii L, Di Donato V, Driul L, Restaino S, Bergamini A, Candotti G, Bocciolone L, Plotti F, Angioli R, Mantovani G, Ceccaroni M, Cassani C, Dominoni M, Giambanco L, Amodeo S, Leo L, Thomasset R, Raimondo D, Seracchioli R, Malzoni M, Gorlero F, Di Luca M, Busato E, Kilzie S, Dell'acqua A, Scarfone G, Vercellini P, Petrillo M, Dessole S, Capobianco G, Ciavattini A, Delli Carpini G, Giannella L, Mereu L, Tateo S, Sorbi F, Fambrini M, Cicogna S, Romano F, Ricci G, Trojano G, Consonni R, Cantaluppi S, Lippolis A, Tinelli R, D'ippolito G, Aguzzoli L, Mandato VD, Palomba S, Calandra D, Rosati M, Gallo C, Surico D, Remorgida V, Ruscitto F, Beretta P, Panici PB, Raspagliesi F. Characteristics and patterns of care of endometrial cancer before and during COVID-19 pandemic. *J Gynecol Oncol.* 2022;33(1):e10.

[50] Vitale SG, Riemma G, Alonso Pacheco L, Carugno J, Haimovich S, Tesarik J, De Angelis MC, Di Spiezio Sardo A, De Franciscis P. Hysteroscopic endometrial biopsy: from indications to instrumentation and techniques. A call to action. *Minim Invasive Ther Allied Technol. 2021*;30(5):251–62.

[51] Vitale SG, Riemma G, Carugno J, Perez-Medina T, Alonso Pacheco L, Haimovich S, Parry JP, Di Spiezio Sardo A, De Franciscis P. Postsurgical barrier strategies to avoid the recurrence of intrauterine adhesion formation after hysteroscopic adhesiolysis: a network meta-analysis of randomized controlled trials. *Am J Obstet Gynecol.* 2022;226(4):487-498.e8.

[52] Vitale SG, Saponara S, Sicilia G, Klarić M, Sorrentino F, D'Alterio MN, Nappi L, Angioni S. Hysteroscopic diode laser myolysis: from a case series to literature review of incisionless myolysis techniques for managing heavy menstrual bleeding in premenopausal women. *Arch Gynecol Obstet.* 2024;309(3):949–59.

[53] Vitale SG, Moore O, Riemma G, Carugno J, Yarto ML, Haimovich S. Hysteroscopic laser ablation of symptomatic uterine fibroids: insights from a prospective study. *Climacteric.* 2023;26(5):497–502.

[54] Erkanli S, Ayhan A. Fertility-Sparing Therapy in Young Women With Endometrial Cancer. *Int J Gynecol Cancer.* 2010;20(7):1170–87.

[55] Mazzon I, Corrado G, Morricone D, Scambia G. Reproductive preservation for treatment of stage IA endometrial cancer in a young woman: hysteroscopic resection. *Int J Gynecol Cancer.* 2005;15(5):974–8.

[56] Zhang Q, Qi G, Kanis MJ, Dong R, Cui B, Yang X. Comparison among fertility-sparing therapies for well differentiated early-stage endometrial carcinoma and complex atypical hyperplasia. *Oncotarget.* 2017;8(34).

[57] Vitale SG, Parry JP, Carugno J, Cholkeri-Singh A, Della Corte L, Cianci S, Schiattarella A, Riemma G, De Franciscis P. Surgical and Reproductive Outcomes after Hysteroscopic Removal of Retained Products of Conception: A Systematic Review and Meta-analysis. *J Minim Invasive Gynecol.* 2021;28(2):204–17.

[58] Yang BY, Gulinazi Y, Du Y, Ning CC, Cheng YL, Shan WW. Metformin plus Megestrol Acetate (MA) compared with MA alone as fertility-sparing treatment in patients with atypical endometrial hyperplasia and well differentiated endometrial cancer: a randomised controlled trial. *BJOG.* 2020;127(7):848–57.

[59] Bilir E, Kahramanoğlu İ. The role of hysteroscopy in fertility preservation in endometrial cancer and atypical endometrial hyperplasia: a semi-systematic literature review. *Arch Gynecol Obstet.* 2023;308(4):1113–26.

[60] Chiofalo B, Palmara V, Vilos GA, Pacheco LA, Lasmar RB, Shawki O, Giacobbe V, Alibrandi A, Di Guardo F, Vitale SG. Reproductive outcomes of infertile women undergoing "see and treat" office hysteroscopy: a retrospective observational study. *Minim Invasive Ther Allied Technol.* 2021;30(3):147–53.

[61] Alonso S, Castellanos T, Lapuente F, Chiva L. Hysteroscopic surgery for conservative management in endometrial cancer: A review of the literature. *Ecancermedicalscience.* 2015;9:505.

[62] Gallos ID, Yap J, Rajkhowa M, Luesley DM, Coomarasamy A, Gupta JK. Regression, relapse, and live birth rates with fertility-sparing therapy for endometrial cancer and atypical complex endometrial hyperplasia: a systematic review and metaanalysis. *Am J Obstet Gynecol.* 2012;207(4):266.e1-.e12.

[63] Vitale SG, Laganà AS, Török P, Lasmar RB, Carugno J, Palumbo M, Tesarik J. Virtual sonographic hysteroscopy in assisted reproduction: A retrospective cost-effectiveness analysis. *Int J Gynaecol Obstet.* 2022;156(1):112–8.

[64] Vitale SG, Laganà AS, Caruso S, Garzon S, Vecchio GM, La Rosa VL, Casarin J, Ghezzi F. Comparison of three biopsy forceps for hysteroscopic endometrial biopsy in postmenopausal patients (HYGREB-1): A multicenter, single-blind randomized clinical trial. *Int J Gynaecol Obstet.* 2021;155(3):425–32.

[65] Vitale SG, Caruso S, Rapisarda AMC, Valenti G, Rossetti D, Cianci S, Cianci A. Biocompatible porcine dermis graft to treat severe cystocele: impact on quality of life and sexuality. *Arch Gynecol Obstet.* 2016;293(1):125–31.

[66] Giannini A, D'Oria O, Vizza E, Congiu MA, Cuccu I, Golia D'Augè T, Saponara S, Capalbo G, Di Donato V, Raspagliesi F, Bogani G. Robotic-assisted, laparoscopic, and vaginal hysterectomy in morbidly obese patients with endometrial hyperplasia and endometrial cancer. *Minim Invasive Ther Allied Technol.* 2024;33(6):358–64.

[67] Corrado G, Vizza E, Perrone AM, Mereu L, Cela V, Legge F, Hilaris G, Pasciuto T, D'Indinosante M, La Fera E, Certelli C, Bruno V, Kogeorgos S, Fanfani F, De Iaco

P, Scambia G, Gallotta V. Comparison Between Laparoscopic and Robotic Surgery in Elderly Patients With Endometrial Cancer: A Retrospective Multicentric Study. *Front Oncol.* 2021;11:724886.

[68] Atallah D, El Kassis N, Safi J, El Hachem H, Chahine G, Moubarak M. The use of hysteroscopic endometrectomy in the conservative treatment of early endometrial cancer and atypical hyperplasia in fertile women. *Arch Gynecol Obstet.* 2021;304(5):1299–305.

[69] Shiwani H, Clement NS, Daniels JP, Atiomo W. Metformin for endometrial hyperplasia. *Cochrane Database Syst Rev.* 2024;2024(5).

[70] Vitale SG, Laganà AS, Noventa M, Giampaolino P, Zizolfi B, Butticè S, La Rosa VL, Gullo G, Rossetti D. Transvaginal Bilateral Sacrospinous Fixation after Second Recurrence of Vaginal Vault Prolapse: Efficacy and Impact on Quality of Life and Sexuality. *Biomed Res Int.* 2018;2018:5727165.

Chapter 8

Endometrial Cancer

Paolo Scollo[1,*], MD
Benito Chiofalo[1], MD, PhD
Ilenia Paterniti[2], MD
Francesco Sgalambro[3], MD
Basilio Pecorino[4], MD
and Giuseppe Scibilia[5], MD

[1]Maternal and Child Department, Obstetrics and Gynecology
Cannizzaro Hospital of Catania, Kore University of Enna, Enna, Italy
[2]Obstetrics and Gynecology Unit, Department of Human Pathology,
University of Messina, Messina, Italy
[3]Obstetrics and Gynecology Unit, "*Gaspare Rodolico*" University Hospital,
Department of General Surgery and Medical Surgical Specialties,
University of Catania, Catania, Italy
[4]Gynecology and Obstetrics, "*Umberto I*" Hospital, Kore University of Enna,
Enna, Italy
[5]Gynecology and Obstetrics "*Giovanni Paolo II*" Hospital, Ragusa,
Kore University of Enna, Enna, Italy

Abstract

Endometrial cancer is one of the most common gynecological malignancies and a significant public health concern, with a rising global incidence influenced by geographic, lifestyle, and demographic factors. Its pathogenesis is closely linked to obesity, reproductive patterns, and genetic predispositions, such as Lynch syndrome, which significantly

* Corresponding Author's Email: paolo.scollo@unikore.it

In: Endometrium and Related Endouterine Pathologies
Editors: Liliana Mereu and Salvatore Giovanni Vitale
ISBN: 979-8-89530-818-9

elevate the risk. Clinical manifestations often include abnormal uterine bleeding as a hallmark symptom, accompanied by other systemic and local signs as the disease progresses.
The classification of endometrial cancer has evolved, incorporating both traditional dualistic models and advanced molecular subtyping, which defines four distinct groups with unique prognostic and therapeutic implications. Diagnostic strategies combine advanced imaging techniques, such as transvaginal ultrasound and MRI, with hysteroscopic and histopathological evaluations. The updated FIGO staging system integrates anatomical, histological, and molecular characteristics to refine prognosis and guide treatment planning.
Management primarily involves surgical intervention, often complemented by tailored adjuvant therapies, including radiotherapy, chemotherapy, and immunotherapy, depending on the stage and molecular profile of the tumor. Recent advancements, such as sentinel lymph node mapping, minimally invasive surgical techniques, and fertility-preserving treatments, have further improved outcomes. Breakthroughs in systemic therapies, particularly immune checkpoint inhibitors, are transforming care for advanced and recurrent cases.
Future perspectives emphasize the integration of artificial intelligence, multi-omics approaches, and personalized medicine to optimize early diagnosis, risk stratification, and treatment. Ongoing clinical trials and emerging technologies hold the potential to revolutionize therapeutic options, addressing disparities in access to care and improving the prognosis and quality of life for affected women globally.

Keywords: endometrial cancer, molecular classification, immunotherapy, FIGO staging, sentinel lymph node mapping

Introduction

Endometrial cancer represents a significant challenge in modern gynecological oncology, not only due to its rising incidence but also because of the complex interplay of factors influencing its development and progression. While the disease is often associated with postmenopausal women, shifts in global health trends, such as the obesity epidemic and delayed childbirth, are reshaping its epidemiology. Additionally, hereditary conditions, particularly Lynch syndrome, underscore the importance of genetic predisposition in certain populations [1].

The diversity of endometrial cancer in terms of clinical presentation, histopathological subtypes, and molecular characteristics necessitates a multifaceted approach to its diagnosis and management. From early-stage disease, often presenting with clear symptoms like abnormal uterine bleeding, to aggressive forms that demand advanced diagnostic tools and treatment modalities, the spectrum of clinical scenarios highlights the need for precise strategies [2].

As our understanding of the disease expands, so too do the tools available to combat it. Recent advancements in imaging, surgical techniques, and systemic therapies are providing clinicians with more effective means of intervention. Furthermore, the integration of molecular insights into staging and treatment planning marks a pivotal step toward personalized medicine, offering the potential for improved outcomes and reduced overtreatment [3–5].

The complexity of endometrial cancer also extends to its global impact, with disparities in access to care and diagnosis shaping outcomes across different regions [6] Addressing these challenges requires a concerted effort to bridge gaps in healthcare delivery while continuing to innovate in the realms of research and treatment development. This chapter explores these aspects, providing a detailed examination of the current state and future directions in the management of endometrial cancer.

8.1. Epidemiology and Pathogenesis

Endometrial cancer stands out as a significant public health concern, being one of the most commonly diagnosed gynecological cancers worldwide. It ranks as the sixth most common cancer among women, with a growing number of cases reported each year. In 2020 alone, approximately 417,000 new cases were identified globally, representing a substantial proportion of cancers affecting women. However, the distribution and prevalence of this disease vary markedly across different regions of the world, influenced by a combination of lifestyle, environmental, and healthcare-related factors [7].

In more developed countries, such as those in North America, Western Europe, and Australia, endometrial cancer incidence rates are notably higher. For instance, in the United States, it is recognized as the most frequently occurring gynecological malignancy, with over 60,000 new cases diagnosed annually [7]. The elevated rates in these regions are largely attributed to lifestyle patterns characterized by sedentary behavior, poor dietary habits, and a high prevalence of obesity, all of which are known to significantly increase the risk of endometrial cancer [8]. In these areas, an aging population also plays a crucial role, as the disease predominantly affects postmenopausal women, particularly those between the ages of 55 and 65 years [1].

Conversely, in developing regions, including parts of Africa, South-Central Asia, and Southeast Asia, the incidence of endometrial cancer tends to be much lower. This difference may stem from distinct reproductive patterns, such as higher parity (having more children), which is protective against the disease [9]. However, it is also important to consider the role of underdiagnosis and limited access to healthcare services in these regions, which might result in fewer reported cases rather than an actual lower prevalence. Additionally, lifestyle factors such as lower obesity rates and higher levels of physical activity may contribute to the reduced risk observed in these populations [9].

One of the most alarming aspects of the global incidence of endometrial cancer is the steady increase in cases, particularly in developed nations. This trend is driven largely by the rising obesity epidemic, which is a well-established risk factor for the disease [10]. Obesity increases estrogen levels, promoting abnormal growth of the endometrial lining, and its prevalence has reached worrying levels in many parts of the world. Furthermore, changes in reproductive behavior, such as having fewer children and delaying childbirth, are thought to contribute to the increasing rates. The aging population also adds to the burden, as longer life expectancy means more women are reaching the age range at which endometrial cancer is most likely to develop [2, 11].

Looking ahead, the future presents significant challenges. Projections suggest that by 2040, the global burden of endometrial cancer could rise by around 40%. This increase is expected to be driven not only by population growth and aging but also by the continued global adoption of Westernized lifestyles that favor sedentary behavior and high-calorie diets. Addressing this growing problem requires a multifaceted approach [12]. Public health initiatives aimed at promoting healthy lifestyles, reducing obesity, and increasing awareness of risk factors could play a pivotal role in prevention. Moreover, improving access to healthcare and encouraging early detection in underserved regions are critical steps toward reducing the impact of this disease on a global scale [12].

Pregnancy is a protective factor for endometrial cancer, because high level of progesterone changes the hormonal balance and decidualize the endometrium. Consequently, parous women have a lower risk of developing endometrial cancer compared to nulliparous women because of the relative reduced levels of estrogen in their life [13–15].

Obesity contributes to the increased risk of endometrial cancer in the postmenopausal uterus by a variety of mechanisms. Excessive adipose tissue means excessive aromatase activity, which leads to the conversion of androgens to estrogens. Inappropriate estrogen levels promote excessive proliferation and transcription of proliferative genes [13–15]. Proinflammatory adipokines associated with visceral adiposity lead to chronic inflammation, hyperinsulinemia, increases in insulin-like growth factor 1 (IGF1), and hyperglycemia. Chronic hyperinsulinemia decreases the concentration of IGF bound to protein 1 and IGF bound to protein 2, which increase bioavailability of free IGF-1 modifying the cellular environment (mitogenesis and anti-apoptosis). It also promotes tumor genesis by reducing the concentration of Sex-Hormone-Binding Globulin (SHBG) in the blood and increasing the bioavailability of estrogens. Scientific evidence indicates that obesity in women is responsible for about 40% of endometrial cancers [13–15].

Recent studies highlighted another risk factor for endometrial hyperplasia and endometrial cancer in young women represented by polycystic ovary syndrome (PCOS) [16]. Women suffering from PCOS are characterized by chronic anovulation and lack of progesterone releasing post ovulation, with high levels of unopposed estrogen which could cause endometrial thickening, increasing the risk of hyperplasia and, in some cases of endometrial cancer [17].

North America and Europe have the highest incidence of endometrial cancer. Endometrial cancer mainly affects menopausal women. The median age of patients at diagnosis is 63 years. Most cases are diagnosed in women aged 55 to 64 years [18].

In women with Lynch syndrome, the risk related to the onset of malignant tumors is 40-80% for colon cancer, 40-60% for endometrial cancer and 10-12% for ovarian cancer. The onset of endometrial neoplasia in a young woman can be considered as a sentinel event of a Lynch syndrome [19].

8.2. Clinical Manifestations

The clinical manifestations of endometrial cancer can range from subtle symptoms in its early stages to more pronounced and distressing signs as the disease progresses. One of the most common and hallmark symptoms is abnormal uterine bleeding (AUB) [20]. This often presents as postmenopausal bleeding, which is the most significant red flag for this condition.

Postmenopausal women who experience even a single episode of vaginal bleeding should seek immediate medical attention, as this symptom is strongly associated with endometrial cancer. In women who have not yet reached menopause, the condition may manifest as heavy, prolonged, or irregular menstrual bleeding, which may initially be attributed to hormonal imbalances or other benign gynecological conditions [20].

The abnormal vaginal bleeding could be of different entity during menopause, in young women spotting and menometrorrhagia are the most common symptoms. Usually these are early symptoms and rarely the neoplasm runs asymptomatically, therefore adenocarcinoma of the endometrium is a treatable malignancy because it is diagnosed in an early stage of disease [21].

In addition to abnormal bleeding, some patients may report a watery or blood-tinged vaginal discharge, which is typically non-menstrual in nature. While this discharge may be odorless initially, in cases where infection sets in or the cancer has progressed, the discharge can become foul-smelling [22]. Furthermore, as the disease advances, patients may experience pelvic or lower abdominal pain that is persistent or occurs intermittently. This discomfort may be accompanied by a feeling of pressure or fullness in the pelvic region [23].

Other symptoms of advanced disease may include painful urination (dysuria), difficulty emptying the bladder, or even the presence of blood in the urine if the cancer has invaded adjacent structures such as the bladder [24–26]. Women may also report pain during sexual intercourse (dyspareunia), which can significantly affect their quality of life [27]. Systemic symptoms like unexplained weight loss, fatigue, and general malaise may arise in more advanced stages of the disease. If the cancer metastasizes, additional symptoms may include shortness of breath, bone pain, or other signs indicative of spread to distant organs. Significant lymph node involvement can lead to edema in the lower limbs. Finally, abdominal-pelvic pain and pressure and sub-occlusive syndromes, are late signs of carcinosis [20].

8.3. Classification and Diagnosis

Endometrial cancer (EC) has traditionally been classified into type I and type II according to etiology, histology, and prognosis. Type I represents the estrogen-related tumors (about 80% of cases) that usually occurs on a background of obesity arising from endometrial atypical hyperplasia and that usually has favorable prognosis. Type II are the non-estrogen-related cancers that mainly arises from polyps or Endometrial Intraepithelial Carcinoma (EIC) in a context of endometrial atrophy. Type I, that is known as endometrioid type because of its histotype, is usually moderate to well differentiated (Figure 1). Type 2 is represented by Papillary serous carcinoma and clear cell carcinoma and it is usually poorly differentiated and it has an aggressive clinical behaviour [3].

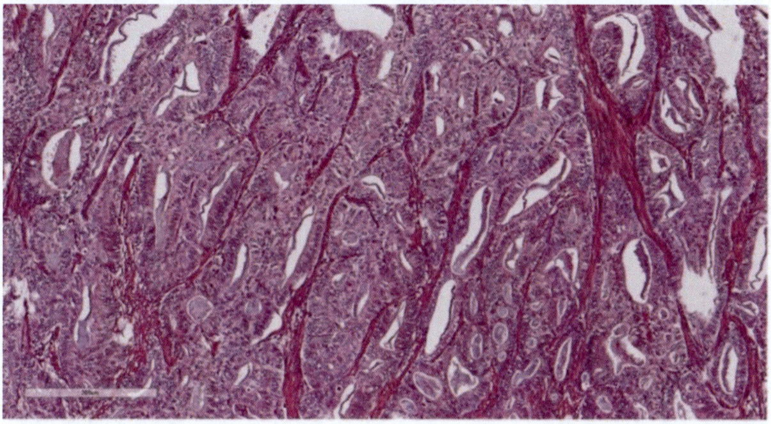

Figure 1. Histological appearance of endometrioid carcinoma of the endometrium.

Different histological types of endometrial cancer, according to a dualistic model, are described in Table 1.

According to this dualistic model the molecular origin and carcinogenesis of type I tumors results from impaired DNA Mismatch Repair system of cells, condition that is called "microsatellite instability," resulting in the accumulation of mutations in oncogenes and in tumor suppressor genes [28]. On the contrary, type II tumors carcinogenesis is due to the alterations of p53 that lead to chromosomal instability with loss or amplification of large chromosomal regions characterized by genes encoding important proteins such as E-Caderin [29]. Reduced expression of E caderin is associated with invasiveness and poor prognosis of the neoplasm. Most of tumors with a high grade of differentiation express estrogen receptors but not the p53 mutation [29]. In contrast, most tumors with low grade of differentiation do not have immunoreactivity for the receptors of estrogens but they are strongly positive for immunoreaction for p53, without evidence of microsatellite instability [29]. Although these evidences in many cases there is an overlap in the immunohistochemical and molecular characteristics of tumors. In recent years this dualistic model firstly ideated by Bockman in 1983 has been considered insufficient to adequately represents the heterogeneity of these neoplasms while the attention has been focused on genomic, transcriptomic and proteomic researches, until 2013 when the hormonal classification was replaced by the molecular classification proposed by The Cancer Genome Atlas [3–5].

Table 1. Different histological types of endometrial cancer, according to a dualistic model

Hystological subtypes type I	Hystological subtypes type II
Endometrioid Adenocarcinoma: Most common type (~80-90% of cases). Resembles normal endometrial glands. Typically, well-differentiated and lower grade. Often associated with mutations in PTEN, PIK3CA, KRAS, and microsatellite instability.	Serous Carcinoma: Represents 5-10% of cases. Characterized by papillary structures and high nuclear atypia. Frequently associated with TP53 mutations. High-grade and aggressive, with a tendency to spread early.
Villoglandular Adenocarcinoma: Rare variant of endometrioid cancer. Characterized by a papillary growth pattern with glandular features. Generally, has a favorable prognosis.	Clear Cell Carcinoma: Rare, comprising ~5% of cases. Features clear cytoplasm and hobnail cells. Aggressive behavior with poor prognosis.
	Carcinosarcoma (Malignant Mixed Müllerian Tumor): Contains both epithelial and mesenchymal components. Highly aggressive and often metastatic at diagnosis.
	Mucinous Adenocarcinoma: Contains cells with abundant mucin. Rare, typically less aggressive.
	Squamous Cell Carcinoma: Extremely rare as a primary endometrial tumor.
	Undifferentiated/Dedifferentiated Carcinoma: Composed of poorly differentiated or completely undifferentiated cells. Highly aggressive with poor outcomes.

This molecular classification is based on four subgroups, which best reflect the heterogeneity of this tumor:

- POLE gene-ultramutated (POLE mutated), in which cells are characterized by high mutagenicity (in particular mutations in the exonuclease domain of POLE 58-subunit-e of DNA polymerases involved in the DNA replication process, mutations in PTEN, PIK3R1, PIK3CA, FBXW7, and KRAS) and excellent prognosis;

- MSI hypermutated (MSI-H), with microsatellite instability related to defects in mismatch repair genes, secondary to MLH1 promoter methylation, with high mutagenicity, recurrent frameshift deletions of RPL22, and mutations in KRAS and PTEN. MSI-H cancers are commonly seen in Lynch syndrome;
- low-copy number, or endometrioid-like group, is the most common, characterized by the absence of a specific molecular profile, low mutagenicity and intermediate outcomes;
- high-copy number, also known as serous-like group, is associated with TP53 mutations and is characterized by poor outcomes.

Talhouk et al. suggested a simplified and pragmatic molecular-based classification called Proactive Molecular Risk Classifier Endometrial Cancer (ProMise), which is obtained by immunohistochemical evaluation of proteins made on formalin-embedded and paraffin-fixed tissues [30].

This classification distinguishes POLE mutated tumors (5-15%), tumors with MSI-H/mismatch repair-deficient (25-30%), tumors with abnormal p53 (5-15%), and tumors without specific molecular alterations (30-40%). The presence of MSIH/MMR-d should refer the woman for genetic evaluation for Lynch syndrome screening. This molecular characteristic has been identified as a potential predictive factor of good response to immunotherapies [4, 5].

For patients and family members with Lynch syndrome a prophylactic endometrial biopsy is recommended to assess for cancer and to preserve fertility in selected patients, deferring surgical menopause until childbearing is complete, then hysterectomy and bilateral salpingo-oophorectomy is recommended. In addition, annual colonoscopy is recommended to decrease the risk from colorectal cancer [31].

In consideration of the variability of the prognosis that exists within the different types of cancer described in the aforementioned classification it is essential to carry out tests on the biopsies for the immunohistochemical markers P53 and MMR, and a molecular analysis for POLE mutations in order to select the best management of the patient; adjuvant therapies may be tailored on molecular subtypes, knowing that POLE-mutated cancers often require less aggressive treatment because of their behaviour [32].

Endometrial adenocarcinoma behaviour depends also on the grade of differentiation the cancer cells. There are 3 grades which reflect cell differentiation and their rate of division and multiplication (tumor growth).

The lower is the grade, the better the prognosis. Serous and clear cell carcinoma are always a grade 3. Poor prognosis and mortality may be related to high-risk histologies (eg, serous carcinomas) or high-grade diseases, to patients being diagnosed at an age ≥ 65 years, to neoplasms with >50% depth of myometrial invasion, to lymph node involvement, tumor size, lymphovascular space invasion (LVSI ≥5 vessels), and cervical stromal invasion. Recent studies underlined the prognostic role of LVSI; it seems that the presence of lymphovascular space invasion increases the risk of tumor recurrence [33].

Currently, there are no validated screening tests for endometrial carcinoma. The first exam to perform in any woman who complains of abnormal vaginal blood loss is Trans-Vaginal Ultrasonography. This study technique provides a way to evaluate endometrial thickness (suspicious if it is thicker than 4 mm in postmenopausal age that are not under tamoxifen treatment, whereas in fecund age the evaluation of endometrium depends on the phase of the ovarian cycle) [34, 35].

Other characteristics are the homogeneity of endometrium and the vascularization. The analysis of the blood perfusion of the endometrium is performed using colour and power Doppler [36]. Ultrasound evaluation is essential to hypothesize endometrial abnormalities and possible hyperplasia or cancer, but the diagnosis can only be obtained from targeted biopsies, carried out by hysteroscopy, and then from histopathology with a false-negative rate of about 10% [37, 38]. Transvaginal ultrasound is also useful for the evaluation of myometrial and cervical stroma infiltration [39–41]. Pelvic masses may be identified during a physical examination in case of advanced tumors [42]. Hysteroscopy is the gold standard for the identification of abnormal endometrium and for the collection of a sample for histological examination [43–47].

The sample can be collected with outpatient hysteroscopy using miniaturized grasps or with operative resectoscopy under general or local anaesthesia using operative hysteroscopes [48–52].

Preoperative imaging is recommended to tailor surgery and adjuvant treatments [53]. Magnetic resonance imaging (MRI) with paramagnetic contrast is useful to stage the carcinoma of the endometrium, it allows to suppose the depth of myometrial infiltration, the infiltration of the stroma of the cervix and of the walls of the vagina, the infiltration of adipose tissue of the parameters and it is able to demonstrate the presence of pelvic or lumbo-aortic enlarged lymph nodes [54]. Computed Tomography (CT scan) and positron emission tomography-CT (PET-CT) have poor diagnostic accuracy compared to MRI in the evaluation of the local uterine neoplasm, but they are useful in the evaluation of any sites of extra-uterine disease (abdominal lymph nodes, liver, lungs) [55]. Scintigraphy bone scan is an investigation limited to clinically suspected cases of bone localization of the disease.

Staging of endometrial cancer is based on the anatomical-pathological and non-clinical evaluation of the illness. Staging can be done after the patient has undergone surgery.

Two classifications have been drawn up: the FIGO (International Federation of Gynecology and Obstetrics) and the American Joint Committee on Cancer (AJCC) staging [5, 56].

The AJCC system classifies cancer of the uterus on three factors: extension of the tumor (T); lymph node involvement (N) and presence of metastases (M).

The new 2023 FIGO staging of endometrial cancer is based on the stratification of different stages basing on different prognostic factors like myometrial invasion, lymphovascular space involvement, grading of cell differentiation, histology and distant spread. Furthermore, the integration of molecular factors is encouraged, and molecular information can be recorded in the FIGO stage by the addition of "m" for molecular classification, and a subscript indicating the specific molecular subtype [3, 57].

Table 2. 2009 FIGO staging [58]

2009 FIGO STAGING:	
STAGE I	Tumor confined to the corpus uteri
STAGE IA	No or less than half myometrial invasion
STAGE IB	Invasion equal to more than half myometrium
STAGE II	Invasion of cervical stroma, not beyond the uterus
STAGE III	Local spread of the tumor
STAGE IIIA	Invasion of the serosa uteri and/or adnexa
STAGE IIIB	Vaginal and/or parametrial involvement
STAGE IIIC	Metastases to pelvic (IIIC1) and/or para-aortic lymph-nodes (IIIC2)
STAGE IV	Invasion of bladder and/or bowel, and/or distant metastases
STAGE IVA	Bladder or bowel mucosa involvement
STAGE IVB	Distant metastases including intra-abdominal metastases or inguinal lymph-nodes

The 2023 FIGO staging compared to the previous one diffused in 2009 [58] is changed from a traditional purely anatomical description of tumor size, borders, invasion of adjacent tissues and metastases to an integrated staging system with tumor-biology and molecular characteristics, providing important information for the cancer treatment: the changes made have significant implications regarding the systemic and radiotherapy treatments and the selection of patients for surgery at both the primary diagnosis and at relapse (Table 2-3) [59].

Table 3. 2023 FIGO staging [59]

2023 FIGO STAGING	
STAGE I	Tumor confined to the corpus uteri
STAGE IA	POLEmut confined to uterine corpus +/- cervical invasion, regardless of LVSI or histotype
STAGE IA1	Low-grade endometrioid, limited to polyp/endometrium without myoinvasion
STAGE IA2	Low-grade endometrioid, myoinvasion <50%, no or focal LVSI
STAGE IA3	Low-grade endometrioid carcinoma of the endometrium and ovary
STAGE IB	Low-grade endometrioid, myoinvasion ≥50%, no or focal LVSI
STAGE IC	Aggressive histotypes, limited to polyp or endometrium
STAGE II	Confined to the uterus
STAGE IIA	Low grade endometrioid, invasion of the cervical stroma
STAGE IIB	Low grade endometrioid substantial LVSI
STAGE IIC	Aggressive histotypes, myoinvasion mp53 abn confined to uterus+/-cervical invasion+ myoinvasion regardless of LVSI or histologies
STAGE III	Local spread
STAGE IIIA1	Spread to ovary or fallopian tube (except when meeting stage IA3 criteria)
STAGE IIIA2	Involvement of uterine subserosa or spread through the uterine serosa
STAGE IIIB1	Spread to the vagina and/or the parametria
STAGE IIIB2	Metastasis to the pelvic peritoneum
STAGE IIIC	Pelvic lymph node metastasis
STAGE IIIC1 I	Micrometastasis (0.2-2mm and/or >200 cells)
STAGE IIIC1 II	Macrometastasis (>2mm in size)
STAGE IIIC2	Para-aortic lymph node metastasis (up to renal vessels) Micro IIIC2 I or macrometastases IIIC2 II
STAGE IV	Advanced disease
STAGE IVA	Invasion of the bladder and/or the intestinal mucosa
STAGE IVB	Peritoneal metastasis beyond the pelvis
STAGE IVC	Distant metastasis

Knowledge of the histological subtype and grade is essential for treatment decision making in endometrial cancer. The 2023 FIGO staging system describes the different prognosis of high-grade (aggressive: serous, clear cell, high-grade endometrioid, mesonephric-like, gastrointestinal-type mucinous endometrial, undifferentiated carcinomas, and carcinosarcomas) histological subtypes compared to low-grade (G1/G2) endometrioid (non-aggressive) histological subtypes [59].

According to the 2009 FIGO staging system, all metastases of endometrial cancer to the ovary were considered as stage IIIA, whereas the new FIGO 2023 differentiates low-grade endometrioid carcinoma of the endometrium and the ovary (if specific criteria are met: <50% myometrial invasion, absence of LVSI, no other metastases and the ovarian tumor is equivalent to pT1a) from other metastatic tumors to the ovary (2023 FIGO IIIA1). This new differentiation is based on the favorable biological behavior and good prognosis of low-grade endometroid carcinomas of the endometrium and ovary [59].

Though actually the most underlined concept is the relevance of the recent molecular classification, helpful to esteem the endometrial cancer prognosis, considered as a new field of research and a key to improve the management and treatment of women.

The 2023 FIGO staging system describes two different and interesting scenarios of two molecularly different substages in early stage: 1) Uterus confined (corpus+/−cervical invasion) disease with a pathogenic POLE-mutation is defined as 2023 FIGO IA m POLEmut, and 2) Uterus confined (corpus+/−cervical invasion) disease with myometrial invasion with a p53 abnormality that is defined as 2023 FIGO IIC m p53abn. It is nowadays known that POLEmut early-stage disease has an excellent prognosis, and European Guidelines suggest omitting adjuvant treatment for this reason, whereas it is well known that p53 abnormal cases with myometrial invasion have a poor prognosis, even in previously defined stage I disease [59, 60].

The new 2023 FIGO stage distinguishes between micro and macro pelvic (IIIC1) and para-aortic (IIIC2) metastases, by the addition of “i” for micro (0.2-2 mm in size) and “ii” for macro-metastases (>2 mm) to underline the significant prognostic difference related to the size of the lymph nodes involved [61]. Furthermore, the new FIGO 2023 staging system describes in a different way from the previous one, metastases involving pelvic lymph nodes, extrapelvic lymph nodes or peritoneal metastases rather than distant organs due to their different prognosis and disease’s behavior. Peritoneal carcinomatosis limited to the pelvis only now is considered stage IIIB2 (downgraded from the previous stage IVB 2009) and peritoneal carcinomatosis beyond the pelvis now forms a separate substage (2023 IVB) rather than others abdominal metastases (stage IVC 2023) [62].

8.4. Appropriate Management According to International Clinical Guidelines

The appropriate management of endometrial cancer is described by the European Society for Medical Oncology (ESMO), European Society of Gynaecological Oncology (ESGO) and the National Comprehensive Cancer Network (NCCN) and it is based on stage, histological type and molecular profile of the tumour [63].

Total hysterectomy, bilateral salpingo-oophorectomy and lymph node assessment is the primary treatment for apparent uterine-confined endometrial carcinoma, unless patients desire for fertility-sparing (Figure 2) [64, 65].

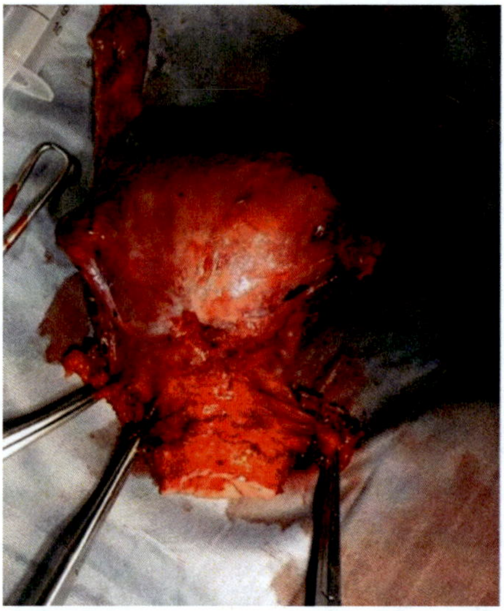

Figure 2. Surgical specimen of Classe A sec. Querlew-Morrow radical hysterectomy for endometrial cancer.

Total or radical hysterectomy, bilateral salpingo-oophorectomy and lymph node assessment may be performed by any surgical route (eg, laparoscopic, robotic, vaginal, abdominal), although nowadays the surgical way considered the gold standard is the abdominal minimally invasive approach (laparoscopy or robotic surgery), due to a lower rate of surgical site infection, transfusion, venous thromboembolism, decreased hospital stay and costs [66–68]. During surgical exploration the surgeon may excise any suspicious nodule, bulk, fibrosis or necrosis on omentum, peritoneum, diaphragm for tumour staging [69]. Intraperitoneal morcellation of uterus should be avoided or made safely into specific bags. No specific contraindications are known about uterine manipulation during surgery. A fundamental procedure to be carried out is the Lymph node assessment. The evaluation of the nodal vessels that drain the uterus provided important information that influence current surgical strategies [70].

In past years, a full standard pelvic lymphadenectomy (with or without para-aortic nodal dissection up to the infrarenal region) has been recommended for all patients [71, 72]. The sentinel lymph node biopsy after mapping (SLN) is a possible more selective approach recommended also by international guidelines. Different randomized clinical trials reported that routine lymph node dissection does not improve oncologic outcomes of patients with endometrial cancer. Prospective and retrospective studies demonstrate that compared to systemic lymphadenectomy, SLN mapping with ultrastaging may increase the detection of lymph node tiny metastasis with low false-negative rates: it may also be used in high risk histologies [73]. Lymph nodes should be processed using ultrastaging that consists of serial sectioning with review of multiple hematoxylin and eosin stained slides, and with or without cytokeratin immunohistochemistry staining [74]. A variety of dyes, such as Methylene Blue 1%, and Patent Blue 2.5% sodium, are available to detect sentinel nodes. Indocyanine green recently emerged as an efficient imaging dye that requires an-infrared camera for localization of metastasis. This technology is now available using the laparoscopic technique or the robotic platform, with different intraoperative features (Figure 3-4).

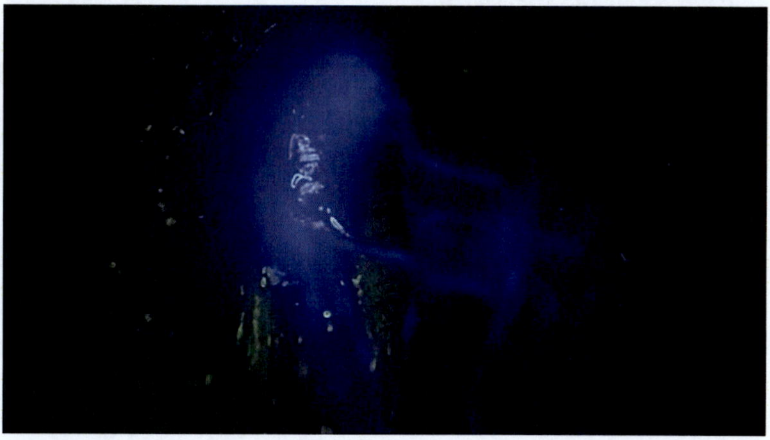

Figure 3. Laparoscopic lymph nodal mapping of the left pelvis using indocyanine green.

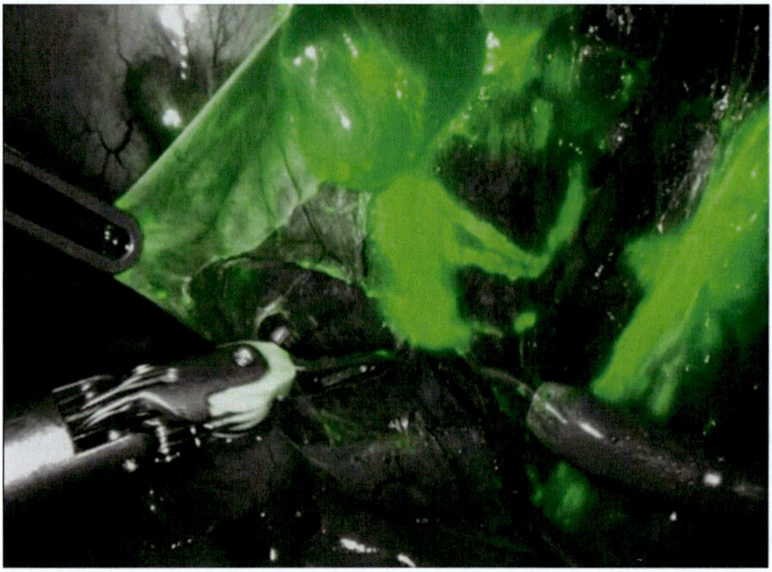

Figure 4. Lymph nodal mapping in the right pelvis using the Da Vinci Xi robotic platform.

Indocyanine green allows also a complete visualization of the lymphatic drainage of the uterus, thus providing a great advantage for the surgeon [75].

Lymph nodes mapping should be done prior to hysterectomy, except in cases where a bulky uterus must be removed to allow the access to the obliterated pelvis (Figure 5) [70].

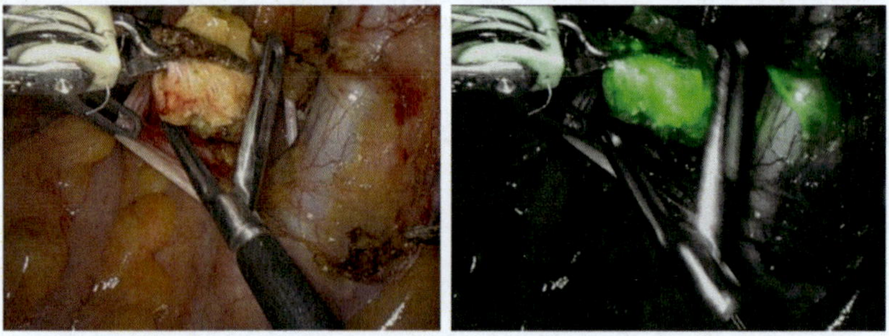

Figure 5. Surgical excision of pelvic sentinel lymph node using the robotic Da Vinci Xi platform.

Decide where to inject the tracer in patients with endometrial cancer has been controversial. Evidence suggests that in endometrial carcinoma, cervical injection with ICG (immunochromatographic assay) results in a higher detection rate than hysteroscopic injection and that the nodal anatomical distribution is similar. The dye is usually injected into the cervix both at the surface (1 to 3 mm) and in depth (1 to 2 cm) at 3 and 9 o'clock. With this technique, the tracer penetrates the uterine lymphatic trunks (which meet in the parameters) and appears in the wide ligament leading to pelvic sentinel lymph nodes and occasionally paraortic [75].

If the mapping is not clear, re-injection and then a systematic pelvic nodal dissection is the better surgical choice.

After surgery the disease assessment includes hysterectomy type, tumour site and size, histologic type (endometrioid, serous, clear cell, carcinosarcoma, or undifferentiated) and grade, myometrial invasion (depth of invasion in mm), cervical stromal involvement, and lymphovascular invasion (4 or more involved vessels in at least one hematoxylin and eosin section when LVSI is considered "focal," 5 or more positive vessels to consider a "substantial" LVSI) and possible distant organ involvement [76]. FIGO 2023 stages IA and IB include low-grade endometrioid cancers with no or focal LVSI, whereas the presence of substantial LVSI, in low-grade endometrioid cancers confined to the uterus automatically upshifts these cases to a stage IIB. Extensive literature has documented that substantial LVSI represents an independent prognostic factor for pelvic regional recurrence and for distant metastasis [77].

For staging goal omentectomy should be performed in serous carcinoma.

Adjuvant therapies are indicated according to FIGO stage and molecular classification.

In patients with low-risk endometrial cancer (endometrioid stage I, grade 1-2, myometrial invasion <50%, LVSI negative), no adjuvant treatment is indicated. In patients with intermediate risk endometrioid cancer (endometrioid stage I, grade 1-2, ≥50% myometrial invasion, LVSI negative, >60 years), adjuvant brachytherapy is recommended to reduce the risk of vaginal recurrence. In patients with intermediate-high risk endometrial cancer (stage I endometrioid, grade 3): adjuvant brachytherapy is recommended to reduce vaginal recurrence of cancer, adjuvant external beam radiotherapy (EBRT) is recommended for positive LVSI cases to decrease pelvic recurrence [78].

For patients with cervical involvement (endometrioid histologies stage II), suitable for primary surgery, a radical class A (Querleu Morrow classification) hysterectomy is recommended with bilateral salpingo-ovariectomy and lymph node assessment. More radical hysterectomy does not improve oncological outcomes of these patients. In case of positive nodes external beam radiotherapy + brachytherapy and chemotherapy are recommended.

In case of extrauterine disease (endometrioid histologies stage III) total hysterectomy, bilateral salpingo-oophorectomy and surgical debulking are necessary (with or without neoadjuvant chemotherapy) with the goal to have no measurable residual disease, followed by chemotherapy, external beam radiotherapy and vaginal brachytherapy as adjuvant treatment. For distant visceral metastasis (e.g., liver metastasis), recommended options include systemic therapy with (or without) EBRT [79]. Patients that are not in clinical conditions to undergo surgery or with unresectable extrauterine pelvic disease are typically treated with EBRT with (or without) brachytherapy with (or without) systemic therapy, followed by re-evaluation of tailored surgery [80].

In case of stage IV disease with distant metastasis the possible therapies are:

1) Platinum-based chemotherapy (carboplatin+paclitaxel),
2) hormonal therapy in hormone receptor-positive tumors,
3) immunotherapy (pembrolizumab for MSI-H or dMMR tumors).

Although the primary treatment of endometrial cancer is the hysterectomy and salpingo-oophorectomy, fertility sparing may be considered for selected patients with grade 1 stage IA1/2. The preserving fertility treatment may consist in a continuous progestin-based therapy, such as megestrol acetate, medroxyprogesterone, or an intrauterine device (IUD) containing levonorgestrel associated or not with hysteroscopic resection of pathologic endometrium [81–83]. Patients should receive a counselling with medical doctors with proven experience in oncofertility, as this therapy is not the standard of care for endometrial carcinomas. Progestins should be carefully prescribed considering any risk factors and contraindications such as previous breast cancer, stroke, myocardial infarction, pulmonary embolism, deep vein thrombosis, and smoking. NCCN Guidelines suggests close monitoring with endometrial biopsies every 3 to 6 months [57, 80, 84].

Hysterectomy and salpingo-oophorectomy with surgical staging is recommended:

1) after childbearing is complete;
2) if patients have documented progression on biopsy;

3) if endometrial cancer is still present after 6 to 12 months of progestin-based therapy.

Preservation of the ovaries may be considered in patients under 45 years old in case of grade 1 neoplasm with myometrial invasion <50%, without evidence of ovarian disease or other ectopic disease to avoid iatrogenic menopause. In the case of ovarian preservation, bilateral salpingectomy must be performed. Preservation of the ovaries is contraindicated in patients with BRCA mutations or Lynch syndrome [57, 80].

8.5. Updates in Endometrial Cancer Treatments

For many years, the only possibility of treatment for endometrial cancer was represented by megestrol acetate and platinum-based chemotherapy. The therapeutic management began to change and improve since 2020 with the introduction of immunotherapy, a valid opportunity especially for those women who had not had an optimal response to the frontline chemotherapy [6].

Recently, several studies such as RUBY, NRG-GY018 or DUO-E have shown encouraging results on the use of PD-(L)1 inhibitors in combination with chemotherapy especially, but not only, for advanced or recurrent endometrial cancer. During ESMO 2023, investigators presented updated findings from the phase 3 RUBY trial, a double-blind, multicenter trial in which patients with advanced or first recurrent endometrial cancer randomly have received the anti–PD-1 antibody Dostarlimab or placebo, plus carboplatin and paclitaxel. Results have shown that Dostarlimab gave benefit over placebo in terms of progression-free survival and overall survival especially but not only in patients with mismatch repair–deficient (dMMR)/microsatellite instability–high (MSI-H) disease [85].

The Food and Drug Administration (FDA) in 2024 has approved three new immunotherapy drugs that act like immune checkpoint inhibitor. The first approval, announced on June 14, is for durvalumab (Imfinzi) given in combination with chemotherapy to treat people with advanced endometrial cancer with mismatch repair deficiency. The DUO-E trial indicated that the combination of durvalumab with chemotherapy reduced the risk of disease progression or death by 58% compared to chemotherapy alone.

The second approval, announced on June 17, is for pembrolizumab (Keytruda) given along with chemotherapy, and on August 1, FDA approved dostarlimab (Jemperli) plus carboplatin and paclitaxel followed by maintenance dostarlimab for people with advanced endometrial cancers regardless of dMMR status [86]. Dostarlimab had previously been approved, in 2023, for advanced endometrial cancers that are dMMR.

Continuous research is focused on new therapeutic targets and combination strategies to further enhance treatment efficacy and patient quality of life.

8.6. Integrated Approaches and Future Perspectives

In recent years the treatment of endometrium carcinoma is one of the most controversial topics in oncology. New technologies, biomolecular knowledge and targeted immunotherapies are rapidly overturning the established knowledge regarding this frequent but still lethal disease [87].

Artificial intelligence integrated with ultrasound and with hysteroscopes could help in early diagnosis and in planning the proper therapeutic management, distinguishing specific characteristics of each different type of endometrial cancer [88]. Integration between artificial intelligence and next-generation robotic platform will guide the surgeon for a tailored surgical treatment [89].

Endometrial cancer risk classification necessitates for larger and more diverse patient cohorts, giving the right weight to the different risk factors and molecular pathways. Data are expected from numerous ongoing clinical trials exploring treatment escalation and de-escalation within the four molecular subtypes as well as matching targeted therapies to specific mutational or biomarker profiles [90].

Organoids derived from endometrial cancer cells could help in choosing target therapies, especially for patients choosing fertility sparing strategies.

Finally, the rapid development of multi-omics in endometrial cancer opens several fields of study for novel therapeutic targets, including non-coding RNAs such as miRNAs and long non-coding RNAs as important regulators of gene expression [91].

Conclusion

Endometrial cancer remains a significant challenge in women's health, with its rising global incidence demanding continued advancements in prevention, diagnosis, and treatment. While early-stage disease often benefits from timely diagnosis and effective interventions, more aggressive subtypes and advanced stages pose considerable therapeutic challenges. The integration of molecular classification into clinical practice has revolutionized the approach to staging and management, enabling more precise and personalized treatment strategies.

Emerging therapeutic options, such as immunotherapy and targeted therapies, represent a paradigm shift, particularly for patients with advanced or recurrent disease. Additionally, minimally invasive surgical techniques and fertility-preserving options offer improved outcomes and quality of life for selected patient populations. Despite these advancements, disparities in access to care and the rising burden in developing regions underscore the need for global efforts to enhance healthcare infrastructure and accessibility.

Future progress hinges on harnessing cutting-edge technologies such as artificial intelligence, multi-omics, and organoid models, which promise to refine risk stratification, early diagnosis, and tailored treatments. Collaborative research and large-scale clinical trials will be pivotal in addressing the heterogeneity of the disease and optimizing therapeutic outcomes.

Ultimately, a multidisciplinary and patient-centered approach, supported by ongoing innovation and global cooperation, is essential to mitigate the burden of endometrial cancer and improve prognosis and survival for women worldwide.

References

[1] Raglan O, Kalliala I, Markozannes G, Cividini S, Gunter MJ, Nautiyal J, Gabra H, Paraskevaidis E, Martin-Hirsch P, Tsilidis KK, Kyrgiou M. Risk factors for endometrial cancer: An umbrella review of the literature. *Int J cancer.* 2019;145(7):1719–30.

[2] Crosbie EJ, Kitson SJ, McAlpine JN, Mukhopadhyay A, Powell ME, Singh N. Endometrial cancer. *Lancet.* 2022;399(10333):1412–28.

[3] Li JJX, Ip PPC. Endometrial Cancer: An Update on Prognostic Pathologic Features and Clinically Relevant Biomarkers. *Surg Pathol Clin.* 2022;15(2):277–99.

[4] Rios-Doria E, Momeni-Boroujeni A, Friedman CF, Selenica P, Zhou Q, Wu M, Marra A, Leitao MM, Iasonos A, Alektiar KM, Sonoda Y, Makker V, Jewell E, Liu Y, Chi D, Zamarin D, Abu-Rustum NR, Aghajanian C, Mueller JJ, Ellenson LH, Weigelt B. Integration of clinical sequencing and immunohistochemistry for the molecular classification of endometrial carcinoma. *Gynecol Oncol.* 2023;174:262–72.

[5] Berek JS, Matias-Guiu X, Creutzberg C, Fotopoulou C, Gaffney D, Kehoe S, Lindemann K, Mutch D, Concin N, Berek JS, Wilailak S, Kehoe S, Anorlu R, Cain J, Creutzberg C, Fotopoulou C, Lindeque G, Matias-Guiu X, McNally O, Okamoto A, Pareja R, Pomerantz T, Scambia G, Schmalfeld B, Tahlak MA, Berek J, Concin N, Creutzberg C, Fotopoulou C, Gaffney D, Kehoe S, Lindemann K, Matias-Guiu X. FIGO staging of endometrial cancer: 2023. *Int J Gynaecol Obstet.* 2023;162(2):383–94.

[6] Bogani G, Scambia G, Cimmino C, Fanfani F, Costantini B, Loverro M, Ferrandina G, Landoni F, Bazzurini L, Grassi T, Vitobello D, Siesto G, Perrone AM, Zanagnolo V, De Iaco P, Multinu F, Ghezzi F, Casarin J, Berretta R, Capozzi VA, Zupi E, Centini G, Pellegrino A, Corso S, Stevenazzi G, Montoli S, Boschi AC, Comerci G, Greco P, Martinello R, Sopracordevole F, Giorda G, Simoncini T, Caretto M, Sartori E, Ferrari F, Cianci A, Sarpietro G, Matarazzo MG, Zullo F, Bifulco G, Morelli M, Ferrero A, Biglia N, Barra F, Ferrero S, Maggiore ULR, Cianci S, Chiantera V, Ercoli A, Sozzi G, Martoccia A, Schettini S, Orlando T, Cannone FG, Ettore G, Puppo A, Borghese M, Martinelli C, Muzii L, Di Donato V, Driul L, Restaino S, Bergamini A, Candotti G, Bocciolone L, Plotti F, Angioli R, Mantovani G, Ceccaroni M, Cassani C, Dominoni M, Giambanco L, Amodeo S, Leo L, Thomasset R, Raimondo D, Seracchioli R, Malzoni M, Gorlero F, Di Luca M, Busato E, Kilzie S, Dell'acqua A, Scarfone G, Vercellini P, Petrillo M, Dessole S, Capobianco G, Ciavattini A, Delli Carpini G, Giannella L, Mereu L, Tateo S, Sorbi F, Fambrini M, Cicogna S, Romano F, Ricci G, Trojano G, Consonni R, Cantaluppi S, Lippolis A, Tinelli R, D'ippolito G, Aguzzoli L, Mandato VD, Palomba S, Calandra D, Rosati M, Gallo C, Surico D, Remorgida V, Ruscitto F, Beretta P, Panici PB, Raspagliesi F. Characteristics and patterns of care of endometrial cancer before and during COVID-19 pandemic. *J Gynecol Oncol.* 2022;33(1).

[7] Sung H, Ferlay J, Siegel RL, Laversanne M, Soerjomataram I, Jemal A, Bray F. Global Cancer Statistics 2020: GLOBOCAN Estimates of Incidence and Mortality Worldwide for 36 Cancers in 185 Countries. *CA Cancer J Clin.* 2021;71(3):209–49.

[8] Aune D, Navarro Rosenblatt DA, Chan DSM, Vingeliene S, Abar L, Vieira AR, Greenwood DC, Bandera E V., Norat T. Anthropometric factors and endometrial cancer risk: a systematic review and dose–response meta-analysis of prospective studies. *Ann Oncol.* 2015;26(8):1635–48.

[9] Zhang S, Gong TT, Liu FH, Jiang YT, Sun H, Ma XX, Zhao YH, Wu QJ. Global, Regional, and National Burden of Endometrial Cancer, 1990–2017: Results From the Global Burden of Disease Study, 2017. *Front Oncol.* 2019;9:497602.

[10] Corrado G, Mereu L, Bogliolo S, Cela V, Gardella B, Sperduti I, Certelli C, Pellegrini A, Posar G, Zampa A, Tateo S, Gadducci A, Spinillo A, Vizza E. Comparison between single-site and multiport robot-assisted hysterectomy in obese patients with endometrial cancer: An Italian multi-institutional study. *Int J Med Robot.* 2020;16(2):e2066.

[11] World Cancer Research Fund/American Institute for Cancer Research. *Food, Nutrition, Physical Activity, and the Prevention of Cancer: a Global Perspective.* Washington DC: AICR; 2007.

[12] Bizuayehu HM, Dadi AF, Hassen TA, Ketema DB, Ahmed KY, Kassa ZY, Amsalu E, Kibret GD, Alemu AA, Alebel A, Shifa JE, Assefa Y, Tessema GA, Sarich P, Gebremedhin AF, Bore MG. Global burden of 34 cancers among women in 2020 and projections to 2040: Population-based data from 185 countries/territories. *Int J cancer.* 2024;154(8):1377–93.

[13] Renehan AG, Tyson M, Egger M, Heller RF, Zwahlen M. Body-mass index and incidence of cancer: a systematic review and meta-analysis of prospective observational studies. *Lancet* (London, England). 2008;371(9612):569–78.

[14] Crosbie EJ, Zwahlen M, Kitchener HC, Egger M, Renehan AG. Body mass index, hormone replacement therapy, and endometrial cancer risk: a meta-analysis. *Cancer Epidemiol Biomarkers Prev.* 2010;19(12):3119–30.

[15] Onstad MA, Schmandt RE, Lu KH. Addressing the Role of Obesity in Endometrial Cancer Risk, Prevention, and Treatment. *J Clin Oncol.* 2016;34(35):4225–30.

[16] Ali DES, Shah M, Ali A, Malik MO, Rehman F, Badshah H, Ehtesham E, Vitale SG. Treatment with Metformin and Combination of Metformin plus Pioglitazone on Serum Levels of IL-6 and IL-8 in Polycystic Ovary Syndrome: A Randomized Clinical Trial. *Horm Metab Res.* 2019;51(11):714–22.

[17] Teede HJ, Tay CT, Laven JSE, Dokras A, Moran LJ, Piltonen TT, Joham AE. Recommendations from the 2023 International Evidence-based Guideline for the Assessment and Management of Polycystic Ovary Syndrome. *Eur J Endocrinol.* 2023;189(2):G43--G64.

[18] National Cancer Institute. Surveillance, Epidemiology, and End Results Program. *Cancer stat facts: uterine cancer.* [Internet]. National Cancer Institute. 2024 [cited 2025 Jan 10]. Available from: https://seer.cancer.gov/statfacts/html/corp.html.

[19] Garg K, Soslow RA. Endometrial carcinoma in women aged 40 years and younger. *Arch Pathol Lab Med.* 2014;138(3):335–42.

[20] Bakkum-Gamez JN, Gonzalez-Bosquet J, Laack NN, Mariani A, Dowdy SC. Current issues in the management of endometrial cancer. *Mayo Clin Proc.* 2008;83(1):97–112.

[21] Pessoa JN, Freitas ACL, Guimaraes RA, Lima J, Reis HLB dos, Filho AC. Endometrial Assessment: When is it Necessary? *J Clin Med Res.* 2013;6(1):21.

[22] Shi Y, Zhu Y, Fan S, Vitagliano A, Liu X, Liao Y, Liang Y, Vitale SG. Clinical Characteristics and Antifungal Susceptibility of Candida nivariensis from Vulvovaginal Candidiasis. *Gynecol Obstet Invest.* 2020;85(1):88–93.

[23] Makker V, MacKay H, Ray-Coquard I, Levine DA, Westin SN, Aoki D, Oaknin A. Endometrial cancer. *Nat Rev Dis Prim.* 2021;7(1).

[24] Vitale SG, Saponara S, Succu AG, Sicilia G, Martsidis K, D'Alterio MN, Angioni S. Efficacy and Safety of Non-Ablative Dual Wavelength Diode Laser Therapy for Genitourinary Syndrome of Menopause: A Single-Center Prospective Study. *Adv Ther.* 2024;41(12):4617–27.

[25] Cai T, Mazzoli S, Migno S, Malossini G, Lanzafame P, Mereu L, Tateo S, Wagenlehner FM, Pickard RS, Bartoletti R. Development and validation of a

nomogram predicting recurrence risk in women with symptomatic urinary tract infection. *Int J Urol.* 2014;21(9):929–34.
[26] Vitale SG, Laganà AS, Noventa M, Giampaolino P, Zizolfi B, Butticè S, La Rosa VL, Gullo G, Rossetti D. Transvaginal Bilateral Sacrospinous Fixation after Second Recurrence of Vaginal Vault Prolapse: Efficacy and Impact on Quality of Life and Sexuality. *Biomed Res Int.* 2018;2018:5727165.
[27] Vitale SG, Caruso S, Rapisarda AMC, Valenti G, Rossetti D, Cianci S, Cianci A. Biocompatible porcine dermis graft to treat severe cystocele: impact on quality of life and sexuality. *Arch Gynecol Obstet.* 2016;293(1):125–31.
[28] Llobet D, Pallares J, Yeramian A, Santacana M, Eritja N, Velasco A, Dolcet X, Matias-Guiu X. Molecular pathology of endometrial carcinoma: practical aspects from the diagnostic and therapeutic viewpoints. *J Clin Pathol.* 2009;62(9):777–85.
[29] Mell LK, Meyer JJ, Tretiakova M, Khramtsov A, Gong C, Yamada SD, Montag AG, Mundt AJ. Prognostic Significance of E-Cadherin Protein Expression in Pathological Stage I-III Endometrial Cancer. *Clin Cancer Res.* 2004;10(16):5546–53.
[30] Talhouk A, McConechy MK, Leung S, Yang W, Lum A, Senz J, Boyd N, Pike J, Anglesio M, Kwon JS, Karnezis AN, Huntsman DG, Gilks CB, McAlpine JN. Confirmation of ProMisE: A simple, genomics-based clinical classifier for endometrial cancer. *Cancer.* 2017;123(5):802–13.
[31] Seppälä TT, Latchford A, Negoi I, Sampaio Soares A, Jimenez-Rodriguez R, Evans DG, Ryan N, Crosbie EJ, Dominguez-Valentin M, Burn J, Kloor M, Knebel Doeberitz M von, Duijnhoven FJB va., Quirke P, Sampson JR, Møller P, Möslein G. European guidelines from the EHTG and ESCP for Lynch syndrome: an updated third edition of the Mallorca guidelines based on gene and gender. *Br J Surg.* 2021;108(5):484–98.
[32] Ottolina J, Ferrandina G, Gadducci A, Scollo P, Lorusso D, Giorda G, Breda E, Savarese A, Candiani M, Zullo F, Mangili G. Is the endometrial evaluation routinely required in patients with adult granulosa cell tumors of the ovary? *Gynecol Oncol.* 2015;136(2):230–4.
[33] Abu-Rustum NR. Updates to the Management of Endometrial Cancer. *J Natl Compr Cancer Netw.* 2024;22(Supplement).
[34] Chiofalo B, Mazzon I, Di Angelo Antonio S, Amadore D, Vizza E, Laganà AS, Vocaturo G, Calagna G, Favilli A, Palmara V, Maranto M, Vitale SG, Cucinella G, Granese R, Ghezzi F, Sperduti I, Triolo O. Hysteroscopic Evaluation of Endometrial Changes in Breast Cancer Women with or without Hormone Therapies: Results from a Large Multicenter Cohort Study. *J Minim Invasive Gynecol.* 2020;27(4):832–9.
[35] Vitale SG, Riemma G, Haimovich S, Carugno J, Alonso Pacheco L, Perez-Medina T, Parry JP, Török P, Tesarik J, Della Corte L, Cobellis L, Di Spiezio Sardo A, De Franciscis P. Risk of endometrial cancer in asymptomatic postmenopausal women in relation to ultrasonographic endometrial thickness: systematic review and diagnostic test accuracy meta-analysis. *Am J Obstet Gynecol.* 2023;228(1):22-35.e2.

[36] Haldorsen IS, Salvesen HB. What Is the Best Preoperative Imaging for Endometrial Cancer? *Curr Oncol Rep.* 2016;18(4):1–11.

[37] Vitale SG. The Biopsy Snake Grasper Sec. VITALE: A New Tool for Office Hysteroscopy. *J Minim Invasive Gynecol.* 2020;27(6):1414–6.

[38] Vitale SG, Angioni S, Saponara S, Sicilia G, Etrusco A, D'Alterio MN, Cobellis L, De Franciscis P, Riemma G. TikTok as a platform for hysteroscopy information: An analytical video-based cross-sectional study to assess quality, reliability, and accuracy. *Int J Gynecol Obstet.* 2025;168(1):353–61.

[39] Vitale SG, Angioni S, D'Alterio MN, Ronsini C, Saponara S, De Franciscis P, Riemma G. Risk of endometrial malignancy in women treated for breast cancer: the BLUSH prediction model–evidence from a comprehensive multicentric retrospective cohort study. *Climacteric.* 2024;25(5):482–8.

[40] Florio P, Puzzutiello R, Filippeschi M, D'Onofrio P, Mereu L, Morelli R, Marianello D, Litta P, Mencaglia L, Petraglia F. Low-dose spinal anesthesia with hyperbaric bupivacaine with intrathecal fentanyl for operative hysteroscopy: a case series study. *J Minim Invasive Gynecol.* 2012;19(1):107–12.

[41] Vitale SG, De Angelis MC, Della Corte L, Saponara S, Carugno J, Laganà AS, Török P, Tinelli R, Pérez-Medina T, Ertas S, Urman B, Angioni S. Uterine cervical stenosis: from classification to advances in management. Overcoming the obstacles to access the uterine cavity. *Arch Gynecol Obstet.* 2024;309(3):755–64.

[42] Petrone M, Bergamini A, Tateo S, Castellano LM, Pella F, Rabaiotti E, Bocciolone L, Mereu L, Candiani M, Mangili G. Transvaginal ultrasound in evaluation and follow-up of ovarian granulosa cell tumors. *Int J Gynecol Cancer.* 2020;30(9):1384–9.

[43] Vitale SG, Angioni S, Saponara S, Sicilia G, Mignacca A, Caiazzo A, De Franciscis P, Riemma G. Hysteroscopic metroplasty and its reproductive impact among the social networks: A cross-sectional analysis on video quality, reliability and creators' opinions on YouTube, TikTok and Instagram. *Int J Med Inform.* 2025;195:105776.

[44] Vitale SG, Riemma G, Carugno J, Chiofalo B, Vilos GA, Cianci S, Budak MS, Lasmar BP, Raffone A, Kahramanoglu I. Hysteroscopy in the management of endometrial hyperplasia and cancer in reproductive aged women: new developments and current perspectives. *Transl Cancer Res.* 2020;9(12):7767–77.

[45] Török P, Molnár S, Herman T, Jashanjeet S, Lampé R, Riemma G, Vitale SG. Fallopian tubal obstruction is associated with increased pain experienced during office hysteroscopy: a retrospective study. *Updates Surg.* 2020;72(1):213–8.

[46] Vitale SG, Parry JP, Carugno J, Cholkeri-Singh A, Della Corte L, Cianci S, Schiattarella A, Riemma G, De Franciscis P. Surgical and Reproductive Outcomes after Hysteroscopic Removal of Retained Products of Conception: A Systematic Review and Meta-analysis. *J Minim Invasive Gynecol.* 2021;28(2):204–17.

[47] Vitale SG, Saponara S, Sicilia G, Klarić M, Sorrentino F, D'Alterio MN, Nappi L, Angioni S. Hysteroscopic diode laser myolysis: from a case series to literature review of incisionless myolysis techniques for managing heavy menstrual bleeding in premenopausal women. *Arch Gynecol Obstet.* 2024;309(3):949–59.

[48] Chiofalo B, Calandra M, Bruno V, Tarantino V, Esposito G, Vizza E, Corrado G, Scambia G, Catena U. Outpatient Hysteroscopic Polypectomy-A Retrospective Study Comparing Rigid and Semirigid Office Hysteroscopes. *Diagnostics* (Basel, Switzerland). 2023;13(5).

[49] Vitale SG, Bruni S, Chiofalo B, Riemma G, Lasmar RB. Updates in office hysteroscopy: a practical decalogue to perform a correct procedure. *Updates Surg.* 2020;72(4):967–76.

[50] Vitale SG, Di Spiezio Sardo A, Riemma G, De Franciscis P, Alonso Pacheco L, Carugno J. In-office hysteroscopic removal of retained or fragmented intrauterine device without anesthesia: a cross-sectional analysis of an international survey. *Updates Surg.* 2022;74(3):1079–85.

[51] Vitale SG, Laganà AS, Caruso S, Garzon S, Vecchio GM, La Rosa VL, Casarin J, Ghezzi F. Comparison of three biopsy forceps for hysteroscopic endometrial biopsy in postmenopausal patients (HYGREB-1): A multicenter, single-blind randomized clinical trial. *Int J Gynecol Obstet.* 2021;155(3):425–32.

[52] Vitale SG, Moore O, Riemma G, Carugno J, Yarto ML, Haimovich S. Hysteroscopic laser ablation of symptomatic uterine fibroids: insights from a prospective study. *Climacteric.* 2023;26(5):497–502.

[53] Savelli L, Ceccarini M, Ludovisi M, Fruscella E, DE Iaco PA, Salizzoni E, Mabrouk M, Manfredi R, Testa AC, Ferrandina G. Preoperative local staging of endometrial cancer: transvaginal sonography vs. magnetic resonance imaging. *Ultrasound Obstet Gynecol.* 2008;31(5):560–6.

[54] Manfredi R, Mirk P, Maresca G, Margariti PA, Testa A, Zannoni GF, Giordano D, Scambia G, Marano P. Local-regional staging of endometrial carcinoma: role of MR imaging in surgical planning. *Radiology.* 2004;231(2):372–8.

[55] Suga T, Nakamoto Y, Saga T, Higashi T, Hamanaka Y, Tatsumi M, Hayashida K, Hara T, Konishi I, Fujii S, Togashi K. Clinical value of FDG-PET for preoperative evaluation of endometrial cancer. *Ann Nucl Med.* 2011;25(4):269–75.

[56] Edge SB, Compton CC. The American Joint Committee on Cancer: the 7th edition of the AJCC cancer staging manual and the future of TNM. *Ann Surg Oncol.* 2010;17(6):1471–4.

[57] National Comprehensive Cancer Network. NCCN Clinical Practice Guidelines in Oncology: Uterine Neoplasms. Version 2.2024 [Internet]. 2024 [cited 2025 Jan 12]. Available from: https://www.nccn.org/guidelines/guidelines-detail?category=1&id=1473.

[58] Pecorelli S. Revised FIGO staging for carcinoma of the vulva, cervix, and endometrium. *Int J Gynaecol Obstet.* 2009;105(2):103–4.

[59] Gaffney D, Matias-Guiu X, Mutch D, Scambia G, Creutzberg C, Fotopoulou C, Berek JS, Concin N. 2023 FIGO staging system for endometrial cancer: The evolution of the revolution. *Gynecol Oncol.* 2024;184:245–53.

[60] Leon-Castillo A, De Boer SM, Powell ME, Mileshkin LR, Mackay HJ, Leary A, Nijman HW, Singh N, Pollock PM, Bessette P, Fyles A, Haie-Meder C, Smit VTHBM, Edmondson RJ, Putter H, Kitchener HC, Crosbie EJ, De Bruyn M, Nout RA, Horeweg N, Creutzberg CL, Bosse T. Molecular Classification of the

PORTEC-3 Trial for High-Risk Endometrial Cancer: Impact on Prognosis and Benefit From Adjuvant Therapy. *J Clin Oncol.* 2020;38(29):3388–97.

[61] Matsuo K, Klar M, Song BB, Roman LD, Wright JD. Validation of the 2023 FIGO staging schema for advanced endometrial cancer. *Eur J Cancer.* 2023;193:113316.

[62] Haight PJ, Riedinger CJ, Backes FJ, O'Malley DM, Cosgrove CM. The right time for change: A report on the heterogeneity of IVB endometrial cancer and improved risk-stratification provided by new 2023 FIGO staging criteria. *Gynecol Oncol.* 2023;175:32–40.

[63] Concin N, Matias-Guiu X, Vergote I, Cibula D, Mirza MR, Marnitz S, Ledermann J, Bosse T, Chargari C, Fagotti A, Fotopoulou C, Gonzalez Martin A, Lax S, Lorusso D, Marth C, Morice P, Nout RA, O'Donnell D, Querleu D, Raspollini MR, Sehouli J, Sturdza A, Taylor A, Westermann A, Wimberger P, Colombo N, Planchamp F, Creutzberg CL. ESGO/ESTRO/ESP guidelines for the management of patients with endometrial carcinoma. *Int J Gynecol Cancer.* 2021;31(1):12–39.

[64] Chiofalo B, Valenti G, Madeo D, Vizza E, Ciancio F. A step-by-step decalogue for performing a simplified type A total laparoscopic hysterectomy using fewer accesses and tools. *Gynecol Pelvic Med.* 2023;6(0):28–28.

[65] Angioni S, Pontis A, Pisanu A, Mereu L, Roman H. Single-port access subtotal laparoscopic hysterectomy: A prospective case-control study. *J Minim Invasive Gynecol.* 2015;22(5):807–12.

[66] Giannini A, D'Oria O, Vizza E, Congiu MA, Cuccu I, Golia D'Augè T, Saponara S, Capalbo G, Di Donato V, Raspagliesi F, Bogani G. Robotic-assisted, laparoscopic, and vaginal hysterectomy in morbidly obese patients with endometrial hyperplasia and endometrial cancer. *Minim Invasive Ther Allied Technol.* 2024;33(6):358–64.

[67] Corrado G, Vizza E, Cela V, Mereu L, Bogliolo S, Legge F, Ciccarone F, Mancini E, Gallotta V, Baiocco E, Monterossi G, Perri MT, Zampa A, Pasciuto T, Scambia G. Laparoscopic versus robotic hysterectomy in obese and extremely obese patients with endometrial cancer: A multi-institutional analysis. *Eur J Surg Oncol.* 2018;44(12):1935–41.

[68] Mereu L, Carri G, Khalifa H. Robotic single port total laparoscopic hysterectomy for endometrial cancer patients. *Gynecol Oncol.* 2012;127(3):644.

[69] ACOG practice bulletin, clinical management guidelines for obstetrician-gynecologists, number 65, August 2005: management of endometrial cancer. *Obstet Gynecol.* 2005;106(2):413–25.

[70] Khoury-Collado F, Murray MP, Hensley ML, Sonoda Y, Alektiar KM, Levine DA, Leitao MM, Chi DS, Barakat RR, Abu-Rustum NR. Sentinel lymph node mapping for endometrial cancer improves the detection of metastatic disease to regional lymph nodes. *Gynecol Oncol.* 2011;122(2):251–4.

[71] Imboden S, Mereu L, Siegenthaler F, Pellegrini A, Papadia A, Tateo S, Mueller MD. Oncological safety and perioperative morbidity in low-risk endometrial cancer with sentinel lymph-node dissection. *Eur J Surg Oncol.* 2019;45(9):1638–43.

[72] Tateo S, Nozza A, Del Pezzo C, Mereu L. Robotic single-site pelvic lymphadenectomy. *Gynecol Oncol.* 2014;134(3):631.

[73] Buda A, Gasparri ML, Puppo A, Mereu L, De Ponti E, Di Martino G, Novelli A, Tateo S, Muller M, Landoni F, Papadia A. Lymph node evaluation in high-risk early stage endometrial cancer: A multi-institutional retrospective analysis comparing the sentinel lymph node (SLN) algorithm and SLN with selective lymphadenectomy. *Gynecol Oncol.* 2018;150(2):261–6.

[74] Mereu L, Berlanda V, Surico D, Gardella B, Pertile R, Spinillo A, Tateo S. Evaluation of quality of life, body image and surgical outcomes of robotic total laparoscopic hysterectomy and sentinel lymph node mapping in low-risk endometrial cancer patients – A Robotic Gyne Club study. *Acta Obstet Gynecol Scand.* 2020;99(9):1238–45.

[75] Chiofalo B, Laganà AS, Ghezzi F, Certelli C, Casarin J, Bruno V, Sperduti I, Chiantera V, Peitsidis P, Vizza E. Beyond Sentinel Lymph Node: Outcomes of Indocyanine Green-Guided Pelvic Lymphadenectomy in Endometrial and Cervical Cancer. *Int J Environ Res Public Health.* 2023;20(4).

[76] Schipa C, Ripa M, Gallotta V, Russo A, Polidori L, Fanfani F, Capomacchia FM, Corrado G, Vizza E, Perrone AM, Mereu L, Cela V, Legge F, Hilaris G, Pasciuto T, D'Indinosante M, La Fera E, Certelli C, Bruno V, Kogeorgos S, De Iaco P, Lathouras K, Sollazzi L, Scambia G, Aceto P. Can the Modified Frailty Index (mFI) Predict Intraoperative and Postoperative Complications in Older Women with Endometrial Cancer Undergoing Laparoscopic or Robotic Surgery? A Multicenter Observational Study. *J Clin Med.* 2023;12(23).

[77] Marchetti C, Ferrandina G, Cormio G, Gambino A, Cecere S, Lorusso D, De Giorgi U, Bogliolo S, Fagotti A, Mammoliti S, Narducci F, Bergamini A, Scollo P, Biglia N, Breda E, Tamberi S, Marinaccio M, Angioli R, Salerno L, Eusebi MC, Loizzi V, Scambia G, Panici PB. Brain metastases in patients with EOC: Clinico-pathological and prognostic factors. A multicentric retrospective analysis from the MITO group (MITO 19). *Gynecol Oncol.* 2016;143(3):532–8.

[78] Pignata S, Ferrandina G, Scarfone G, Scollo P, Odicino F, Cormio G, Katsaros D, Frigerio L, Mereu L, Ghezzi F, Manzione L, Lauria R, Breda E, Alletti DG, Ballardini M, Vernaglia A, Sorio R, Tumolo S, Musso P, Magni G, Pisano C, Morabito A. Poor outcome of elderly patients with platinum-sensitive recurrent ovarian cancer: results from the SOCRATES retrospective study. *Crit Rev Oncol Hematol.* 2009;71(3):233–41.

[79] Prisco MG, Zannoni GF, De Stefano I, Vellone VG, Tortorella L, Fagotti A, Mereu L, Scambia G, Gallo D. Prognostic role of metastasis tumor antigen 1 in patients with ovarian cancer: a clinical study. *Hum Pathol.* 2012;43(2):282–8.

[80] Concin N, Matias-Guiu X, Vergote I, Cibula D, Mirza MR, Marnitz S, Ledermann J, Bosse T, Chargari C, Fagotti A, Fotopoulou C, Gonzalez Martin A, Lax S, Lorusso D, Marth C, Morice P, Nout RA, O'Donnell D, Querleu D, Raspollini MR, Sehouli J, Sturdza A, Taylor A, Westermann A, Wimberger P, Colombo N, Planchamp F, Creutzberg CL. ESGO/ESTRO/ESP guidelines for the management of patients with endometrial carcinoma. *Int J Gynecol Cancer.* 2021;31(1):12–39.

[81] Urman B, Yakin K, Ertas S, Alper E, Aksakal E, Riemma G, Angioni S, Vitale SG. Fertility and anatomical outcomes following hysteroscopic adhesiolysis: An 11-year retrospective cohort study to validate a new classification system for

intrauterine adhesions (Urman-Vitale Classification System). *Int J Gynecol Obstet.* 2024;165(2):644–54.

[82] Chiofalo B, Palmara V, Vilos GA, Pacheco LA, Lasmar RB, Shawki O, Giacobbe V, Alibrandi A, Di Guardo F, Vitale SG. Reproductive outcomes of infertile women undergoing "see and treat" office hysteroscopy: a retrospective observational study. *Minim Invasive Ther Allied Technol.* 2021;30(3):147–53.

[83] Vitale SG, Laganà AS, Török P, Lasmar RB, Carugno J, Palumbo M, Tesarik J. Virtual sonographic hysteroscopy in assisted reproduction: A retrospective cost-effectiveness analysis. *Int J Gynaecol Obstet.* 2022;156(1):112–8.

[84] Vitale SG, Riemma G, Carugno J, Perez-Medina T, Alonso Pacheco L, Haimovich S, Parry JP, Di Spiezio Sardo A, De Franciscis P. Postsurgical barrier strategies to avoid the recurrence of intrauterine adhesion formation after hysteroscopic adhesiolysis: a network meta-analysis of randomized controlled trials. *Am J Obstet Gynecol.* 2022;226(4):487-498.e8.

[85] Mirza MR, Sharma S, Herrstedt J, Shahin MS, Cibula D, Fleming E, Raspagliesi F, Buscema J, Hanker LC, Coleman RL, Boere IA, Schneider K, Gilbert L, Slomovitz BM, Teneriello MG, Powell MA, Ghosh S, Stevens S, Ring K, Stuckey A. 740MO Dostarlimab + chemotherapy for the treatment of primary advanced or recurrent endometrial cancer (pA/rEC): Analysis of progression free survival (PFS) and overall survival (OS) outcomes by molecular classification in the ENGOT-EN6-NSGO/GOG-3031/RUBY trial. *Ann Oncol.* 2023;34:S507.

[86] Joly Lobbedez F, Leary A, Ray-Coquard IL, Asselain B, Rodrigues MJ, Gladieff L, Bazan F, Abadie Lacourtoisie S, Lebreton C, Bengrine Lefevre L, Leroy K, Leman R, Fournel P, Largillier R, Selle F, Frenel JS, Fernandez Y, Foa C, You B, Alexandre J. LBA42 Olaparib vs placebo as maintenance therapy after platinum-based chemotherapy in advanced/metastatic endometrial cancer patients: The GINECO randomized phase IIb UTOLA trial. *Ann Oncol.* 2023;34:S1283–4.

[87] Greggi S, Franchi M, Aletti G, Biglia N, Ditto A, Fagotti A, Giorda G, Mangili G, Odicino F, Salerno MG, Vizza E, Scaffa C, Scollo P. Management of endometrial cancer in Italy: a national survey endorsed by the Italian Society of Gynecologic Oncology. *Int J Surg.* 2014;12(10):1038–44.

[88] Saponara S, Angioni S, Parry JP, Pacheco LA, Carugno J, Moawad N, Haimovich S, Lasmar RB, Dealberti D, Aksakal E, Urman B, Nappi L, Vitale SG. The Pivotal role of hysteroscopy in diagnosing subtle uterine lesions in infertile patients: Seeing the unseen can make the difference. *Eur J Obstet Gynecol Reprod Biol.* 2025;305:132–41.

[89] Corrado G, Vizza E, Perrone AM, Mereu L, Cela V, Legge F, Hilaris G, Pasciuto T, D'Indinosante M, La Fera E, Certelli C, Bruno V, Kogeorgos S, Fanfani F, De Iaco P, Scambia G, Gallotta V. Comparison Between Laparoscopic and Robotic Surgery in Elderly Patients With Endometrial Cancer: A Retrospective Multicentric Study. *Front Oncol.* 2021;11:724886.

[90] Bruno V, Betti M, D'Ambrosio L, Massacci A, Chiofalo B, Pietropolli A, Piaggio G, Ciliberto G, Nisticò P, Pallocca M, Buda A, Vizza E. Machine learning endometrial cancer risk prediction model: integrating guidelines of European

Society for Medical Oncology with the tumor immune framework. *Int J Gynecol Cancer.* 2023;33(11):1708–14.

[91] Bagnoli M, Canevari S, Califano D, Losito S, Maio M Di, Raspagliesi F, Carcangiu ML, Toffoli G, Cecchin E, Sorio R, Canzonieri V, Russo D, Scognamiglio G, Chiappetta G, Baldassarre G, Lorusso D, Scambia G, Zannoni GF, Savarese A, Carosi M, Scollo P, Breda E, Murgia V, Perrone F, Pignata S, De Cecco L, Mezzanzanica D. Development and validation of a microRNA-based signature (MiROvaR) to predict early relapse or progression of epithelial ovarian cancer: a cohort study. *Lancet Oncol.* 2016;17(8):1137–46.

Index

D

E

F

G

J

K

L

M

N

O

P

Q

R

S

T

U

V

W